CARDIOLOGY RESEARCH AND CLINICAL DEVELOPMENTS

OFF-PUMP CORONARY ARTERY BYPASS GRAFTING

OUTCOMES, CONCERNS AND CONTROVERSIES

CARDIOLOGY RESEARCH AND CLINICAL DEVELOPMENTS

Additional books in this series can be found on Nova's website under the Series tab.

Additional E-books in this series can be found on Nova's website under the E-book tab.

CARDIOLOGY RESEARCH AND CLINICAL DEVELOPMENTS

OFF-PUMP CORONARY ARTERY BYPASS GRAFTING

OUTCOMES, CONCERNS AND CONTROVERSIES

SHAHZAD G. RAJA
AND
MOHAMED AMRANI
EDITORS

NOVA BIOMEDICAL

New York

For permission to use material from this book please contact us:
Telephone 631-231-7269; Fax 631-231-8175
Web Site: http://www.novapublishers.com

Library of Congress Cataloging-in-Publication Data

ISBN 978-1-62081-575-5

Library of Congress Control Number: 2012935714

Published by Nova Science Publishers, Inc. † New York

To my mother for her sacrifices and struggle, for her devotion to her family and dedication to her profession, and above all, for being a role model for all those around her.

To my father for his honesty and humility, for his dedication to his profession, and above all, for reminding his children that words are the most powerful weapon used by mankind.

SGR

CONTENTS

Preface

Conventional coronary artery bypass (CABG) using cardiopulmonary bypass (CPB) and cardioplegic arrest has been the gold standard for surgical treatment of coronary artery disease for the last four decades. In the last 20 years, however, interest has re-emerged in performing CABG without the use of CPB, termed off-pump coronary artery bypass grafting or simply OPCAB. The technique of OPCAB surgery following its resurgence has been extensively scrutinized and remains to this day one of the most debated and polarized issues in cardiac surgery. *Off-pump Coronary Artery Bypass Grafting: Outcomes, Concerns & Controversies* provides in-depth insight into the subject of OPCAB grafting. The book is divided into three sections and as suggested by the title the chapters in these sections discuss in detail the current outcomes, focus on concerns and attempt to resolve controversies associated with OPCAB in an evidence-based manner. The text coherently describes various issues and is a valuable resource for those in the early stages of cardiac surgical training as well as practicing surgeons.

The chapters are written by established experts and are well referenced. Tables, algorithms, diagrams, and figures have been extensively used to highlight key aspects of OPCAB grafting. The idea behind this book is to make it a highly practical, user-friendly reference and learning text so that it becomes a resource of great value to a wide variety of staff working with patients undergoing OPCAB grafting. In addition, the systematic and structured format of the book makes it an ideal revision aid for postgraduate trainees in cardiac surgery preparing for certification and fellowship examination. The editors hope that this book will prove to be an ideal source for mastering all of the most important current knowledge and techniques in OPCAB surgery - whether for specialty board review or day-to-day practice.

As in any publication of this magnitude we are indebted to many people. First and foremost, to all the chapter authors, who are some of the busiest physicians in the world; their time and energy have enabled us to produce this superb volume in a timely fashion. Special thanks to our secretary, Elaine Pert, for acting as a link between us and the numerous contributing authors and to our families for their support and understanding during the production of this edition. Finally, and last but not least, we would like to thank the entire

Editorial and Production team at Nova Science Publishers who have been towers of strength and encouragement. We are grateful to them for their ideas, their patience and their gentle but regular persistence without which we would never have got this far.

S G Raja
M Amrani
January 2012
London

SECTION 1: INDICATIONS, CONTRAINDICATIONS AND OUTCOMES

In: Off-Pump Coronary Artery Bypass Grafting
Editors: S.G. Raja and M. Amrani
ISBN 978-1-62081-575-5

Chapter 1

INDICATIONS AND CONTRAINDICATIONS OF OFF-PUMP CORONARY ARTERY BYPASS GRAFTING

***Marco Moscarelli*[1], *Nishith N. Patel*[2] *and Gianni D. Angelini*[3]**
[1]Clinical Fellow Cardiothoracic Surgery,
Imperial College NHS Trust, London, UK
[2]NIHR Academic Clinical Fellow in Cardiac Surgery, University of Bristol, UK
[3]British Heart Foundation Professor of Cardiac Surgery,
Imperial College London and University of Bristol, UK

ABSTRACT

Off-pump coronary artery bypass grafting (OPCAB) has emerged as an important surgical technique with the potential to avoid the harmful effects of cardiopulmonary bypass (ONCAB). Its uptake worldwide, however, has been slow due to the poor understanding of the vast evidence surrounding this technique and this is reflected in the lack of clear guidelines from learned societies. Six systematic reviews of over 50 randomized controlled trials have clearly demonstrated that OPCAB is as safe as ONCAB in low risk patients. Concerns remain, however, of incomplete revascularization and greater rates of graft occlusion. Large observational studies from expert centers demonstrate that OPCAB has a clear benefit in terms of reduced mortality and morbidity with rates of revascularization and graft patency comparable to ONCAB surgery. Moreover, the greatest benefit of OPCAB is seen in high risk patients such as the elderly, women and patients with co-morbidities. Unfortunately, there are currently no randomized controlled trials comparing OPCAB to ONCAB in this high risk group of patients. The second major reason for the poor uptake of OPCAB is the lack of training in this technique. Several observational studies have shown that OPCAB can be safely incorporated into routine clinical practice and training programmes without any adverse effects. However, it is important to recognize that OPCAB is a specialized technique requiring dedication, infrastructure, and expertise to achieve proficiency and good results. This chapter provides an in-depth insight into evidence-based indications and contraindications of OPCAB and focuses on authors' experience of how the uptake of

OPCAB can be increased in different units including the training of surgical trainees in this procedure.

Introduction

Off-pump coronary artery bypass grafting (OPCAB) has evolved during the past two decades with the aim of avoiding the harmful effects of cardiopulmonary bypass (CPB). Despite favorable evidence from both prospective randomized trials and large observational studies, however, the adoption of OPCAB has been variable. There is a general ambiguity in the minds of surgeons and expert bodies of the robust evidence surrounding this clinically and cost effective technique. Many surgeons still believe that OPCAB cannot guarantee complete revascularization in all patients because fewer grafts are performed on the lateral wall, and most importantly, that it is associated with decreased vein graft patency. However, the accumulating wealth of evidence emphasizes the potential of reducing mortality and morbidity especially in high-risk patients.

The aims of this chapter are therefore to review the guidelines and evidence concerning OPCAB, determine the patient subpopulations that will most benefit from OPCAB surgery and lastly provide our own experience of how the uptake of OPCAB can be increased in different units including the training of surgical trainees in this procedure.

Indications and Contraindications: Finding Evidence from Literature

Guidelines

Comprehensive guidelines defining the indications and contraindications for OPCAB are sparse. The most recent guidelines were issued as a joint statement from the European Society of Cardiology (ESC) and the European Association for Cardio-Thoracic Surgery (EACTS) [1]. They state that for patients with mild or moderate chronic kidney disease, an off-pump approach may be considered when surgical revascularization is needed.

Recommendations have also been provided by the American Heart Association Council on Cardiovascular Surgery and Anesthesia[2] and the National Institute for Health and Clinical Excellence (NICE), UK [3].

The American Heart Association Council on Cardiovascular Surgery and Anesthesia in collaboration with the interdisciplinary working group on quality of care and outcomes research has stated that patients may achieve an excellent outcome with either type of procedure, and that individual outcomes probably depend on factors other than use of CPB [2].

The recent NICE (3) guidance for OPCAB states that:

1. Current evidence on the safety and efficacy of OPCAB is adequate to support the use of this procedure provided that normal arrangements are in place for clinical governance, consent and audit.

2. During the consent process, patients should be informed that they will be offered OPCAB rather than ONCAB, but that ONCAB may be a possibility. They should be informed about the uncertainties in relation to longer-term risks of graft occlusion and mortality, as well as the likely advantages of OPCAB, including the lower incidence of stroke.
3. Patient selection and treatment should be carried out by cardiac surgical teams who are skilled in both procedures.
4. NICE encourages clinicians to submit data on patients having OPCAB to the UK Central Cardiac Audit Database (www.ccad.org.uk), with a view to ultimately providing information about longer-term outcomes by linking the database to national statistics records.

The new NICE guidance made evidence-based statements mainly from one randomized trial [4], one meta-analysis of RCTs [5], one meta-analysis of RCTs and non-RCTs [6], the National Registry of UK [7], two non-randomized trial [8, 9], one non-randomized controlled study [10], and one case series study [11].

It is clear the currently available guidelines are vague, incomplete and do not encompass the vast body of evidence available.

Systematic Reviews and Randomized Controlled Trials

To date, six systematic reviews have been published of RCTs comparing OPCAB with ONCAB surgery and these have been summarized in Table 1.

Table 1. Systematic reviews comparing off-pump and on-pump coronary artery bypass grafting

Author year, reference	RCTs	Patients	Early Mortality	Late Mortality	AMI	Stroke	AF	Infection	Repeat revascu-larization
Takagi, 2010 (12)	12	4326	-	1.37 (1.04, 1.81)	-	-	-	-	-
Feng, 2009 (13)	10	2018	1.00 (0.56, 1.77)	1.10 (0.46, 2.65)	0.61 (0.31, 1.17)	0.56 (0.21, 1.47)	-	-	1.38 (0.72, 2.67)
Møller, 2008 (5)	66	5537	0.98 (0.66, 1.44)	-	0.95 (0.65, 1.37)	0.53 (0.31, 0.91)	0.69 (0.57, 0.83)	-	1.34 (0.83, 2.18)
Sedrakyan, 2006 (14)	41	3996	0.96 (0.58, 1.60)	-	0.80 (0.54, 1.19)	0.50 (0.27, 0.93)	0.70 (0.57, 0.84)	0.52 (0.37, 0.74)	1.90 (0.92, 3.90)
Cheng, 2005 (15)	37	3369	1.02 (0.58, 1.80)	-	0.77 (0.48, 1.26)	0.68 (0.33, 1.40)	0.58 (0.44, 0.77)	0.41 (0.23, 0.74)	1.61 (0.71, 3.65)
Wijeysundera, 2005 (6)	37	3449	0.91 (0.45, 1.83)	-	0.79 (0.50, 1.25)	0.52 (0.25, 1.05)	0.59 (0.46, 0.77)	-	1.72 (0.78, 3.94)

Effect measures reported as odds ratios (95% confidence intervals) Key: AMI = acute myocardial infarction ; AF = atrial fibrillation

These systematic reviews of RCTs in low-risk patients demonstrate similar outcomes for both interventions in terms of mortality, myocardial infarction, and need for repeat revascularization at 1 and 2 years. They also demonstrate that OPCAB is associated with reductions in the risks for stroke, atrial fibrillation, wound infection, and acute kidney injury. OPCAB also reduces transfusion and inotrope requirements, ventilation time, intensive care unit and hospital stays, and in-hospital and 1-year direct costs. The systematic review by Takagi et al. [12] reported worse long term outcomes with OPCAB. However, their meta-analysis was heavily weighted by the recent ROOBY trial, a prospective, multi- center trial with 2000 patients randomly assigned to undergo OPCAB or ONCAB during a 6-year period [4]. They reported a 33% increase in the risk of the primary long-term composite end point of death from any cause, nonfatal myocardial infarction, or repeat revascularization within 1 year for patients undergoing OPCAB (relative risk, 1.33; 95% CI, 1.01–1.76; P= 0.04; number needed to cause 1 harmful event, 71). This study, however, had several major limitations. More than 70% of eligible patients (scheduled for urgent or elective coronary artery bypass grafting) were excluded because of clinical reservations of the surgical team or small target vessels. This suggests inexperience of surgeons in the trial, who were required to have performed just 20 OPCAB procedures to participate. Conversion to ONCAB, which is known to increase morbidity and mortality [16, 17], occurred in more than 12% of cases, much greater than the 1% to 3% reported by centers specializing in OPCAB [17, 18]. In the OPCAB group, more than 50% of patients received red blood cell transfusions, which contrasts with the 30% in previous randomized trials [15]. Finally, only a small minority of the studied population were high-risk patients, a group more likely to benefit from OPCAB. Removal of this trial from the meta-analysis demonstrates no-difference between both surgical techniques (OR 1.344 (95% CI 0.952 – 1.896).

Our group has recently reported long term follow-up at 6 to 8 years among survivors of the BHACS-1 and BHACS-2 trials [19, 20]. We found no difference in the likelihoods of graft occlusion (odds ratio [OR], 1.00; 95% confidence interval [CI], 0.55–1.81), death (hazard ratio [HR], 1.24; 95% CI, 0.72–2.15), major adverse cardiac-related events (HR, 0.84; 95% CI, 0.58–1.24) or health-related quality of life outcomes between the OPCAB and ONCAB groups.

We can therefore conclude that the routine application of OPCAB is as safe as ONCAB in low risk patients based upon Level 1A evidence arising from 6 systematic reviews.

Observational Studies

Although RCTs are the gold standard for evaluating new interventions, they are underpowered to demonstrate a difference in hard end points. Detecting a postoperative mortality reduction from 3 to 2% with 80% power would require more than 8000 patients. As can be readily imagined, no trials have enrolled so many patients. Observational studies, although confounded by uncontrollable variables, provide data from very large groups of patients with long-term follow-up. Observational studies from high-volume, expert centres are especially valuable as they provide evidence from an "all-comers" policy (overcoming selection bias) and from surgeons who specialize in the technique of OPCAB. Several large propensity-matched retrospective series and meta-analyses from centers proficient in OPCAB have provided compelling evidence in favor of the technique.

A retrospective analysis of 49,830 patients from the New York state registry reported lower 30-day mortality, incidence of postoperative stroke and respiratory failure in risk-adjusted isolated OPCAB versus ONCAB surgery [21]. Three-year follow-up revealed that OPCAB patients had a higher rate of repeat revascularization, but survival was equivalent between the two groups [21]. A similar intention to-treat analysis of 42,477 patients from the Society of Thoracic Surgeons National Adult Cardiac Surgery database showed a reduction in risk-adjusted mortality, stroke, perioperative myocardial infarction, renal failure, mediastinitis, need for reoperation, atrial fibrillation, and prolonged ventilation in OPCAB versus ONCAB patients [22]. A meta-analysis of 22 risk-adjusted (logistic regression or propensity-score) observational studies (n=293,617) showed OPCAB to be associated with reduced 30-day mortality (OR 0.72; 95% CI 0.66 to 0.78), stroke (OR 0.62; 95% CI 0.55 to 0.69), myocardial infarction (OR 0.66; 95% CI 0.50 to 0.88), and atrial fibrillation (OR 0.78; 95% CI 0.74 to 0.82) [6]. At one to two years, OPCAB was associated with trends toward reduced mortality, but also increased repeat revascularization (OR 1.35, 95% CI 0.76 to 2.39).

The UK national register report of 86,047 patients treated since 1999 concluded that 1-year survival for patients treated in the period 2004 to 2008 was 97% for off-pump CABG and 96% for on-pump CABG [7]. The 5-year follow-up (for patients who had reached that time point), showed that survival was 89% for off-pump CABG and 89% for on-pump CABG.

Kuss and colleagues [23] in a propensity score analyses comparing off- and on-pump surgery found OPCAB superior in virtually all the assessed short-term outcomes. This benefit was statistically significant for mortality [OR: 0.69, 95%-CI: 0.60-0.75], stroke, renal failure, RBC transfusion, wound infection, prolonged ventilation, inotropic and intra-aortic balloon pump (IABP) support.

OPCAB: Identifying Patients that will Benefit the Most

In 2004, the International Society for Minimally Invasive Cardiothoracic Surgery (ISMICS) issued a consensus statement saying that OPCAB should be considered in patients with EuroSCORE greater than 5, age greater than 75, diabetes, renal failure, left ventricular dysfunction, left main disease, and in patients undergoing reoperation [24]. Evidence was drawn from observational studies and propensity scored meta-analysis, but there are no prospective randomized trials comparing OPCAB and ONCAB in high-risk patients.

The following sections discuss studies of patients with older age, at risk of acute renal failure (ARF) or at high risk of neurological morbidity, patients with poor left ventricular function, atheromatous aorta, female, re-operative patients, patients who have had acute coronary syndrome and those who are at high risk by virtue of multiple comorbidities.

Elderly Patients

Hoff and colleagues [25] compared outcomes in patients 80 years and older who underwent non emergent coronary artery bypass with (N = 169) and without (N = 60) cardiopulmonary bypass from January 1999 through June 2001. Both groups were at increased perioperative risk based on the Society of Thoracic Surgeons risk model (7.7% OPCAB vs. 5.8% CAB, $p = 0.03$). There were no operative deaths in the OPCAB group but there were eight (4.7%) in the ONCAB group (p = NS). Perioperative stroke (0% OPCAB vs. 7.1% ONCAB, $p = 0.04$), prolonged ventilation (1.7% OPCAB vs. 11.8% ONCAB, $p = 0.02$), and transfusion rate (33% OPCAB vs. 70.4% ONCAB, $p < 0.001$) were all lower in the OPCAB group. A shorter hospital stay (6.3 days OPCAB vs. 11.5 days ONCAB, $p < 0.001$) resulted in lower hospital cost in the OPCAB group. They concluded that off-pump coronary artery bypass grafting in elderly patients was associated with fewer complications, a shorter hospital stay, and lower hospital cost.

Hirose and colleagues conducted a retrospective chart review for patients who underwent isolated off-pump and on-pump CABG between January 1997 and December 2000 [26]. The OPCAB group consisted of 60 men and 44 women with a mean age of 78.8 years, and the ONCAB group consisted of 54 men and 20 women with a mean age of 77.6 years. Distal anastomoses were significantly fewer in the OPCAB group (2.4 in off-pump group versus 3.7 in on-pump group), but total arterial bypass was more frequently achieved in the OPCAB group (82.7% versus 25.7%). Intubation time (8.4 versus 18.4 hours), intensive care unit stay (2.2 versus 3.5 days), and postoperative stay (13.8 versus 20.0 days) were significantly shorter in the OPCAB than in the ONCAB group. The frequency of the occurrence of major complications was significantly lower in the off-pump group than the on-pump group, especially in regard to postoperative stroke and respiratory failure. Multivariate analysis showed that off-pump CABG significantly reduced patients' recovery period and the incidence of postoperative complications. Early follow-up results, cardiac event-free and survival rates did not significantly differ between the two groups.

In a retrospective analysis of octogenarians undergoing OPCAB versus ONCAB, Nagpal et al. found similar rates of perioperative myocardial infarction, renal dysfunction and mortality although OPCAB patients had a significantly lower incidence of stroke (1.5% OPCAB versus 7.6% ONCAB) and lower prolonged ventilation [27].

Jensen et al. evaluated 3-month neurocognitive outcomes in elderly patients (mean age 76 years) in a randomized trial of OPCAB versus ONCAB. In this study, no difference was seen in stroke rate or cognitive outcome as evaluated by four different neuropsychological tests [28].

On the other hand, Athanasiou performed a meta-analysis of nine clinical trials examining the incidence of stroke in patients over the age of 70 and found a benefit in the OPCAB group [29].

In a similar meta-analysis of OPCAB versus ONCAB in elderly patients (>70 years), Panesar and associates [30] found a reduction in mortality, stroke, and atrial fibrillation in the OPCAB group. The benefit was even more evident in octogenarians with respect to stroke and mortality.

Renal Dysfunction

Postoperative acute renal failure (ARF) in patients undergoing CABG has been associated with high morbidity and mortality. Chertow et al. reported a mortality of 63% at 30 days for those patients requiring hemodialysis compared with 4.3% for those without renal dysfunction [31].

Mangano and colleagues identified similar mortality rates among patients with postoperative renal failure [32].

The injurious effect of CPB on renal function is multifactorial, mainly related to non-pulsatile perfusion, renal hypoperfusion, hypothermia, microembolisation, anemia and increased levels of circulating catecholamines, and cytokines.

There is evidence from several studies that OPCAB can reduce morbidity and mortality in patients with normal renal function, in those with renal dysfunction not yet on hemodialysis as well as in those with end-stage renal failure on dialysis.

Ascione and colleagues [33] in a cohort of 50 patients randomly assigned to receive OPCAB and ONCAB found no deaths, myocardial infarctions or acute renal failure in either group. Glomerular filtration as assessed by creatinine clearance and the urinary microalbumin/creatinine ratio was significantly worse in the OPCAB group. Renal tubular function was also impaired in the OPCAB group as assessed by increased N-acetyl glucosaminidase activity.

Several authors have reported a favorable effect of OPCAB in high-risk patients in terms of potential prevention of ARF [34].

Sajja et al. found a significant reduction of ARF in patients with preoperative renal impairment undergoing OPCAB compared to ONCAB [35].

Dewey et al. showed improved operative mortality in favor of OPCAB among patients with dialysis-dependent renal failure; this early benefit, however, did not translate into improved long- term survival [36]. Abu-Omarand and colleagues in a cohort of 60 patients equally randomized into OPCAB and ONCAB found that avoidance of CPB reduced renal injury mainly in patients with pre-existing renal dysfunction [37].

Neurological Injuries

Neurological injuries range from stroke to neurocognitive dysfunction. ONCAB is associated with an increased risk of stroke. CPB has been advocated as a main risk for cerebral injuries related to micro- and macro-embolizations from aortic manipulation and systemic hypoperfusion. OPCAB therefore promised to reduce the incidence of cerebral injuries.

In a recent meta-analysis, Sedrakyan et al.14 assessed data from 3996 patients enrolled in 41 RCTs comparing OPCAB with ONCAB. OPCAB was associated with a 50% reduction in the relative risk of stroke (95% CI, 7% to 73%), 30% reduction in atrial fibrillation (95% CI, 16% to 43%) and 48% reduction in wound infection (95% CI, 26% to 63%). This translated into avoidance of 10 strokes per 1000 CABG.

Atherosclerosis of the ascending aorta is another important risk factor for stroke and it is well known that manipulation of the aorta increases the risk of neurologic complication [38]. OPCAB allows coronary revascularisation using an anaortic technique.

Calafiore reported a stroke rate of less than 0.3% in more than 1000 anaortic OPCAB procedures [39], similar to results by Vallely in a much larger cohort of patients [40].

In a recent meta-analysis Misfeld and colleagues found that the avoidance of aortic manipulation during off-pump decreases neurologic complications relative to standard techniques [41]. Mishra et al. performed a propensity matched comparison of OPCAB versus ONCAB of 991 patients with atheromatous aortic disease and found a significant decrease in in-hospital mortality (1.4 versus .3%; P<0.001) and stroke incidence (0.50 versus 0.97%, p<0.05), with OPCAB being the only independent predictor of decreased stroke rate [8].

Depressed Left Ventricular Function

Shennib and colleagues retrospectively collected data on demographics, preoperative risk factors, operative and postoperative outcomes of patients who had undergone isolated CABG between January 1, 1998, and October 31, 2001 [42]. A total of 77 patients (31 OPCAB/46 ONCAB) were identified as having an ejection fraction (EF) of less than 0.35. Operative mortality was 3.2% after the OPCAB procedure versus 10.9% for the ONCAB. The OPCAB procedure resulted in significantly fewer requirements for blood transfusions, fewer distal anastomoses per patient, and a higher incidence of atrial fibrillation compared with ONCAB. They concluded that patients with poor left ventricular function may undergo surgical revascularization using off-pump technique with relatively good results and low mortality levels. The lower number of grafts performed in the OPCAB group did not seem to affect clinical outcomes.

Ascione and colleagues analyzed data of 5,195 consecutive patients undergoing coronary artery bypass grafting (CABG) alone from April 1996 to August 2002 [43]. Two hundred and fifty patients (median age 65 years) with preoperative left ventricular ejection fraction less than 30% (74 OPCAB; 29.6%) were identified and early and midterm clinical outcomes were assessed. After adjustment for consultant team and propensity scores no differences between groups with regard to in-hospital mortality and morbidity were found. The only in-hospital outcome to show a significant difference after adjustment was the need for intraoperative inotropic support, which was higher in the ONCAB group (OR 5.1; 95% CI 2.55 to 10.2; $p <$ 0.001). The median follow-up times for the on- and off-pump groups were 3.4 years and 1.4 years respectively. Three-year survival was higher with ONCAB (87% ONCAB versus 73% OPCAB) but this difference did not reach statistical significance after adjustment for prognostic variables (HR 0.54, 95% CI 0.22 to 1.26, $p = 0.16$). Conversely, Al-Ruzzeh in a cohort of 305 consecutive patients, who underwent primary isolated coronary artery bypass grafting (199 patients ONCAB / 106 OPCAB) for multivessel disease with depressed left ventricular function did not find that using CPB was an independent predictor of operative mortality [44]. Darwazah and Youn found a reduction in perioperative morbidity in OPCAB patients, specifically in terms of lowering the intensive care unit length of stay, respiratory failure, need for intotropes, and need for IABP [45, 46]. Youn et al. also showed similar 6-year survival rates (88% in OPCAB versus 72% in ONCAB) and freedom from major adverse cardiovascular events [46].

Female Gender

Female gender has been recognized as a risk factor for mortality and morbidity after CABG. Puskas et al. recently reported results of 11,413 consecutive patients undergoing isolated CABG over an 8-year period, and among these patients, women undergoing ONCAB were at significantly greater risk of death, stroke, and myocardial infarction compared with men [47]. However, women undergoing OPCAB had statistically similar results to men, suggesting that the latter reduced the gender discrepancy in these outcomes. Similar findings were reported in a larger observational study of 42,477 patients from 63 North American institutions identified from the Society of Thoracic Surgeons (STS) national database [22].

Acute Coronary Syndrome

Few reports are available on the postoperative outcomes of OPCAB in acute coronary syndrome. In 57 patients who underwent OPCAB within the first week of an AMI, Mohr et al. found that CABG without CPB is a relatively low-risk procedure [48].

In a series of 225 patients who underwent CABG within 7 days of AMI, Locker and colleagues showed that the early mortality of patients who underwent operation within the first 48 hours with CPB was significantly higher compared with OPCAB (16.5% vs. 4.3%, $P< 0.044$), but the mortality rate in patients who underwent surgery after 48 hours was similar in both groups (5.8% vs. 3.4%, $P<0.44$) [49]. They concluded that CPB can be used safely for most patients within the first week of AMI, but they advocated avoiding CPB for patients who underwent operation within 48 hours from the onset of symptoms because it was associated with a high operative mortality.

Locker and associates also demonstrated that emergency off-pump CABG for AMI results in a lower mortality compared with conventional CABG (5% vs. 24%); however, the long-term results of patients without CPB were no better than those of patients with CPB, which may have been related to the incomplete revascularization or inferior patency rate of anastomoses performed on the beating heart [49].

Rastan and colleagues studied 638 consecutive patients with acute coronary syndrome who received emergency CABG (240 patients without CPB and 398 patients with CPB) [50]. The authors concluded that the beating heart was associated with an improved hospital outcome and that there were comparable long-term results for high-risk patients presenting with acute coronary syndrome with or without cardiogenic shock.

Recently, Fattouch et al. reported the results of a prospective trial, randomizing patients with acute ST elevation MI (within 48 h of infarction) to OPCAB versus ONCAB [51]. Their findings indicate that OPCAB had a significantly lower mortality, fewer patients with low cardiac output syndrome, decreased ventilator time, and decreased ICU and hospital LOS. In a propensity-matched analysis of 5760 patients undergoing nonelective CABG, Stamou et al. reported a reduction in LOS, and lower rates of postoperative renal failure, need for IABP, and re-exploration for bleeding among OPCAB patients [52].

Reoperative Patients

Few studies compare OPCAB and ONCAB in re-operative patients. Morris found in a propensity-matched comparison a significant reduction in overall postoperative complications, atrial fibrillation, blood transfusion, and hospital length of stay in the OPCAB group [53]. Similar findings were reported by Mishra and colleagues who demonstrated a reduction in the need for prolonged ventilation and inotropic support, and shorter ICU and hospital LOS in favour of redo OPCAB [54]. Vohra et al. found that OPCAB patients, despite having less number of grafts performed, were less likely to need IABP support, had a shorter duration of ventilation, and had similar 5-year survival rates (87% in ONCAB versus 95% in OPCAB) [55].

Kuss and colleagues in an analysis of all randomized trials comparing the on- and off pump technique [56] by means of logistic regression investigated if the effect of OPCAB on mortality, myocardial infarction, stroke, and atrial fibrillation is modified across the range of the three risk factors age, proportion of females and ejection fraction. They found a superiority of the OPCAB in patients with lower EF values for the outcomes of mortality and atrial fibrillation and they concluded that among nearly 10,000 patients from 86 randomized trials, OPCAB was superior in patients with lower EF values, especially for the most valid outcome of mortality.

Multiple Comorbidities

Bittner and colleagues utilizing a Parsonnet risk stratification model analyzed prospectively collected data on a cohort of 57 high-risk coronary artery disease patients, which were operated on with the OPCAB technique [57]. High-risk patients were defined as those with a Parsonnet score of 15 or greater. The average ejection fraction of the patients was 42% (±12.3) and their age ranged from 52 to 85 years (mean 70.6 ± 10.4, 26% women). Unstable angina was present in 42 patients (74%) and 10 patients underwent OPCAB within 24 hours of the occurrence of acute myocardial infarction. In addition to severe coronary artery disease, 32% of the patients presented with congestive heart failure, insulin-dependent diabetes (18%), renal failure (22%), peripheral vascular disease (31%), pulmonary disease (18%), and neurologic disorders (14%). An average of 2.6 ± 0.9 grafts/patient were performed and the posterior descending artery or marginal branches of the circumflex artery or both were grafted in 90%. The 30-day mortality rate was 3.5% (n = 2). They concluded that OPCAB can be performed with a reasonable low morbidity and mortality in high-risk patients.

Chamberlain et al. compared outcomes of 1,570 high-risk patients. Patients in the ONCAB group had fewer high-risk factors, lower Parsonnet scores and were less likely to be 75 years of age or older, to have peripheral vascular disease or hypercholesterolemia, or to have sustained a previous transient ischemic attack [58]. However, they were more likely to be assigned to a higher Canadian Cardiovascular Society class and had more extensive coronary artery disease and were more likely to have unstable angina, to require urgent or emergency operations, and to receive more grafts than those undergoing OPCAB procedures. Unadjusted odds ratios for intensive care unit or high-dependency unit stay, total length of stay, blood loss of more than 1,000 mL, postoperative hemoglobin and transfusion requirement all showed a highly significant benefit for the OPCAB group ($p \leq 0.005$). After adjustment for prognostic variables, odds ratios remained essentially unaltered (adjusted odds ratio estimates 0.36; $p < 0.05$) except for blood loss of more than 1,000 mL (adjusted odds ratio estimate, 0.82; $p = 0.22$). Sensitivity analyses confirmed the robustness of these findings. Authors concluded that OPCAB was safe, effective and associated with reduced morbidity in high-risk patients compared with conventional coronary artery revascularization.

Meharwal et al. evaluated a total of 1,075 patients who underwent OPCAB between October 1996 and June 2001 with one or more of the following risk factors: poor left ventricular function (EF ≤30%), advanced age (>70 years), left main stenosis, acute myocardial infarction, and redo coronary artery surgery [59].These patients were compared with 2,312 similar patients who underwent coronary artery bypass grafting on CPB during the same period. The average number of grafts was 3.0 ± 0.4 and 3.2 ± 0.3 in the OPCAB and ONCAB groups, respectively. Hospital mortality was 3.2% and 4.5% in OPCAB and ONCAB groups respectively ($p = 0.109$). Perioperative myocardial infarction, requirement of inotropic agents, stroke, and renal dysfunction were comparable in two groups. Intubation time (19 ± 5 vs 24 ± 6 hours, $p < 0.001$), mean blood loss (362 ± 53 vs 580 ± 66 mL, $p < 0.001$), atrial fibrillation (14.3 vs 19.7%, $p < 0.001$), and prolonged ventilation (4.6 vs 7.6%, $p = 0.002$) were less in OPCAB group. Intensive care unit stay (20 ± 8 hours) and hospital stay (6 ± 3 days) were significantly less in the OPCAB group ($p < 0.001$). They concluded that in high-risk patients with multivessel coronary artery disease the OPCAB operative mortality is comparable to that associated with ONCAB, and avoidance of CPB is associated with reduced postoperative morbidity in these patients.

Ongoing Prospective Randomized Trials Comparing OPCAB and ONCAB in High Risk Patients

Currently, there are no published prospective randomized comparisons of OPCAB versus ONCAB for the treatment of high-risk patients.

The recently published Best Bypass Surgery Trial claimed to evaluate 30-day outcomes in 341 high-risk patients randomly allocated to undergo either OPCAB or ONCAB [60]. The investigators reported no significant difference in their composite primary outcome of adverse cardiac and cerebrovascular events. Three-year outcome of MACCE was not significantly different found both groups. This trial, however, did not truly recruit high-risk patients. The exclusion criteria were previous heart surgery, left ventricular ejection fraction less than 30%, unstable preoperative condition, and emergency surgery.

Recently, Lemma et al presented their preliminary findings from the On-Off Study at the 2011 Annual Meeting of the American Association of Thoracic Surgeons in Philadelphia. They randomized 411 high-risk patients (EuroSCORE greater than 5) to OPCAB or ONCAB surgery and their composite primary end-point included operative mortality, myocardial infarction, stroke, renal failure, re-operation for bleeding and ARDS, before discharge or within 30 days after surgery. They found that the rate of the composite primary end point was significantly lower in the OPCAB compared to the ONCAB group (OR=0.40 (0.20 – 0.81), p=0.009; number needed to prevent 1 event, 14).

Currently there is a prospective randomized trial underway evaluating the efficacy of OPCAB in high- risk patients, the German Off Pump Coronary Artery Bypass in Elderly Study (GOPCABE, NCT00719667), a multi-center trial randomly allocating 2000 patients older than 75 years (but excluding patients undergoing re-operative surgery) to undergo either OPCAB or ONCAB.

OPCAB: Does Training Mean Broadening the Indications?

If we look carefully through the literature scrutinized above, we would not be surprised to understand that the best outcomes following OPCAB come from high experience / large volume centers, which suggest that this is a specialized technique requiring dedication, infrastructure, and expertise to achieve proficiency and good results.

This in turn raises important questions that relate to the future direction of OPCAB.

How should OPCAB, a specialized technique, be safely introduced into routine clinical practice? Answering this crucial question means broadening the indications of OPCAB.

The adoption of OPCAB has been highly variable. In Asia, the majority of CABG cases are performed off-pump whereas in the United Kingdom OPCAB uptake has plateaued at approximately 17% [7]. The reasons for this include the lack of established training programs, the perception that success with the technique is limited to more proficient surgeons, and a fear of deleterious patient outcomes, especially during the learning curve [61]. In the largest review of the incorporation of OPCAB into a surgical practice (12,540 CABG patients including 1,915 OPCAB procedures), Mack and colleagues [18] reported an increase in OPCAB from 1.2% of cases in 1995 to 34.1% of cases in 2000 (individual surgeon adoption rates ranged from 1% to 96% by 2000). Initially OPCAB case selection considered only elective cases requiring a limited number of grafts (two or three) to the anterior surface of the heart and patients in an unstable condition, those undergoing reoperation, and those requiring multiple bypasses on the lateral surface were generally considered unsuitable. As surgeon experience increased along with developments in stabilizer technology, however, all patients were considered for OPCAB. The OPCAB to on-pump conversion rate in this series was 2.9%. The increased use of OPCAB was associated with a reduction in hospital mortality from 4% to 3.2% and a reduction in procedural morbidity.

In our unit, between 1997 and 2001, the proportion of OPCAB cases increased from 8% to 68% without any increase in procedural morbidity. This was accompanied by a gradual increase in the complexity of cases, number of distal anastomoses, use of multiple arterial conduits, and lateral wall revascularization [62, 63].

Key elements to the adoption of OPCAB are appropriate patient selection, individualized grafting strategy, peer-to-peer training of the entire team, graded clinical experience (preoperative planning, adequate exposure, proximal anastamoses to the aorta, distal anastamoses initially to anterior wall vessels, followed by inferior wall vessels and then lateral wall vessels) [64]. In our experience, the surgeon's learning curve is around 50 to 75 cases and good proficiency with the technique is usually associated with a low 1-2% conversion rate [65, 66].

Where senior surgeons are experienced with the technique, OPCAB can be safely and reproducibly taught to trainees [62, 63, 66]. Careful early case selection with later progression to more complex procedures under the tutelage of experienced trainers has been shown to permit effective training without increased morbidity, even in high risk patients [62, 67]. OPCAB has since the early days been an integral part of our unit training program, with the proportion of OPCAB procedures performed by trainees increased from 18% to 62% between the years 1999 to 2001 [62, 63]. By the end of their third year, residents have performed 40 to 50 multivessel OPCAB revascularizations as first surgeons under direct senior surgeon supervision. An early comparison of outcomes demonstrated no difference between senior surgeon-operated or supervised-trainee operated patients [62]. During the last 2 years of the training program, and after satisfying the senior surgeons that they were proficient in OPCAB techniques, residents are then permitted to perform OPCAB cases without direct supervision. When the results of these unsupervised cases were reviewed, again there was no increase in patient morbidity compared with trainees operating under direct supervision [62].

A major criticism of the ROOBY trial was that 55% of OPCAB cases were performed primarily by residents [4]. However, evidence seems to strongly suggest that, it is not the residents but instead the lack of experienced trainers that resulted in poor outcomes.

CONCLUSION

There is a large wealth of evidence that OPCAB is as safe and effective as ONCAB in low-risk patients undergoing coronary artery surgery. Concerns of incomplete revascularization and graft occlusion are resolved by observational studies from high volume, OPCAB specialized centers. Incorporation of OPCAB into routine clinical practice requires infrastructure and dedication. In addition, OPCAB can be safely taught to trainees. It is likely that the greatest benefit of OPCAB will be seen in high-risk patients and this is supported by numerous observational studies and the recent ON-OFF trial. However, results from the large randomized controlled trials are eagerly awaited. In the meantime, OPCAB can be safely incorporated into routine clinical practice.

REFERENCES

[1] Wijns W., Kolh P., Danchin N. et al. Guidelines on myocardial revascularization: The task force on myocardial revascularization of the European Society of Cardiology (ESC) and the European Association for Cardio-thoracic surgery (EACTS). *Eur Heart J* 2010;31:2501-2555.

[2] Sellke F. W., DiMaio J. M., Caplan L. R. et al. Comparing on-pump and off-pump coronary artery bypass grafting: Numerous studies but few conclusions: A scientific statement from the american heart association council on cardiovascular surgery and anesthesia in collaboration with the interdisciplinary working group on quality of care and outcomes research. *Circulation* 2005;111:2858-2864.

[3] Excellence NIfHaC. *Off-pump coronary artery bypass grafting*. 2011 [cited 30 September 2011]. Available from: http://www.nice.org.uk/nicemedia/live/11034/52580/52580.pdf.

[4] Shroyer A. L., Grover F. L., Hattler B. et al. On-pump versus off-pump coronary-artery bypass surgery. *N Engl J Med* 2009;361:1827-1837.

[5] Møller C. H., Penninga L., Wetterslev J., Steinbruchel D. A., Gluud C. Clinical outcomes in randomized trials of off- vs. On-pump coronary artery bypass surgery: Systematic review with meta-analyses and trial sequential analyses. *Eur Heart J* 2008;29:2601-2616.

[6] Wijeysundera D. N., Beattie W. S., Djaiani G. et al. Off-pump coronary artery surgery for reducing mortality and morbidity: Meta-analysis of randomized and observational studies. *J Am Coll Cardiol* 2005;46:872-882.

[7] Bridgewater B., Keogh B. *Sixth national adult cardiac surgical database report:* Society for Cardiothoracic Surgery in Great Britain & Ireland; 2008.

[8] Mishra M., Malhotra R., Karlekar A., Mishra Y., Trehan N. Propensity case-matched analysis of off-pump versus on-pump coronary artery bypass grafting in patients with atheromatous aorta. *Ann Thorac Surg* 2006;82:608-614.

[9] Magee M. J., Dewey T. M., Acuff T. et al. Influence of diabetes on mortality and morbidity: Off-pump coronary artery bypass grafting versus coronary artery bypass grafting with cardiopulmonary bypass. *Ann Thorac Surg* 2001;72:776-780.

[10] Synnergren M. J., Ekroth R., Oden A., Rexius H., Wiklund L. Incomplete revascularization reduces survival benefit of coronary artery bypass grafting: Role of off-pump surgery. *J Thorac Cardiovasc Surg* 2008;136:29-36.

[11] Agostini M., Fino C., Torchio P. et al. Impact of incomplete revascularization following opcab surgery. *J Card Surg* 2009;24:650-656.

[12] Takagi H., Matsui M., Umemoto T. Off-pump coronary artery bypass may increase late mortality: A meta-analysis of randomized trials. *Ann Thorac Surg*;89:1881-1888.

[13] Feng Z. Z., Shi J., Zhao X. W., Xu Z. F. Meta-analysis of on-pump and off-pump coronary arterial revascularization. *Ann Thorac Surg* 2009;87:757-765.

[14] Sedrakyan A., Wu A. W., Parashar A., Bass E. B., Treasure T. Off-pump surgery is associated with reduced occurrence of stroke and other morbidity as compared with traditional coronary artery bypass grafting: A meta-analysis of systematically reviewed trials. *Stroke* 2006;37:2759-2769.

[15] Cheng D. C., Bainbridge D., Martin J. E., Novick R. J. Does off-pump coronary artery bypass reduce mortality, morbidity, and resource utilization when compared with conventional coronary artery bypass? A meta-analysis of randomized trials. *Anesthesiology* 2005;102:188-203.

[16] Jin R., Hiratzka L. F., Grunkemeier G. L., Krause A., Page US, 3rd. Aborted off-pump coronary artery bypass patients have much worse outcomes than on-pump or successful off-pump patients. *Circulation* 2005;112:I332-337.

[17] Reeves B. C., Ascione R., Caputo M., Angelini G. D. Morbidity and mortality following acute conversion from off-pump to on-pump coronary surgery. *Eur J Cardiothorac Surg* 2006;29:941-947.

[18] Mack M., Bachand D., Acuff T., Edgerton J., Prince S., Dewey T., Magee M. Improved outcomes in coronary artery bypass grafting with beating-heart techniques. *J Thorac Cardiovasc Surg* 2002;124:598-607.

[19] Angelini G. D., Taylor F. C., Reeves B. C., Ascione R. Early and midterm outcome after off-pump and on-pump surgery in beating heart against cardioplegic arrest studies (BHACAS 1 and 2): A pooled analysis of two randomised controlled trials. Lancet 2002;359:1194-1199.

[20] Angelini G. D., Culliford L., Smith D. K, et al. Effects of on- and off-pump coronary artery surgery on graft patency, survival, and health-related quality of life: Long-term follow-up of 2 randomized controlled trials. *J Thorac Cardiovasc Surg* 2009;137:295-303.

[21] Hannan E. L., Wu C., Smith C. R. et al. Off-pump versus on-pump coronary artery bypass graft surgery: Differences in short-term outcomes and in long-term mortality and need for subsequent revascularization. *Circulation* 2007;116:1145-1152.

[22] Puskas J. D., Edwards F. H., Pappas P. A. et al. Off-pump techniques benefit men and women and narrow the disparity in mortality after coronary bypass grafting. *Ann Thorac Surg* 2007;84:1447-1454.

[23] Kuss O., von Salviati B., Borgermann J. Off-pump versus on-pump coronary artery bypass grafting: A systematic review and meta-analysis of propensity score analyses. *J Thorac Cardiovasc Surg* 2010;140:829-835, 835 e821-813.

[24] Puskas J., Cheng D., Knight J. et al. Off-pump versus conventional coronary artery bypass grafting: A meta-analysis and consensus statement from the 2004 ISMICS consensus conference. *Innovations* 2005;1:3-27.

[25] Hoff S. J., Ball S. K., Coltharp W. H., Glassford D. M. Jr., Lea J. W. T. Petracek M. R. Coronary artery bypass in patients 80 years and over: Is off-pump the operation of choice? *Ann Thorac Surg* 2002;74:S1340-1343.

[26] Hirose H., Amano A., Takahashi A. Off-pump coronary artery bypass grafting for elderly patients. *Ann Thorac Surg* 2001;72:2013-2019.

[27] Nagpal A. D., Bhatnagar G., Cutrara C. A. et al. Early outcomes of coronary artery bypass with and without cardiopulmonary bypass in octogenarians. *Can J Cardiol* 2006;22:849-853.

[28] Jensen B. O., Hughes P., Rasmussen L. S., Pedersen P. U., Steinbruchel D. A. Cognitive outcomes in elderly high-risk patients after off-pump versus conventional coronary artery bypass grafting: A randomized trial. *Circulation* 2006;113:2790-2795.

[29] Athanasiou T., Al-Ruzzeh S., Kumar P. et al. Off-pump myocardial revascularization is associated with less incidence of stroke in elderly patients. *Ann Thorac Surg* 2004;77:745-753.

[30] Panesar S. S., Athanasiou T., Nair S. et al. Early outcomes in the elderly: A meta-analysis of 4921 patients undergoing coronary artery bypass grafting--comparison between off-pump and on-pump techniques. *Heart* 2006;92:1808-1816.

[31] Chertow G. M., Lazarus J. M., Christiansen C. L. et al. Preoperative renal risk stratification. *Circulation* 1997;95:878-884.

[32] Mangano C. M., Diamondstone L. S., Ramsay J. G. et al. Renal dysfunction after myocardial revascularization: Risk factors, adverse outcomes, and hospital resource utilization. The multicenter study of perioperative ischemia research group. *Ann Intern Med* 1998;128:194-203.

[33] Ascione R., Lloyd C. T., Underwood M. J., Gomes W. J., Angelini G. D. On-pump versus off-pump coronary revascularization: Evaluation of renal function. *Ann Thorac Surg* 1999;68:493-498.

[34] Bucerius J., Gummert J. F., Walther T. et al. On-pump versus off-pump coronary artery bypass grafting: Impact on postoperative renal failure requiring renal replacement therapy. *Ann Thorac Surg* 2004;77:1250-1256.

[35] Sajja L. R., Mannam G., Chakravarthi R. M. et al. Coronary artery bypass grafting with or without cardiopulmonary bypass in patients with preoperative non-dialysis dependent renal insufficiency: A randomized study. *J Thorac Cardiovasc Surg* 2007;133:378-388.

[36] Dewey T. M., Herbert M. A., Prince S. L. et al. Does coronary artery bypass graft surgery improve survival among patients with end-stage renal disease? *Ann Thorac Surg* 2006;81:591-598.

[37] Abu-Omar Y., Mussa S., Naik M. J. et al. Evaluation of cystatin c as a marker of renal injury following on-pump and off-pump coronary surgery. *Eur J Cardiothorac Surg* 2005;27:893-898.

[38] Bergman P., van der Linden J. Atherosclerosis of the ascending aorta as a major determinant of the outcome of cardiac surgery. *Nat Clin Pract Cardiovasc Med* 2005;2:246-251.

[39] Calafiore A. M., Di Mauro M., Teodori G. et al. Impact of aortic manipulation on incidence of cerebrovascular accidents after surgical myocardial revascularization. Ann Thorac Surg 2002;73:1387-1393.

[40] Vallely M. P., Potger K., McMillan D., Hemli J. M., Brady P. W., Brereton R. J., Marshman D., Mathur M. N., Ross D. E. Anaortic techniques reduce neurological morbidity after off-pump coronary artery bypass surgery. *Heart Lung Circ* 2008;17:299-304.
[41] Misfeld M., Brereton R. J., Sweetman E. A., Doig G. S. Neurologic complications after off-pump coronary artery bypass grafting with and without aortic manipulation: Meta-analysis of 11,398 cases from 8 studies. *J Thorac Cardiovasc Surg* 2011;142:e11-17.
[42] Shennib H., Endo M., Benhamed O., Morin J. F. Surgical revascularization in patients with poor left ventricular function: On- or off-pump? *Ann Thorac Surg* 2002;74:S1344-1347.
[43] Ascione R., Narayan P., Rogers C. A., Lim K. H., Capoun R., Angelini G. D. Early and midterm clinical outcome in patients with severe left ventricular dysfunction undergoing coronary artery surgery. *Ann Thorac Surg* 2003;76:793-799.
[44] Al-Ruzzeh S., Athanasiou T., George S. et al. Is the use of cardiopulmonary bypass for multivessel coronary artery bypass surgery an independent predictor of operative mortality in patients with ischemic left ventricular dysfunction? *Ann Thorac Surg* 2003;76:444-451.
[45] Darwazah A. K., Abu Sham'a R. A., Hussein E., Hawari M. H., Ismail H. Myocardial revascularization in patients with low ejection fraction < or =35%: Effect of pump technique on early morbidity and mortality. *J Card Surg* 2006;21:22-27.
[46] Youn Y. N., Chang B. C., Hong Y. S., Kwak Y. L., Yoo K. J. Early and mid-term impacts of cardiopulmonary bypass on coronary artery bypass grafting in patients with poor left ventricular dysfunction: A propensity score analysis. *Circ J* 2007;71:1387-1394.
[47] Puskas J. D., Kilgo P. D., Kutner M., Pusca S. V., Lattouf O., Guyton R. A. Off-pump techniques disproportionately benefit women and narrow the gender disparity in outcomes after coronary artery bypass surgery. *Circulation* 2007;116:I192-199.
[48] Mohr R., Moshkovitch Y., Shapira I. et al. Coronary artery bypass without cardiopulmonary bypass for patients with acute myocardial infarction. *J Thorac Cardiovasc Surg* 1999;118:50-56.
[49] Locker C., Mohr R., Paz Y. et al. Myocardial revascularization for acute myocardial infarction: Benefits and drawbacks of avoiding cardiopulmonary bypass. *Ann Thorac Surg* 2003;76:771-776.
[50] Rastan A. J., Eckenstein J I., Hentschel B. et al. Emergency coronary artery bypass graft surgery for acute coronary syndrome: Beating heart versus conventional cardioplegic cardiac arrest strategies. *Circulation* 2006;114:I477-485.
[51] Fattouch K., Guccione F., Dioguardi P. et al. Off-pump versus on-pump myocardial revascularization in patients with st-segment elevation myocardial infarction: A randomized trial. *J Thorac Cardiovasc Surg* 2009;137:650-656.
[52] Stamou S. C., Hill P. C., Haile E., Prince S., Mack M. J., Corso P. J. Clinical outcomes of nonelective coronary revascularization with and without cardiopulmonary bypass. *J Thorac Cardiovasc Surg* 2006;131:28-33.
[53] Morris C. D., Puskas J. D., Pusca S. V. et al. Outcomes after off-pump reoperative coronary artery bypass grafting. . Innovations: *Technology & Techniques in Cardiothoracic & Vascular Surgery* 2007;2:29-32.

[54] Mishra Y. K., Collison S. P., Malhotra R., Kohli V., Mehta Y., Trehan N. Ten-year experience with single-vessel and multivessel reoperative off-pump coronary artery bypass grafting. *J Thorac Cardiovasc Surg* 2008;135:527-532.
[55] Vohra H. A., Bahrami T., Farid S. et al. Propensity score analysis of early and late outcome after redo off-pump and on-pump coronary artery bypass grafting. *Eur J Cardiothorac Surg* 2008;33:209-214.
[56] Kuss O., Borgermann J. Do higher-risk patients benefit from off-pump coronary artery bypass grafting? Evidence from an ecologic analysis of randomized trials. *J Thorac Cardiovasc Surg* 2011;142:e117-122.
[57] Bittner H. B., Savitt M. A. Off-pump coronary artery bypass grafting decreases morbidity and mortality in a selected group of high-risk patients. *Ann Thorac Surg* 2002;74:115-118.
[58] Chamberlain M. H., Ascione R., Reeves B. C., Angelini G. D. Evaluation of the effectiveness of off-pump coronary artery bypass grafting in high-risk patients: An observational study. *Ann Thorac Surg* 2002;73:1866-1873.
[59] Meharwal Z. S., Mishra Y. K., Kohli V., Bapna R., Singh S., Trehan N. Off-pump multivessel coronary artery surgery in high-risk patients. *Ann Thorac Surg* 2002;74:S1353-1357.
[60] Moller C. H., Perko M. J., Lund J. T. et al. No major differences in 30-day outcomes in high-risk patients randomized to off-pump versus on-pump coronary bypass surgery: The best bypass surgery trial. *Circulation* 2010;121:498-504.
[61] Murphy G. J., Rogers C. A., Caputo M., Angelini G. D. Acquiring proficiency in off-pump surgery: Traversing the learning curve, reproducibility, and quality control. *Ann Thorac Surg* 2005;80:1965-1970.
[62] Caputo M., Bryan A. J., Capoun R. et al. The evolution of training in off-pump coronary surgery in a single institution. *Ann Thorac Surg* 2002;74:S1403-1407.
[63] Caputo M., Chamberlain M. H., Ozalp F. et al. Off-pump coronary operations can be safely taught to cardiothoracic trainees. *Ann Thorac Surg* 2001;71:1215-1219.
[64] Halkos M. E., Puskas J. D. Teaching off-pump coronary artery bypass surgery. *Semin Thorac Cardiovasc Surg* 2009;21:224-228.
[65] Rogers C. A., Reeves B. C., Caputo M., Ganesh J. S., Bonser R. S., Angelini G. D. Control chart methods for monitoring cardiac surgical performance and their interpretation. *J Thorac Cardiovasc Surg* 2004;128:811-819.
[66] Caputo M., Reeves B. C., Rogers C. A., Ascione R., Angelini G. D. Monitoring the performance of residents during training in off-pump coronary surgery. *J Thorac Cardiovasc Surg* 2004;128:907-915.
[67] Ascione R., Reeves B. C., Pano M., Angelini G. D. Trainees operating on high-risk patients without cardiopulmonary bypass: A high-risk strategy? *Ann Thorac Surg* 2004;78:26-33.

In: Off-Pump Coronary Artery Bypass Grafting
Editors: S.G. Raja and M. Amrani
ISBN 978-1-62081-575-5

Chapter 2

SYSTEMIC INFLAMMATORY RESPONSE AFTER OFF-PUMP CORONARY ARTERY BYPASS GRAFTING

Shahzad G. Raja
Cardiac Surgeon, Harefield Hospital, London, UK

ABSTRACT

It is well documented that cardiopulmonary bypass (CPB) is associated with a systemic inflammatory response, which involves the synthesis of various cytokines and inflammatory mediators. This inflammation sets the stage for initiation of injury of major organs (including multiple organ dysfunction syndrome) as well as amplification of injury induced by alterations in vasoreactivity and organ perfusion. The systemic inflammatory response to cardiac surgery is common, and resultant impairment of multiple organ function is generally mild or subclinical due to physiological reserve within organ systems. Unfortunately, the changing profile of patients, older patients with more co-morbidities and limited physiological reserve, referred for surgery suggests that the systemic inflammatory response may prominently influence surgical outcome in the future. Several strategies including the use of steroids, aprotinin, heparin-coated CPB circuits, and hemofiltration have been reported to reduce the inflammatory reaction induced by CPB and its consequences. A more radical and effective way of counteracting the effects of the inflammatory reaction and oxidative stress may be the omission of CPB itself. The development and application of off-pump coronary artery bypass (OPCAB) technology has largely been driven by this theme of avoiding systemic inflammatory reaction in order to decrease the incidence and/or severity of adverse outcomes. This chapter provides an overview of the influence of CPB on systemic inflammation and attempts to evaluate the current best available evidence on the impact of OPCAB on systemic inflammation.

INTRODUCTION

Cardiac surgery is unique because blood exposed to nonendothelial cell surfaces is collected and continuously recirculated throughout the entire body. This contact with synthetic surfaces in the perfusion circuit and multiple tissues within the wound triggers a massive defense reaction that involves at least five plasma protein systems and five blood cells [1]. This reaction-the inflammatory response to cardiopulmonary bypass (CPB)-initiates a powerful thrombotic stimulus and the production, release, and circulation of a host of microemboli and vasoactive and cytotoxic substances that affect every organ and tissue within the body [1].

Contact and complement plasma protein systems, neutrophils, monocytes, endothelial cells, and to a lesser extent platelets are the principal blood elements involved in the systemic inflammatory response to CPB [2]. Activation of these principal blood elements leads to release of vasoactive and cytotoxic substances; production of cell signaling inflammatory and inhibitory cytokines; expression of complementary cellular receptors that interact with specific cell signaling substances and other cells; and generation of a host of vasoactive and cytotoxic substances that circulate [3].

This systemic inflammatory response to CPB has the potential of engendering a constellation of clinical, biochemical and radiological manifestations of multi-organ dysfunction. Recognition of this fact has resulted in efforts to attenuate this complex multi-faceted response which can have tremendous prognostic implications. Heparin-coated circuits, pulsatile flow, normoxia, normothermia, biventricular bypass without an oxygenator, leukocyte and platelet depletion, and total minimal extracorporeal circulation are some of the modifications and refinements of the technique which have evolved to counteract and possibly eliminate the complications associated with CPB induced systemic inflammatory response [4]. In addition, pharmacological maneuvers such as corticosteroids, aprotinin, phosphodiesterase inhibitors, sodium nitroprusside, antioxidants, monoclonal antibodies for the inhibition of complement, neutrophil adhesion molecule blockade, and the inhibition of nuclear factor kappa B (NF-κB) have also been tried alone or in combination [2]. However the experience with most of these strategies has not been entirely satisfactory and systemic inflammatory response still poses a postoperative management challenge [4].

A more radical and effective way of counteracting the effects of the inflammatory reaction and oxidative stress may be the omission of CPB itself. This idea provided the impetus for reintroduction of off-pump coronary artery bypass (OPCAB) surgery- a technique that predates CPB but was rapidly off staged by on-pump CABG soon after the invention of the heart–lung machine owing to the attraction of operating on a still heart in a bloodless field. Despite tremendous enthusiasm on the part of cardiac surgeons, patients, industry, and the media, skepticism still exists about the actual impact of OPCAB in reducing systemic inflammation. The only means of countering this skepticism is by validating the safety and efficacy of OPCAB through the explicit and conscientious assessment of current best evidence. This chapter provides an overview of CPB-induced systemic inflammation and focuses on the impact of OPCAB on systemic inflammation and its clinical implications.

CPB-Induced Systemic Inflammatory Response

The damaging effects of CPB and the subsequent inflammatory response are the result of the extreme conditions encountered during extracorporeal support, including (1) cell activation on contact with the foreign surfaces of the bypass circuit, (2) mechanical shear stress, (3) tissue ischemia and reperfusion, (4) hypotension, (5) nonpulsatile perfusion, (6) hemodilution with relative anemia, (7) blood product administration, (8) heparin and protamine administration, and (9) hypothermia. A global inflammatory response ensues with the activation of cellular and humoral cascades, including the activation of the complement, coagulation, and fibrinolytic pathways; endotoxin release; cytokine production; endothelial activation with expression of leukocyte adhesion molecules; activation of leukocytes and platelets; and production and release of oxygen-free radicals, nitric oxide, arachidonic acid derivatives, and proteolytic enzymes [5, 6]. The next section provides an insight into these cellular and humoral cascades central to the CPB-induced inflammatory response.

Components of Systemic Inflammatory Response

Complement Activation

Complement activation on CPB occurs through both the alternative (stimulated by foreign surface contact, endotoxin, and kallikrein) and classical (protamine) pathways [6-9] (Figure 1). The exposure of blood to extracorporeal circuits activates the alternative pathway, leading to the formation of C3a and C5a, whereas reversal of heparin with protamine activates the classical pathway with an associated rise in C4a levels and further rise in C3a levels [6-10]. The anaphylatoxins C3a and C5a cause activation, degranulation, and adhesion of neutrophils, and activation of basophils and mast cells with histamine release, as well as platelet aggregation [6, 11-14] (Table 1).

Table 1. The main functions of the complement components & fragments

Components & fragments	Actions
C5a, C3a, $C5a_{desArg}$, C4a	Enhanced vascular permeability
	Smooth muscle contractility
	Mast cells & basophils degranulation
C5a, $C5a_{desArg}$	Neutrophil activation & chemotaxis
	Stimulation of prostaglandins & leukotrienes production
C3b, C4b	Opsonization of bacteria & immune complexes leading to phagocytosis
C3b, C5a, $C5a_{desArg}$	Stimulation of respiratory burst of phagocytes
$C5b678(9)_n$	Lysis of bacteria & foreign cells
C3b, CR1	Solubilization of circulating immune complexes

Neutrophil Activation

Neutrophils are activated by a wide variety of stimuli, including foreign surface contact, endotoxin, cytokines, complement, platelet-activating factor, and ischemia–reperfusion [6]. Once activated, neutrophils begin the process of endothelial adherence and migration with subsequent release of proteases and oxygen-derived free radicals. Endothelial cell barrier dysfunction is impaired, with resultant fluid extravasation [6, 15].

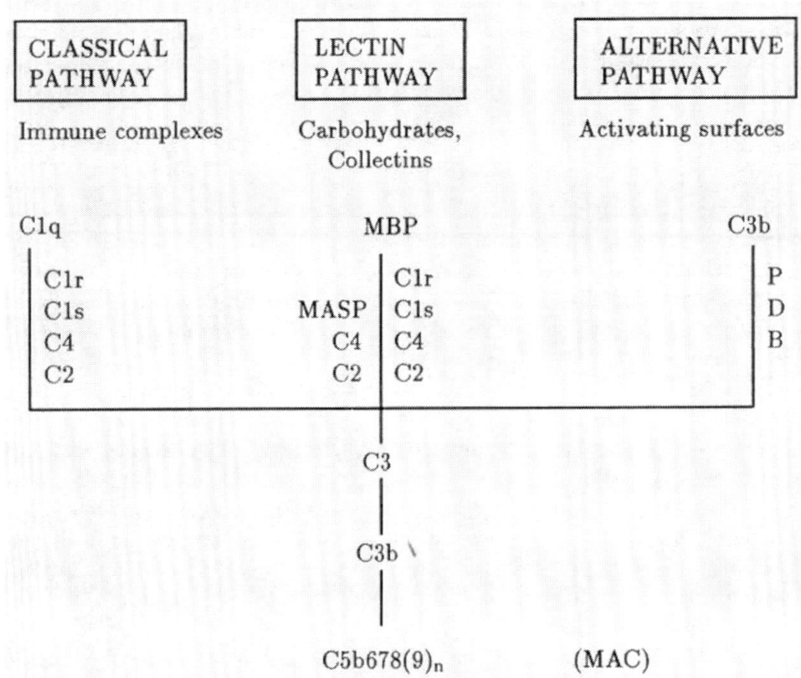

Figure 1. Different activation pathways of the complement system (MBP: mannan-binding protein; MASP: MBP-associated serine protease; B: factor B; D: factor D; P: properdin; MAC: membrane attack complex).

Kinin Production

Kinin peptides are potent vasodilators that also participate in inflammation, leading to increased vascular permeability and neutrophil chemotaxis [6, 16]. The contact activation system is composed of kinin–kallikrein, fibrinolytic-coagulation, and complement systems. During CPB, factor XII is activated by contact with artificial surfaces, producing factor XIIa (Figure 2), which then converts prekallikrein to kallikrein in the presence of high-molecular-weight kininogen. Kallikrein then enters a positive feedback loop with factor XIIa to activate additional factor XII; it also cleaves surface-bound high-molecular-weight kininogen to produce bradykinin [6, 17]. In addition to the response to the CPB circuit, plasma kallikrein levels have been found to significantly increase after the administration of heparin [6, 18]. The biologic effects of kinins are mediated through B_1 and B_2 receptors. B_2 receptors are expressed in many cell types and have a high specific affinity for bradykinin [6, 16].

Activation of B_2 receptors leads to the release of calcium, nitric oxide, eicosanoids, free radicals, and cytokines [6, 19]. Bradykinin can also bind to receptors on endothelial cells, which then produce vasoactive prostaglandins and nitric oxide, leading to vasodilatation and increased capillary permeability. Bradykinin has also been found in the brain parenchyma, with increased levels seen in the brain interstitial space during cerebral ischemia [20]. Mediated by activation of the B_2 receptor, bradykinin can increase the permeability of the blood–brain barrier after ischemia–reperfusion, resulting in plasma extravasation with edema formation and perturbation of the cerebral blood flow [20].

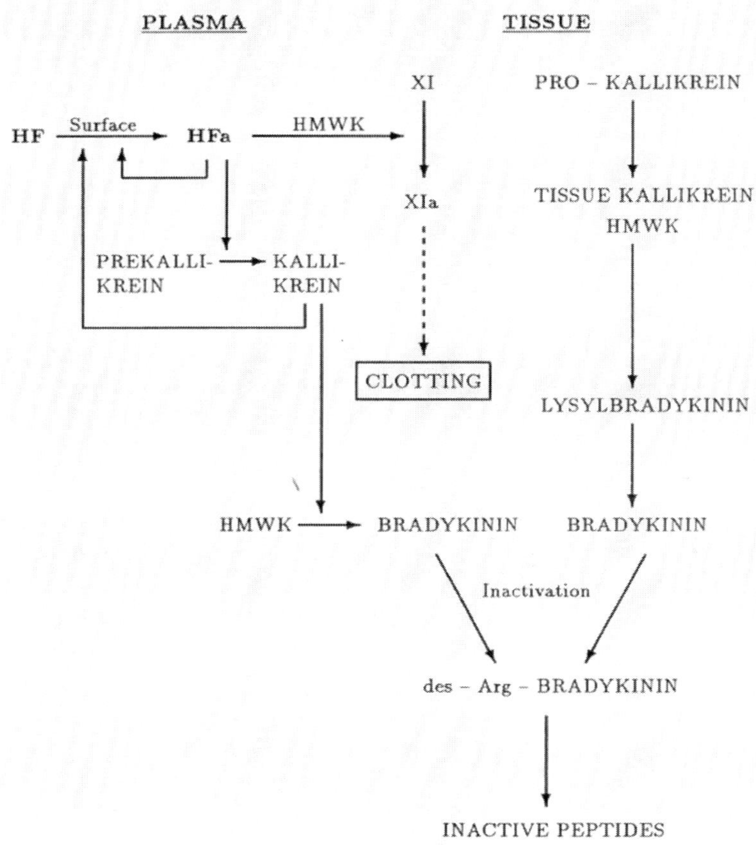

Figure 2. The kinin pathway.

Arachidonic Acid Activation

The arachidonic acid cascade is activated by a number of inflammatory stimuli that result in activation of cyclooxygenase and phospholipase A_2. Arachidonic acid pathway activation results in production of thromboxanes, leukotrienes, and prostaglandins [6, 21] (Figure 3). The neutrophil cell membrane is the primary source of arachidonic acid, but the lung is also a major site of the synthesis, release, and degradation of the eicosanoids. Thromboxane A_2, a strong vasoconstrictor and promoter of platelet aggregation, comes primarily from platelets and release occurs to a great extent in the lungs. Prostaglandin E_1, prostaglandin E_2, and prostacyclin are also released during CPB. These substances have vasodilating and platelet antiaggregant effects that counterbalance the effects of thromboxane A_2. Leukotriene B_4, a strong chemoattractant that promotes plasma leakage and leukocyte adhesion, is also increased during and for a short time after CPB [22].

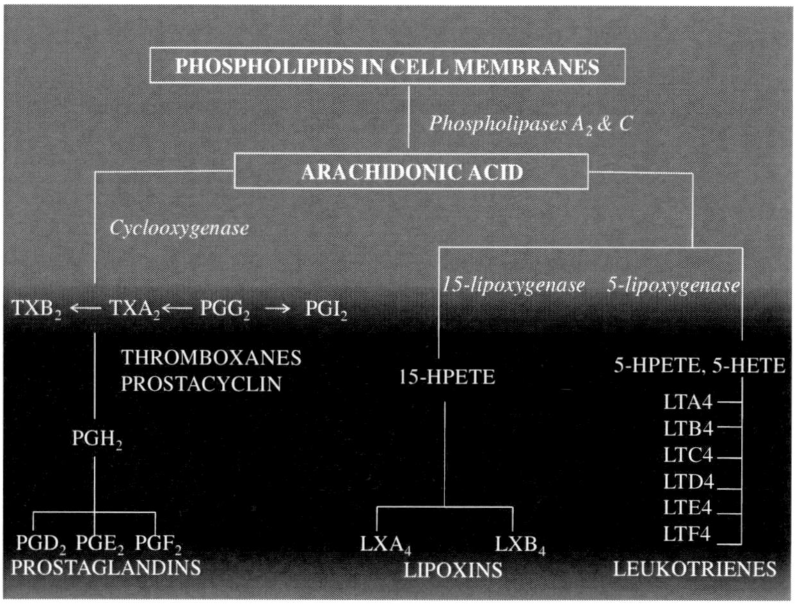

Figure 3. The metabolic pathway of archidonic acid (HPETE: hydroperoxy-eicosatetraenoic acid; HETE: hydroxy-eicosatetraenoic acid; LT: leukotrienes; LX: lipoxins; PG: prostaglandins; PGI: protacyclin; TX: thromboxane).

Cytokines

Cytokines are produced by monocytes, macrophages, lymphocytes, and endothelial cells. Production is stimulated by ischemia–reperfusion, complement activation, and endotoxin release, and is further amplified by the effect of other cytokines [6]. Cytokines can be either protective or damaging depending on their concentration, the cell they are acting on, and the presence of other cytokines [5, 6]. The most important cytokines produced during CPB are the proinflammatory cytokines tumor necrosis factor α (TNFα), interleukin (I L) 1, IL-6, and IL-8, and the antiinflammatory cytokines IL-10 and IL-1 receptor antagonist (IL-1ra) [5, 6]. TNFα, IL-1, IL-6, and IL-8 levels all increase after CPB, and all are participants in the acute inflammatory response. TNFα and IL-1 are early inflammatory cytokines that initiate the inflammatory response and are also pyrogenic. TNFα facilitates leukocyte–endothelial interaction, and elevation of TNFα in postoperative infants has been correlated with capillary leak syndrome [23]. TNFα has also been shown to have a negative inotropic effect in animal studies looking specifically at cardiac function [24]. Interleukin 6 and IL-8 begin to rise near the end of CPB and continue to increase in the first few hours after surgery. Interleukin 6 acts on B cells to differentiate into plasma cells and stimulates hepatocytes to make acute-phase proteins. Increasing IL-6 levels correlate with adverse outcomes [25]. Interleukin 8 stimulates neutrophil chemotaxis, and levels appear to be related to the duration of CPB [26]. Interleukin 10 and IL-1ra are the major antiinflammatory cytokines, whose role is to limit the production of proinflammatory cytokines [5, 6]. They are produced as a response to inflammation and are stimulated in part by the proinflammatory cytokines, especially IL-6.

Cytokines are both participants in inflammation and markers of the ongoing response. The ratio of proinflammatory to antiinflammatory cytokines is predictive of outcome. In patients with the systemic inflammatory response as a result of sepsis, an increased ratio of IL-6 to IL-10 is correlated with poor outcome, and conversely, an elevated ratio of IL-10 to IL-6 in infants undergoing cardiac surgery was predictive of a better outcome [27, 28]. Although the antiinflammatory cytokines limit the extent of the inflammatory response and begin to restore homeostasis, an excessive antiinflammatory cytokine response may follow an excessive proinflammatory response and result in immunocompromise [29, 30].

Platelet-activating Factor

Platelet-activating factor is a phospholipid synthesized by platelets and vascular endothelial cells. Platelet-activating factor receptors are present on platelets as well as neutrophils, monocytes, and endothelial cells. It is a potent neutrophil chemoattractant, activator, and aggregant, and plays an important role in myocardial ischemia–reperfusion injury [6, 31].

Endothelin-1

Endothelin-1 is the most potent endogenous vasoconstrictor involved in the regulation of arterial blood pressure and cardiac output [32]. The lung is an important site for both clearance and production of endothelin-1, and an increase in endothelin concentrations has been correlated with endotoxin levels during CPB [33]. The vasoconstrictor effects of endothelin may lead to intestinal hypoperfusion, resulting in translocation and endotoxin release into the circulation [34].

Thrombin

Cardiopulmonary bypass is a strong procoagulant stimulus [6]. Heparin inhibits the formation of thrombus, but it does not prevent the expression of tissue factor on activated endothelial cells and monocytes, which is central to the extrinsic system of coagulation. Activated endothelial cells and monocytes express tissue factor; when factor VII comes in contact with tissue factor, the coagulation cascade is activated, leading to the conversion of prothrombin to thrombin. The production of thrombin by itself has significant inflammatory and thrombotic properties [35]. Once generated, thrombin leads to increased expression of P-selectin on endothelial cells, which causes neutrophil adherence and activation [35]. Increased activation of thrombin receptors on leukocytes can also lead to the release of chemotactic and inflammatory cytokines [35].

The individual elements of the inflammatory response to CPB ultimately combine through redundancy, positive feedback loops, and amplifying cascades to yield the characteristic, generalized post-CPB injury picture. The end result of this complex inflammatory response is endothelial damage, capillary leak, and end-organ dysfunction.

Off-pump Coronary Artery Bypass Grafting and Systemic Inflammatory Response

Concerns regarding the complications and cost of using CPB have led to renewed interest in OPCAB techniques. By avoidance of aortic crossclamping and CPB, OPCAB may decrease the inflammatory response and improve postoperative organ function and patient outcome, particularly in high-risk patients [36]. Available evidence from a large number of prospective randomized controlled trials [37-44] suggests that OPCAB reduces the elaboration of key mediators of the systemic inflammatory response (Table 2). Use of OPCAB decreases concentrations of cytokines such as TNFα, IL-6, IL-8, IL-10, TNFsr1, and TNFsr2 [36]. It also attenuates the cellular inflammatory response, decreasing neutrophil and monocyte counts, neutrophil elastase, and E-selectin concentrations [36]. Indices of complement activation, such as C3a and C5a, are decreased [36]. In addition, OPCAB attenuates other indices including platelet ß-thromboglobulin and procalcitonin. Finally, OPCAB decreases reactive oxygen-species-induced injury [36]. The next section evaluates in detail the impact of OPCAB on various components of systemic inflammatory response.

Neutrophils and OPCAB

Al-Ruzzeh et al. [45] in a recently published, prospective randomized study compared neutrophil activation in patients undergoing OPCAB (n = 10) versus those undergoing CABG with CPB (n = 10). The results of their study showed that white blood cell (WBC) and neutrophil counts rose in both groups following the operation but were significantly higher in the OPCAB group at 5 hours ($p < .001$ and $p = .002$, respectively). Interleukin 8 concentrations were significantly higher in the CPB group at 5 hours following the initiation of CPB ($p = .034$) while CD11b levels were significantly higher in the CPB group at 60 minutes ($p = .002$). They concluded that that the activation of circulating neutrophils as measured by CD11b expression is lower following OPCAB than in CPB and although OPCAB is associated with significantly higher neutrophil counts, these neutrophils exhibit fewer activation markers. In their opinion the lower postoperative neutrophil counts occurring in the CPB group could be explained by the activation and consequent sequestration of the neutrophils in the CPB circuit and tissues. In another prospective study Okubo et al. [46] utilized a semiquantitative reverse transcription polymerase chain reaction technique to evaluate gene expression of cytokines, adhesion molecules, and vasoactive substances in leukocytes of peripheral blood before and six hours after surgery in patients undergoing OPCAB (n = 10) versus those undergoing CABG with CPB (n = 10). In view of the significantly increased postoperative expression of m-RNA for IL-1, IL-8, and IL-10, TNFα, heme oxygenase (HO)-1, platelet endothelial cellular adhesion molecule (PECAM) and Mac-

1 in the on-pump group but not in the off-pump group ($p<0.05$), they concluded that OPCAB is a less invasive technique than CABG with CPB.

Similarly, Ascione et al. [47] in their prospective RCT showed that showed neutrophil elastase concentrations ($p < 0.0001$) and postoperative WBC, neutrophil, and monocyte counts ($p < 0.01$) were significantly higher in the on-pump than the off-pump group.

Endothelin and OPCAB

In a prospective, randomized study, Dorman et al. [48] measured endothelin (ET) plasma content from patients undergoing CABG using either OPCAB (n = 25) or conventional cardiopulmonary bypass (CPB group, n = 25) before surgery, before and after coronary artery anastomosis, and 6 and 24 hours postoperatively. They also documented specific indices of patient recovery including pulmonary artery pressures, ventilation requirement, and hospital stay. The results of their RCT showed that postoperative systemic arterial ET levels were significantly increased by 200% in the CPB group and 50% in the OPCAB group. ET levels remained significantly higher in the CPB group relative to the OPCAB group throughout the postoperative period of observation ($p < 0.05$). Since pulmonary artery pressures, ventilation requirement, and hospital stay were significantly increased in patients in the CPB group they concluded that increased ET in the postoperative period may contribute to a more complex recovery from coronary artery bypass surgery in patients undergoing cardiopulmonary bypass. Similar results were produced by Wildhirt et al. [49]. The results of their RCT revealed that OPCAB reduces myocardial cell damage and lipid peroxidation and is also associated with a reduced activation of the potent vasoconstrictor peptide endothelin. All of this may contribute to improved myocardial function and faster postoperative recovery from surgical revascularization procedures, particularly in critically ill patients.

Platelets and OPCAB

Gu et al. [50] in their prospective RCT comparing CABG-CPB and minimally invasive direct coronary artery bypass (MIDCAB) showed that the platelet count was similar in both groups at the end of the CABG procedure (from 193 ± 20 to $258 \pm 40 \times 109$ /L in the CPB-CABG group, and from 195 ± 17 to $215 \pm 38 \times 109$/L in the MIDCAB group). However, platelet degranulation, indicated by the release of β-thromboglobulin, was found in the CPB-CABG group (from 446 ± 56 to $1,352 \pm 361$ ng/mL; $p < 0.01$), but not in the MIDCAB group (from 499 ± 76 to 420 ± 77 ng/mL). On the other hand, Moller et al. [51] in their prospective RCT evaluating platelet function four times within the first 24 h (preoperatively, postoperatively, 4 h and 1 day after surgery) after OPCAB and CABG on CPB observed a significant increase of platelet-activating-factor-induced platelet aggregation postoperatively after OPCAB ($p < 0.01$). Platelet aggregation immediately after on-pump CABG was reduced to near half of preoperative values, but within 1 day postoperatively normal platelet aggregation was regained in half of the patients indicating that CABG with CPB resulted in a temporary platelet dysfunction which seemed to be overcome within the first postoperative day. In another prospective nonRCT, comparing the effect of OPCAB and CPB on platelet counts, it was shown that only CABG on CPB was associated with a reduction in platelet counts (76% of baseline, 66–85%, $p = 0.0001$) [52].

Complement and OPCAB

Ascione et al. [47] in their prospective RCT observed that C3a increased significantly in the on-pump group soon after surgery when compared with baseline ($p < 0.0001$) and off-pump group ($p = 0.0197$). Also C5a levels were significantly elevated soon after surgery in the on-pump group when compared with the off-pump group ($p = 0.0116$). However, comparison of data over time (ANOVA) did not show any statistical significance between groups. Matata et al. [53] also showed that the plasma levels of complement C3a, a product of complement activation, were not significantly affected by anesthesia and surgical trauma, however they were rapidly elevated upon the institution of CPB. C3a levels rapidly increased after the initiation of CPB and at 0.5 hours, values were 12 times greater than those observed before anesthesia. Following this, and over the next 2 hours, the C3a levels remained elevated but to a lesser degree, and by 4 hours C3a levels were similar to the values seen before anesthesia. This rise in complement activation was almost completely abolished in the non CPB group patients. In this group, the C3a levels were slightly but significantly elevated 1 and 2 hours after the initiation of bypass grafting, coincidental with the reversion of heparin with protamine. Similarly, Gu et al. [50] observed that complement activation, identified by C3a, increased significantly in the CPB-CABG group at the end of CPB compared with the baseline concentration (from 1,654 ± 202 to 3,503 ± 110 ng/mL; $p < 0.01$), but did not increase in the MIDCAB group (from 789 ± 60 to 725 ± 71 ng/mL). The same group carried out a prospective RCT to examine whether tissue injury caused by chest surgical incision per se contributes to complement activation in CABG patients [54]. They prospectively divided twenty-two patients undergoing CABG without CPB into two groups: a small chest incision via an anterolateral thoracotomy representing a minimized tissue injury (lateral group, $n = 8$), and a conventional median sternotomy representing a large tissue injury (median group, $n = 14$). The results of their study showed that the plasma concentrations of complement 3a increased in both the lateral and median groups right after chest incision ($p < 0.01$ and $p < 0.05$, respectively) and by the end of operation increased only in the median group ($p < 0.01$). The terminal complement complex 5b-9 did not increase in the lateral group, but it did increase in the median group both after incision and by the end of the operation ($p < 0.05$ and $p < 0.05$, respectively). During surgery, complement 4a did not increase, suggesting that it is the alternative rather than the classic pathway that is involved in complement activation by tissue injury. Similar results have been achieved by other investigators [55, 56].

Cytokines and OPCAB

Schulze et al. [57] in their prospective RCT observed that despite comparable surgical trauma coronary revascularization with CPB was associated with a significant expression increase in the TNF-system and sIL-2r when compared to the OPCAB patients. Although IL-6 expression did not differ between both groups, C-reactive protein levels were significantly lower in the OPCAB group. Diegeler et al. [55] showed a significant increased release of IL-8, and IL-10 in patients subjected to CPB during the initial period and for a short time after perfusion (p<0.05). TNFα receptors p55 and p75 showed a prolonged elevation (up to 48 hours) in the CPB group compared with the 2 off-pump groups while IL-6 showed no different release among the 3 surgical groups throughout the entire period. Similar results have been observed by several other investigators [46, 47, 56, 58-61].

Table 2. Randomized controlled trials comparing impact of OPCAB and conventional CABG on systemic inflammatory response

Study	Year	Intervention (n per group)	Main Result
Lin et al, [37]	2010	CABG with CPB (25)[¥] versus OPCAB (20)	Elevated serum IL-8, IL-10, IL-12 were found in all three groups. HSP70 expression within leukocyte was enhanced in CABG patients.s
Onorati et al, [38]	2010	CABG with CPB (40)[€] versus OPCAB (20)	OPCAB was associated with slight endothelial activation and cytokine response. Pulsatile cardiopulmonary bypass CABG significantly attenuates endothelial/cytokine leakage.
Serrano et al, [39]	2010	CABG with CPB (41) versus OPCAB (40)	OPCAB better preserves the myocardium and attenuates inflammation compared to on-pump CABG.
Rasmussen et al, [40]	2007	CABG with CPB (17) versus OPCAB (18)	Oxygenation was more affected by OPCAB. Only part of the systemic inflammatory response (IL-8 & IL-10) was attenuated by OPCAB.
Parolari et al, [41]	2007	CABG with CPB (16) versus OPCAB (14)	The postoperative protracted activation of inflammation is not affected by surgical strategy (on-pump or off-pump).
Tatoulis et al, [42]	2006	CABG with CPB (50) versus OPCAB (50)	The incidence of low SVR, and patterns of SVR changes were similar in both groups, and were clinically unimportant as few patients required vasopressor support. Cardiac outputs and clinical outcomes were excellent in both groups.
Cavalca et al, [43]	2006	CABG with CPB (25) versus OPCAB (25)	OPCAB revealed less perioperative oxidative stress, as reflected by lack of excretion of iPF2alpha-III in urine, by lack of increase of plasma free malondialdehyde, and by lower decreases in plasma total antioxidant status.
Wehlin et al, [44]	2005	CABG with CPB (9) versus OPCAB (11)	Monocyte expression and in vitro mobilization of complement receptors, CD11b and CD35, were similar in both study groups during and after surgery as was the expression of CD62L.
Wan et al, [75]	2004	CABG with CPB (19) versus OPCAB (18)	IL-10, IL-6, IL-8, TNFα, & VCAM-1significantly higher in CABG + CPB group.
Wehlin et al, [76]	2004	CABG with CPB (16) versus OPCAB (21)	Postoperative ET levels were higher in patients who underwent CPB for CABG.
Dorman et al, [48]	2004	CABG with CPB (25) versus OPCAB (25)	Postoperative ET levels were higher in patients who underwent CPB for CABG.
Al-Ruzzeh et al, [45]	2004	CABG with CPB (10) versus OPCAB (10)	Less activation of circulating neutrophils in OPCAB patients.
Moller et al, [51]	2003	CABG with CPB (15) versus OPCAB (15)	Platelets after OPCAB are more easily activated in the early postoperative period. After CABG with CPB there is a temporary platelet dysfunction which improves within the first postoperative day.
Jemielity et al, [77]	2003	CABG with CPB (25) versus OPCAB (25)	Peak IL-6 level significantly lower after OPCAB; CRP higher after CABG; AGP rise comparable.
Okubo et al, [46]	2003	CABG with CPB (10) versus OPCAB (10)	Postoperative expression of m-RNA for IL-1, -8, and -10, TNF-alpha, HO-1, PECAM and Mac-1 increased significantly in the on-pump group but not in the off-pump group (p<0.05).
Wildhirt et al, [58]	2001	CABG with CPB (13) versus OPCAB (13)	Significant reduction in systemic & cardiac adhesion molecule expression after OPCAB.

Table 2. (Continued)

Study	Year	Intervention (n per group)	Main Result
Schulze et al, [57]	2000	CABG with CPB (13) versus OPCAB (13) sternotomy OPCAB	Significant increase in the TNF system & sIL-2r in CABG; no difference in IL-6 levels; CRP & total nitrate/nitrite levels significantly lower in OPCAB.
Wildhirt et al, [49]	2000	CABG with CPB (13) versus OPCAB (13)	OPCAB reduces myocardial cell damage and lipid peroxidation & is also associated with a reduced activation of endothelin.
Gulielmos et al, [61]	2000	CABG with CPB (20) versus OPCAB (20)	The use of CPB was associated with higher levels of troponin-T and CK- MB as signs of myocardial damage. Surgical access was identified as a trigger of inflammatory response, as minithoracotomy wa related to higher levels of IL-6.
Czerny et al, [62]	2000	CABG with CPB (16) versus OPCAB (14)	Significantly lower IL-10, P-selectin, ICAM-1, myoglobin, CK-MB & troponin I release after OPCAB.
Ascione et al, [47]	2000	CABG with CPB (30) versus OPCAB (30)	Neutrophil elastase ($p<0.0001$), IL-8 levels ($p=0.01$), WBC counts ($p<0.01$) & incidence of postop infection ($p<0.0001$) higher in CABG.
Diegeler et al, [55]*	2000	Full sternotomy CABG with CPB (10), full sternotomy OPCAB (10), limited LAT OPCAB (10)	A significant increased release of C3d, C5a, IL-8 IL-10, TNF-α receptors p55 & p75 after CABG.
Matata et al, [53]	2000	CABG with CPB (10) versus OPCAB (10)	Significant increase in lipid H_2O_2 (190% at 4 hours), protein carbonyls (250% at 0.5 hrs) & nitrotyrosine (510% at 0.5 hrs), IL-8, elastase, C3a & sE-selectin in CABG.
Gu et al, [50]	1998	CABG with CPB (31) versus MIDCAB (31)	Leukocyte elastase, platelet beta- thromboglobulin, & C3a levels significantly increased in CABG.

CABG, coronary artery bypass grafting; CPB, cardiopulmonary bypass; OPCAB, off-pump coronary artery bypass surgery; HSP70, heat shock protein 70; IL, interleukin; VCAM-1, vascular cell adhesion molecule-1; ICAM-1, intercellular adhesion molecule-1; TNF, tumor necrosis factor; CRP, C reactive protein; AGP, acid glycoprotein; CK-MB, creatine kinase-MB; LAT, left anterior thoracotomy; MIDCAB, minimally invasive direct coronary artery bypass; SVR, systemic vascular resistance; HO-1, heme oxygenase-1; PECAM, platelet endothelial cellular adhesion molecule; ET, endothelin.

¥ CABG on-pump with cardioplegic arrest = 12, CABG on-pump beating heart = 13.

€ CABG with pulsatile cardiopulmonary bypass = 20, CABG with linear cardiopulmonary bypass.

* The type of operative approach did not influence this immune response.

^ Four surgical techniques were compared: group 1, median sternotomy with CPB in ten patients (eight male, two female; aged 59.6+/-11.0 years (mean+/-SD)); group 2, median sternotomy and off-pump in ten patients (seven male, three female; aged 65.1+/-10.0 years); group 3, minithoracotomy with CPB in ten patients (seven male, three female, aged 61.2+/-10.4 years); group 4, minithoracotomy and off-pump in ten patients (nine male, one female, aged 62.9+/-9.8 years). All patients received a left internal mammary artery graft to the left anterior descending artery (LAD).

Interestingly, Gulielmos et al. [61] in their prospective randomized comparison of four surgical techniques (median sternotomy with CPB, median sternotomy and off-pump, minithoracotomy with CPB and minithoracotomy and off-pump) observed that interleukin-6 (IL-6) levels were significantly higher in minithoracotomy procedures whereas interleukin-1 (IL-1) was significantly increased in all patients compared with the preoperative values. Based on their findings they concluded that surgical access is a trigger of inflammatory response, as minithoracotomy was related to higher levels of IL-6. Furthermore, they were of the view that as IL-1 increased in all procedures and this occurred independently of the surgical access or the use of CPB therefore a potential relationship existed between inflammatory response and anesthesia. Czerny et al. [62] have also observed similar findings.

Endotoxemia and OPCAB

Endotoxin is a lipopolysaccharide from the cell wall of gram-negative bacteria and is recognized to be a major stimulus for the development of the systemic inflammatory response syndrome [63]. Transient endotoxemia in patients undergoing surgery involving CPB has been widely recognized [64]. The endotoxemia associated with cardiac surgery is thought to be dominantly influenced by the use of CPB [65]. Gut translocation has traditionally been perceived as the primary source of endotoxemia [66]. However, the pathogenesis involved in this phenomenon is not entirely clear although leakage of endotoxin into the systemic circulation due to failure of clearance by the hepatic Kupffer cells may be a likely mechanism [67].

Endotoxins have been recognized to have profound biologic effects with the ability to activate different cascade systems, such as complement, coagulation, and white blood cells, and might produce a range of clinical symptoms from headache, chills and myalgia over fever, hypotension, and metabolic acidosis to septic shock and disseminated intravascular coagulation [68, 69].

Aydin et al. [70] in a recently published prospective study have shown that endotoxin and lactate levels were significantly ($p < .05$) lower in the off-pump group at all sampling time points, except after sternotomy. This finding is significant as the relatively lower endotoxin levels observed in off-pump surgery might contribute to improved recovery from surgical revascularization procedures, particularly in critically ill patients.

Other Mediators of Inflammation and OPCAB

C-reactive protein (CRP), one of the major acute phase reactants, enhances phagocytosis of bacteria, viruses and parasites and also activates complement [71]. Levels of CRP were found to be increased in the early days after surgery both in CABG on CPB and OPCAB. However, the increase of CRP levels was greater and persisted for longer time after CABG on CPB with respect to OPCAB [57].

Reactive oxidants, which are cytotoxic inside the phagosome, but act as cytotoxic mediators of acute inflammation outside are produced by neutrophils, monocytes, and macrophages [67]. NADPH (nicotinamide adenine dinucleotide phosphate) oxidase, superoxide dismutase, nitric oxide synthase, and myeloperoxidase produce superoxide (O_2-), hydrogen peroxide (H_2O_2), nitric oxide (NO) and hypochlorous acids respectively [71]. The four products produced by these enzymes, O_2-, H_2O_2, NO, and HOCl, generate all reactive oxidants from nonenzymatic reactions with other molecules or ions resulting in the production of highly cytotoxic substances [71]. Schulze et al. [57] measured systemic nitric oxide production and total nitrate/nitrite (NOx) by using the Griess reaction in their RCT. They showed that systemic NOx levels as the stable end-product of nitric oxide were lower in the OPCAB group.

Increased free radical-induced oxidative stress activity is noticed after CPB [72]. OPCAB is associated with lower degrees of oxidative stress than coronary surgery on CPB [73]. Matata et al. [53] have shown that, in the early hours after surgery, OPCAB patients display significantly lower levels of lipid hydroperoxides, protein carbonyls and nitrotyrosine, all markers of oxidative stress.

In a more recently published RCT, Cavalca et al. [43] randomized 50 low-risk coronary patients to CABG or OPCAB. Urinary isoprostane iPF2alpha-III levels, plasma levels of free malondialdehyde, and total antioxidant status were measured before, during, and up to 24 hours after surgery. The results of the RCT revealed that, in OPCAB, iPF2alpha-III excretion remained unchanged throughout the study. As expected, in CABG, iPF2alpha-III levels significantly increased during surgery and returned at baseline 24 hours later. Free malondialdehyde behaved similarly, with no change in OPCAB and sharp increases during CABG. Conversely, total antioxidant status showed a sharp drop during CABG, followed by a slow recovery, whereas a significantly lower drop occurred in OPCAB. Based on these findings, Cavalca et al. [43] concluded that in low-risk coronary patients, OPCAB revealed less perioperative oxidative stress, as reflected by lack of excretion of iPF2alpha-III in urine, by lack of increase of plasma-free malondialdehyde, and by lower decreases in plasma total antioxidant status.

Correlation between Reduced Systemic Inflammatory Response after OPCAB and Clinical Outcomes

The morbidities of conventional CABG have been attributed to the use of CPB, cardioplegic arrest, and aortic crossclamping resulting in ischemia and reperfusion. The development of off-pump CABG served to eliminate the harmful effects of the heart-lung machine together with cardioplegia [74]. Several clinical trials [75-83] and meta-analyses [84-86] have documented reduced transfusion requirements, shortened length of hospital stay, reduced neurologic complications, and reduced hospital costs for OPCAB recipients compared with those undergoing conventional CABG. Octogenarian patients represent a particularly attractive target for application of OPCAB. The prevalence of comorbid events and the propensity for neurologic dysfunction place octogenarians at higher risk for cardiopulmonary bypass-induced morbidity and mortality. Several studies have shown that OPCAB in elderly patients is associated with fewer complications, a shorter hospital stay, and lower hospital cost [87-90]. These benefits are hypothesized to be the result of reduced CPB-evoked systemic inflammatory response [75].

Although plenty of evidence from RCTs is available to validate that with OPCAB the magnitude of inflammatory response is significantly less (Table 2) yet very few trials [42, 47, 48, 75] have actually correlated or attempted to correlate the biochemical findings with the clinical outcomes. More importantly because of small number of patients neither these trials were powered for clinical conclusions nor any significant difference in clinical outcome between groups was observed. Another significant limitation of most of these trials is the recruitment of low-risk patients. Due to the low-risk nature of the study cohorts in these trials, there were very few deviations from a routine uncomplicated postoperative course, so that no associations between the magnitude of inflammatory response and clinical outcome could be demonstrated. Furthermore, the results of these trials cannot be extrapolated to high-risk patients.

Conclusion

CPB and clinical cardiac surgery produce a broad and intense systemic inflammatory response that varies in degree between patients. The cause is the continuous recirculation of blood that is sequentially in contact with the wound, perfusion circuit, and intravascular compartment to which is added the washout of reperfused ischemic organs and tissues. This systemic inflammatory response together with microembolization is responsible for most of the morbidity of CPB and clinical cardiac surgery.

Evidence from a large number of RCTs indicates that OPCAB reduces the systemic inflammatory response but does not prevent it. In fact, it would be incorrect to expect that OPCAB will abolish the systemic inflammatory response completely. It is worth remembering that while performing OPCAB, the response to surgical trauma, manipulation of the heart, pericardial suction, heparin, protamine, other drugs, and anesthesia are still there and all produce an increase in the markers of acute inflammation. Increasing acceptance to perform OPCAB in elderly patients and those with comorbid conditions is a proof of the fact that this attenuated systemic inflammatory response reduces organ dysfunction. However, an RCT recruiting high-risk population with an adequate sample size correlating inflammatory response and clinical outcome is probably needed to definitely prove the possible associations between the reduced magnitude of the inflammatory response and better clinical outcome in patients undergoing OPCAB surgery.

References

[1] Edmunds LH Jr. Extracorporeal Circulation: Introduction. In: Cohn LH, Edmunds LH Jr. (Eds), *Cardiac Surgery in the Adult*. New York, McGraw-Hill, 2003, p316.

[2] Laffey JG, Boylan JF, Cheng DC. The systemic inflammatory response to cardiac surgery: implications for the anesthesiologist. *Anesthesiology* 2002;97:215-52.

[3] Downing SW, Edmunds LH Jr. Release of vasoactive substances during cardiopulmonary bypass. *Ann Thorac Surg* 1992;54:1236-43.

[4] Ngaage D. L. Off-pump coronary artery bypass grafting: the myth, the logic and the science. *Eur J Cardiothorac Surg* 2003;24:557-70.

[5] Brix-Christensen V. The systemic inflammatory response after cardiac surgery with cardiopulmonary bypass in children. *Acta Anaesthesiol Scand* 2001;45:671-679.

[6] Kozik DJ, Tweddell JS. Characterizing the inflammatory response to cardiopulmonary bypass in children. *Ann Thorac Surg* 2006;81:S2347-54.

[7] Chenoweth DE, Cooper SW, Hugli TE, et al. Complement activation during cardiopulmonary bypass. Evidence for generation of C3a and C5a anaphylatoxins, *N Engl J Med* 1981;304:497-503.

[8] Kirklin J K, Westaby S, Blackstone EH et al. Complement and the damaging effects of cardiopulmonary bypass. *J Thorac Cardiovasc Surg* 1983;86:845-857.

[9] Kirklin JK, Chenoweth DE, Naftel DC, et al. Effects of protamine administration after cardiopulmonary bypass on complement, blood elements, and the hemodynamic state. *Ann Thorac Surg*. 1986;41:193-199.
[10] Steinberg JB, Kapelanski DP, Olson JD, et al. Cytokine and complement levels in patients undergoing cardiopulmonary bypass. *J Thorac Cardiovasc Surg* 1993;106:1008-1016.
[11] Moat NE, Shore DF, Evans TW. Organ dysfunction and cardiopulmonary bypassthe role of complement and complement regulatory proteins. *Eur J Cardiothorac Surg* 1993;7:563-573.
[12] Wachtfogel YT, Kucich U, Greenplate J, et al. Human neutrophil degranulation during extracorporeal circulation. *Blood* 1987;69:324-330.
[13] Polley MJ, Nachman RL. Human platelet activation by C3a and C3a des-arg. *J Exp Med* 1983;158:603-615.
[14] Antonsen S, Brandslund I, Clemensen S, et al. Neutrophil lysosomal enzyme release and complement activation during cardiopulmonary bypass. *Scand J Thorac Cardiovasc Surg* 1987;21:47-52.
[15] Boyle EM Jr, Pohlman TH, Johnson MC, et al. Endothelial cell injury in cardiovascular surgerythe systemic inflammatory response. *Ann Thorac Surg* 1997;63:277-284.
[16] Campbell DJ, Dizon B, Kladis A, et al. Activation of the kallikrein-kinin system by cardiopulmonary bypass in humans. *Am J Physiol* 2001;281:R1059-R1070.
[17] Mojcik CF, Levy JH. Aprotinin and the systemic inflammatory response after cardiopulmonary bypass. *Ann Thorac Surg* 2001;71:745-754.
[18] Saatvedt K, Lindberg H, Michelsen S, et al. Activation of the fibrinolytic, coagulation and plasma kallikrein-kinin systems during and after open heart surgery in children. *Scan J Clin Lab Invest* 1995;55:359-367.
[19] Hellal F, Pruneau D, Palmier B, et al. Detrimental role of bradykinin B_2 receptor in a murine model of diffuse brain injury. *J Neurotrauma* 2003;20:841-851.
[20] Abbott NJ. Inflammatory mediators and modulation of blood-brain barrier permeability. *Cell Mol Neurobiol* 2000;20:131-147.
[21] Downing SW, Edmunds LH Jr. Release of vasoactive substances during cardiopulmonary bypass. *Ann Thorac Surg* 1992;54:1236-1243.
[22] Jansen NJ, van Oeveren W, van den Brock L, et al. Inhibition by dexamethasone of the reperfusion phenomena in cardiopulmonary bypass. *J Thorac Cardiovasc Surg* 1991;102:515-525.
[23] Chew MS, Brandslund I, Brix-Christensen V, et al. Tissue injury and the inflammatory response to pediatric cardiac surgery with cardiopulmonary bypass. A descriptive study *Anesthesiology* 2001;94:745-753.
[24] Hansen PR, Svendsen JH, Hoyer S, et al. Tumor necrosis factor-alpha increases myocardial microvascular transport in vivo. *Am J Physiol* 1994;266:H60-H67.
[25] Oka Y, Murata A, Nishijima J, et al. Circulating interleukin 6 as useful marker for predicting postoperative complications. *Cytokine* 1992;4:298-304.
[26] Finn A, Naik S, Klein N, et al. Interleukin-8 release and neutrophil degranulation after pediatric cardiopulmonary bypass. *J Thorac Cardiovasc Surg* 1993;105:234-241.
[27] Taniguchi T, Koido Y, Aiboshi J, et al. Change in the ratio of interleukin-6 to interleukin-10 predicts a poor outcome in patients with systemic inflammatory response syndrome. *Crit Care Med* 1999;27:1262-1264.
[28] Hovels-Gurich HH, Schumacher K, Vazquez-Jimenez JF, et al. Cytokine balance in infants undergoing cardiac operation. *Ann Thorac Surg* 2002;73:601-608.

[29] Brix-Christensen V, Petersen TK, Ravn HB, et al. Cardiopulmonary bypass elicits a pro- and anti-inflammatory cytokine response and impaired neutrophil chemotaxis in neonatal pigs. *Acta Anaesthesiol Scand* 2001;45:407-413.
[30] Adib-Conquy M, Asehnoune K, Moine P, et al. Long-term-impaired expression of nuclear factor-kappa B and I kappa B alpha in peripheral blood mononuclear cells of trauma patients. *J Leukoc Biol* 2001;70:30-38.
[31] Kubes P, Ibbotson G, Russell J, et al. Role of platelet-activating factor in ischemia/reperfusion-induced leukocyte adherence. *Am J Physiol* 1990;259:G300-G305.
[32] Wan S, LeClerc JL, Vincent JL. Inflammatory response to cardiopulmonary bypassmechanisms involved and possible therapeutic strategies. *Chest* 1997;112:676-692.
[33] te Velthuis H, Jansen PGM, Oudemans-van Straaten HM, et al. Circulating endothelin in cardiac operationsinfluence of blood pressure and endotoxin. *Ann Thorac Surg* 1996;61:904-908.
[34] Boyle EM Jr, Verrier ED, Spiess BD. Endothelial cell injury in cardiovascular surgerythe procoagulant response. *Ann Thorac Surg* 1996;62:1549-1557.
[35] Levy JH, Tanaka KA. Inflammatory response to cardiopulmonary bypass. *Ann Thorac Surg* 2003;75(*Suppl*):S715-S720.
[36] Raja SG, Dreyfus GD. Modulation of systemic inflammatory response after cardiac surgery. Asian Cardiovasc *Thorac Ann* 2005;13:382-95.
[37] Lin CY, Yang TL, Hong GJ, et al. Enhanced intracellular heat shock protein 70 expression of leukocytes and serum interleukins release: comparison of on-pump and off-pump coronary artery surgery. *World J Surg* 2010;34:675-81.
[38] Onorati F, Rubino AS, Nucera S, et al. Off-pump coronary artery bypass surgery versus standard linear or pulsatile cardiopulmonary bypass: endothelial activation and inflammatory response. *Eur J Cardiothorac Surg* 2010;37:897-904.
[39] Serrano CV Jr, Souza JA, Lopes NH, et al. Reduced expression of systemic proinflammatory and myocardial biomarkers after off-pump versus on-pump coronary artery bypass surgery: a prospective randomized study. *J Crit Care* 2010;25:305-12.
[40] Rasmussen BS, Laugesen H, Sollid J, et al. Oxygenation and release of inflammatory mediators after off-pump compared with after on-pump coronary artery bypass surgery. *Acta Anaesthesiol Scand* 2007;51:1202-10.
[41] Parolari A, Camera M, Alamanni F, et al. Systemic inflammation after on-pump and off-pump coronary bypass surgery: a one-month follow-up. *Ann Thorac Surg* 2007;84:823-8.
[42] Tatoulis J, Rice S, Davis P, et al. Patterns of postoperative systemic vascular resistance in a randomized trial of conventional on-pump versus off-pump coronary artery bypass graft surgery. *Ann Thorac Surg* 2006;82:1436-44.
[43] Cavalca V, Sisillo E, Veglia F, et al. Isoprostanes and oxidative stress in off-pump and on-pump coronary bypass surgery. *Ann Thorac Surg* 2006;81:562-7.
[44] Wehlin L, Vedin J, Vaage J, Lundahl J. Peripheral blood monocyte activation during coronary artery bypass grafting with or without cardiopulmonary bypass. *Scand Cardiovasc J* 2005;39:78-86.
[45] Al-Ruzzeh S, Hoare G, Marczin N, et al. Off-pump coronary artery bypass surgery is associated with reduced neutrophil activation as measured by the expression of CD11b: a prospective randomized study. *Heart Surg Forum* 2003;6:89-93.
[46] Okubo N, Hatori N, Ochi M, Tanaka S. Comparison of m-RNA expression for inflammatory mediators in leukocytes between on-pump and off-pump coronary artery bypass grafting. *Ann Thorac Cardiovasc Surg* 2003;9:43-9.

[47] Ascione R, Lloyd CT, Underwood MJ, Lotto AA, Pitsis AA, Angelini GD. Inflammatory response after coronary revascularization with or without cardiopulmonary bypass. *Ann Thorac Surg* 2000;69:1198-204.

[48] Dorman BH, Kratz JM, Multani MM, et al. A prospective, randomized study of endothelin and postoperative recovery in off-pump versus conventional coronary artery bypass surgery. *J Cardiothorac Vasc Anesth* 2004;18:25-9.

[49] Wildhirt SM, Schulze C, Conrad N, et al. Reduced myocardial cellular damage and lipid peroxidation in off-pump versus conventional coronary artery bypass grafting. *Eur J Med Res* 2000;5:222-8.

[50] Gu YJ, Mariani MA, van Oeveren W, Grandjean JG, Boonstra PW. Reduction of the inflammatory response in patients undergoing minimally invasive coronary artery bypass grafting. *Ann Thorac Surg* 1998;65:420-4.

[51] Moller CH, Steinbruchel DA. Platelet function after coronary artery bypass grafting: is there a procoagulant activity after off-pump compared with on-pump surgery? *Scand Cardiovasc J* 2003;37:149-53.

[52] Casati V, Gerli C, Franco A, et al. Activation of coagulation and fibrinolysis during coronary surgery: on-pump versus off-pump techniques. *Anesthesiology* 2001;95:1103-9.

[53] Matata BM, Sosnowski AW, Galinanes M. Off-pump bypass graft operation significantly reduces oxidative stress and inflammation. *Ann Thorac Surg* 2000;69:785-91.

[54] Gu YJ, Mariani MA, Boonstra PW, Grandjean JG, van Oeveren W. Complement activation in coronary artery bypass grafting patients without cardiopulmonary bypass: the role of tissue injury by surgical incision. *Chest* 1999;116:892-8.

[55] Diegeler A, Doll N, Rauch T, et al. Humoral immune response during coronary artery bypass grafting: A comparison of limited approach, "off-pump" technique, and conventional cardiopulmonary bypass. *Circulation* 2000;102(19 *Suppl* 3):III95-100.

[56] Struber M, Cremer JT, Gohrbandt B, et al. Human cytokine responses to coronary artery bypass grafting with and without cardiopulmonary bypass. *Ann Thorac Surg* 1999;68:1330-5.

[57] Schulze C, Conrad N, Schutz A, et al. Reduced expression of systemic proinflammatory cytokines after off-pump versus conventional coronary artery bypass grafting. *Thorac Cardiovasc Surg* 2000;48:364-9.

[58] Wildhirt SM, Schulze C, Schulz C, et al. Reduction of systemic and cardiac adhesion molecule expression after off-pump versus conventional coronary artery bypass grafting. *Shock* 2001;16 *Suppl* 1:55-9.

[59] Wan S, Izzat MB, Lee TW, Wan IY, Tang NL, Yim AP. Avoiding cardiopulmonary bypass in multivessel CABG reduces cytokine response and myocardial injury. *Ann Thorac Surg* 1999;68:52-6.

[60] Mazzone A, Gianetti J, Picano E, et al. Correlation between inflammatory response and markers of neuronal damage in coronary revascularization with and without cardiopulmonary bypass. *Perfusion* 2003;18:3-8.

[61] Gulielmos V, Menschikowski M, Dill H, et al. Interleukin-1, interleukin-6 and myocardial enzyme response after coronary artery bypass grafting - a prospective randomized comparison of the conventional and three minimally invasive surgical techniques. *Eur J Cardiothorac Surg* 2000;18:594-601.

[62] Czerny M, Baumer H, Kilo J, et al. Inflammatory response and myocardial injury following coronary artery bypass grafting with or without cardiopulmonary bypass. *Eur J Cardiothorac Surg* 2000 ;17:737-42.

[63] Danner RL, Elin RJ, Hosseini JM, Wesley RA, Reilly JM, Parillo JE. Endotoxemia in human septic shock. *Chest* 1991;99:169-75.
[64] Andersen LW, Baek L, Degn H, Lehd J, Krasnik M, Rasmussen JP. Presence of circulating endotoxins during cardiac operations. *J Thorac Cardiovasc Surg* 1987;93:115-9.
[65] Rocke DA, Gaffin SL, Wells MT, Koen Y, Brock-Utine JG. Endotoxemia associated with cardiopulmonary bypass. *J Thorac Cardiovasc Surg* 1987;93:832-7.
[66] Riddington DW, Venkatesh B, Boivin CM, et al. Intestinal permeability, gastric intramucosal pH, and systemic endotoxemia in patients undergoing cardiopulmonary bypass. *JAMA* 1996;275:1007-12.
[67] Raja SG, Berg GA. Impact of off-pump coronary artery bypass surgery on systemic inflammation: current best available evidence. *J Card Surg* 2007;22:445-55.
[68] Morrison DC, Kline LF. Activation of the classical and properdin pathways of complement by bacterial lipopoysaccharide (LPS). *J Immunol* 1977;118:362-8.
[69] Morrison DC, Ryan JL. Endotoxins and disease mechanisms. *Annu Rev Med* 1987;38:417-32.
[70] Aydin NB, Gercekoglu H, Aksu B, et al. Endotoxemia in coronary artery bypass surgery: a comparison of the off-pump technique and conventional cardiopulmonary bypass. *J Thorac Cardiovasc Surg* 2003;125:843-8.
[71] Backes JM, Howard PA, Moriarty PM. Role of C-reactive protein in cardiovascular disease. *Ann Pharmacother* 2004;38:110-8.
[72] Maier RV. Pathogenesis of multiple organ dysfunction syndrome - endotoxin, inflammatory cells, and their mediators: cytokines and reactive oxygen species. *Surg Infect (Larchmt)* 2000;1:197-205.
[73] Ulus AT, Aksoyek A, Ozkan M, et al. Cardiopulmonary bypass as a cause of free radical-induced oxidative stress and enhanced blood-borne isoprostanes in humans. *Free Radic Biol Med* 2003;34:911-7.
[74] Gerritsen WB, van Boven WJ, Driessen AH, et al. Off-pump versus on-pump coronary artery bypass grafting: oxidative stress and renal function. *Eur J Cardiothorac Surg* 2001;20:923-9.
[75] Wan IY, Arifi AA, Wan S, et al. Beating heart revascularization with or without cardiopulmonary bypass: evaluation of inflammatory response in a prospective randomized study. *J Thorac Cardiovasc Surg* 2004;127:1624-31.
[76] Wehlin L, Vedin J, Vaage J, Lundahl J. Activation of complement and leukocyte receptors during on- and off pump coronary artery bypass surgery. *Eur J Cardiothorac Surg* 2004;25:35-42.
[77] Jemielity MM, Perek B, Buczkowski P, et al. Inflammatory response following off-pump and on-pump coronary artery bypass grafting. *Heart Surg Forum* 2003;6(*Suppl* 1):S40-1.
[78] Angelini GD, Taylor FC, Reeves BC, Ascione R. Early and midterm outcome after off-pump and on-pump surgery in Beating Heart Against Cardioplegic Arrest Studies (BHACAS 1 and 2): A pooled analysis of two randomised controlled trials. *Lancet* 2002;359:1194-9.
[79] Nathoe HM, van Dijk D, Jansen EW, et al. A comparison of on-pump and off-pump coronary bypass surgery in low-risk patients. *N Engl J Med* 2003;348:394-402.
[80] Gerola LR, Buffolo E, Jasbik W, et al. Off-pump versus on-pump myocardial revascularization in low-risk patients with one or two vessel disease: Perioperative results in a multicenter randomized controlled trial. *Ann Thorac Surg* 2004;77:569-73.

[81] van Dijk D, Nierich AP, Jansen EW, et al. Early outcome after off-pump versus on-pump coronary bypass surgery: Results from a randomized study. *Circulation* 2001;104:1761-6.

[82] Straka Z, Widimsky P, Jirasek K, et al. Off-pump versus on-pump coronary surgery: Final results from a prospective randomized study PRAGUE-4. *Ann Thorac Surg* 2004;77:789-93.

[83] Lee JD, Lee SJ, Tsushima WT, et al. Benefits of off-pump bypass on neurologic and clinical morbidity: A prospective randomized trial. *Ann Thorac Surg* 2003;76:18-26.

[84] Parolari A, Alamanni F, Cannata A, et al. Off-pump versus on-pump coronary artery bypass: meta-analysis of currently available randomized trials. *Ann Thorac Surg* 2003;76:37-40.

[85] van der Heijden GJ, Nathoe HM, Jansen EW, Grobbee DE. Meta-analysis on the effect of off-pump coronary bypass surgery. *Eur J Cardiothorac Surg* 2004;26:81-4.

[86] Reston JT, Tregear SJ, Turkelson CM. Meta-analysis of short-term and mid-term outcomes following off-pump coronary artery bypass grafting. *Ann Thorac Surg* 2003 ;76:1510-5.

[87] Hoff SJ, Ball SK, Coltharp WH, et al. Coronary artery bypass in patients 80 years and over: is off-pump the operation of choice? *Ann Thorac Surg* 2002;74:S1340-3.

[88] Demaria RG, Carrier M, Fortier S, et al. Reduced mortality and strokes with off-pump coronary artery bypass grafting surgery in octogenarians. *Circulation* 2002;106(12 *Suppl* 1):I5-10.

[89] Beauford RB, Goldstein DJ, Sardari FF, et al. Multivessel off-pump revascularization in octogenarians: early and midterm outcomes. *Ann Thorac Surg* 2003;76:12-7.

[90] Stamou SC, Dangas G, Dullum MK, et al. Beating heart surgery in octogenarians: perioperative outcome and comparison with younger age groups. *Ann Thorac Surg* 2000;69:1140-5.

In: Off-Pump Coronary Artery Bypass Grafting
Editors: S.G. Raja and M. Amrani
ISBN 978-1-62081-575-5

Chapter 3

Postoperative Bleeding and Transfusion Requirements after Off-Pump Coronary Artery Bypass Grafting

Shahzad G. Raja
Cardiac Surgeon, Harefield Hospital, London, UK

Abstract

Excessive postoperative bleeding continues to play a key role as an important cause of morbidity and mortality after surgery on cardiopulmonary bypass. Multiple etiologies lead to bleeding after cardiac surgery. The contact activation with the extracorporeal circuit, shear forces, activation of the complement system, fibrinolysis, and extrinsic factors, such as the use of newer, longer-acting antiplatelet or antithrombotic agents all contribute to increased postoperative bleeding. Because of the decreased hemostatic function and the resultant blood loss, patients undergoing surgery on cardiopulmonary bypass often receive allogeneic blood transfusions. Transfusion of allogeneic blood products may expose the patient to additional risks (transfusion reactions, viral transmissions, immunosuppression, and increased mortality) and increased cost. Surgical re-exploration of the mediastinum resulting from postoperative hemorrhage occurs in 3% to 5% of patients. Morbidity, mortality, and hospital costs increase significantly with the re-exploration of the mediastinum.

Coronary artery bypass surgery without the utilization of cardiopulmonary bypass termed off-pump coronary artery bypass grafting has been gaining in popularity in the last few years. Resurgence of interest in off-pump coronary artery bypass grafting is associated with the expectation that avoiding deleterious effects of the cardiopulmonary bypass leads to better outcomes and possibly decreased costs and resource utilization. This chapter provides an overview of normal hemostasis focuses on cardiopulmonary bypass-induced derangements in hemostasis and evaluates the impact of off-pump coronary artery bypass grafting on postoperative blood loss and transfusion requirements.

Introduction

The refinement of extracorporeal circulation during the past 30 years has allowed surgeons to treat various cardiac pathologies. The quiet, motionless, and essentially bloodless field that is provided with the diversion of circulation has allowed surgeons to have unparalleled access to intracardiac and extracardiac structures [1].

Limitations once thought insurmountable no longer exist with the evolution of myocardial protective measures and cardioplegia[1]. However, the price of a still and bloodless field is ultimately paid by the patients in the form of sequelae of negative effects of cardiopulmonary bypass (CPB) including blood trauma, activation of a series of inflammatory responses, nonpulsatile flow, and possible embolization of air or debris—most particularly embolization of atherosclerotic debris from the aorta [2].

Approximately 5% to 7% of patients undergoing cardiac surgery lose more than 2 L of chest tube drainage during the first 24 hours postoperatively, and up to 5% require reexploration for bleeding, resulting in an increased length of stay and higher mortality [3,5]. About half of these bleeding episodes are due to an identifiable surgical bleeding source, whereas the other 50% are presumably due to a coagulopathy. Hemostatic changes may result from both CPB and non–CPB-related variables, as well as pharmacologic modulation of the hemostatic system in the perioperative period.

Despite improvements in the construction of CPB circuits and advances in both surgical and blood conservation techniques, there is still a substantial demand for perioperative blood product transfusion. This may be due to the changing demographics of the cardiac surgical population. More complex operations are being performed on older, sicker patients. Due to the complexities of the coagulation system, of the cardiac surgical procedures, the materials used in the CPB circuits, and a number of uncontrollable variables, we do not yet have a complete understanding of what causes the coagulopathy of bypass [6]. This chapter provides an overview of the pathophysiologic effects of CPB on hemostasis and focuses on the impact of off-pump coronary artery bypass grafting on bleeding and transfusion requirements.

Normal Hemostasis

Blood clotting is a host defense mechanism that, in a coordinated response with the inflammatory and repair responses, helps protect the integrity of the vascular tissue after injury. The system becomes activated immediately after injury, involving a complex interaction between platelets, leukocytes, plasma proteins, and endothelial cells. This coordinated response leads to the formation of a platelet plug, the generation of a fibrin clot, the deposition of white blood cells in the area of injury, and the initiation of inflammation and repair [6, 7].

The coagulation cascade may be thought of as an amplification system in which, upon exposure to damaged tissue or foreign surfaces, trace plasma proteins become activated and initiate reactions leading to the conversion of relatively large amounts of prothrombin to thrombin [6]. This then converts significant amounts of fibrinogen to fibrin (Figure 1).

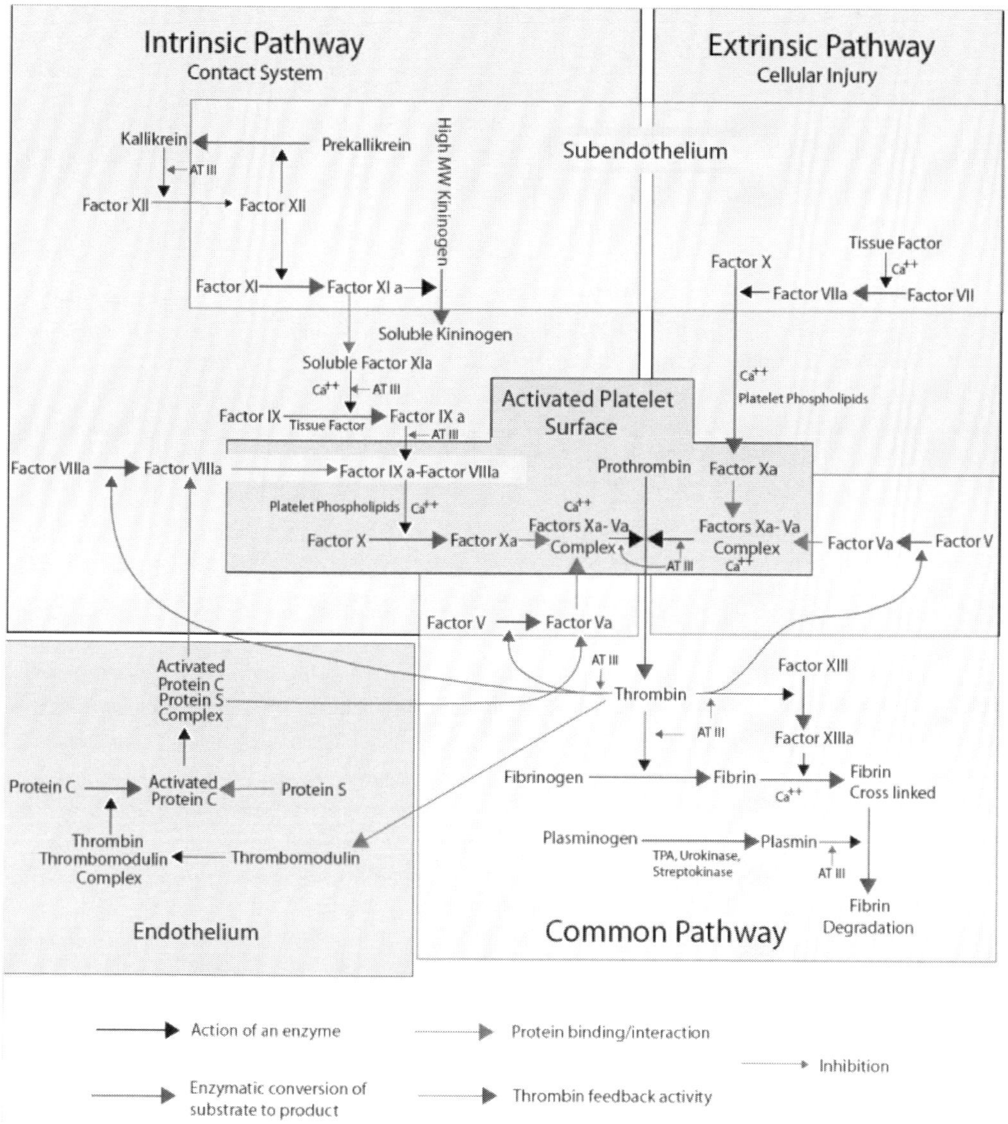

Figure 1. The coagulation cascade.

There are many amplifiers, controls, and feedback loops along the way. The generation of thrombin is a key regulatory step in the hemostatic cascade. Its production not only results in fibrin formation and platelet activation, but also stimulates fibrinolysis.

A balance between coagulation and fibrinolysis is important for hemostatic homeostasis, thereby preventing excessive clotting or bleeding. The coagulation cascades do not function in a vacuum, but depend on interaction with platelets and the endothelium. Cell membranes, especially those of platelets and endothelial cells, play an integral role in the formation and expression of procoagulant complexes [6,8,9].

Historically, the coagulation cascade was divided into the intrinsic pathway beginning with contact activation of factor XII (FXII), the extrinsic pathway initiated by tissue factor (TF) and FVII, and the common pathway of activation of prothrombin to thrombin and subsequent generation of a fibrin clot. Today, we know that there is interaction and feedback between the cascade systems and that they do not function independently [6, 10].

There are several regulatory reactions in the coagulation system that help limit coagulation to the site of injury. In addition to stimulating the fibrinolytic pathway, thrombin activates the regulatory proteins C and S. Protein C is, normally, adherent to the endothelial cell surface. When activated by thrombin, protein C activates its cofactor protein S and inhibits factors V and VIII [6,11]. Antithrombin III (ATIII), a plasma protease inhibitor, serves as a scavenger of any residual coagulation proteases. Its activity is accelerated by heparan sulfate found on the endothelial surface or by circulating heparin [7]. The heparin-ATIII complex scavenges thrombin and inhibits factors IXa and Xa [12,13]. Platelets are metabolically active, nonnucleated blood cells with multiple functions in hemostasis.

They adhere to the site of vascular injury, release procoagulant substances, aggregate with each other to form a hemostatic plug, and provide a procoagulant surface for coagulation proteins to work [6,14,15].

Endothelial cells lining the vascular tree are actively involved in the regulation of hemostasis. In the resting state, the endothelium promotes anticoagulation, but in response to injury or stress, the endothelium will take on a procoagulant role [6,12]. The endothelial surface contains heparan sulfate, which binds circulating ATIII and potentiates its function as a thrombin scavenger. The endothelial cell membrane contains the glycoprotein thrombomodulin, which, when bound to thrombin, inhibits its ability to cleave fibrinogen to fibrin [12,16]. Endothelial cells release TF pathway inhibitor (TFPI), which inhibits the extrinsic coagulation pathway, and produce tissue plasminogen activator (t-PA). Furthermore, endothelial cells inhibit platelet function through their release of nitric oxide, prostaglandins, and adenosine, which impair adhesion and aggregation [6,12]. When endothelial cells are stimulated by the stress of hypoxia or by circulating mediators such as thrombin, they take on a procoagulant state. Thrombomodulin expression and t-PA production are decreased, while plasminogen activator inhibitor type 1 (PAI-1) production is increased. Platelet activating factor (PAF) and von Willebrand factor (vWF) are released. The stressed endothelial cells can release TF, thus activating the extrinsic coagulation pathway. At the same time, the endothelial cells will express phospholipid-binding sites for the coagulation protein complexes to function on. Membrane microparticles are shed into the bloodstream to provide even greater surface area for assembly of coagulation complexes [12,17].

To prevent excessive clotting and systemic thrombosis, the fibrinolytic system is activated. In addition to its role in the formation of the fibrin clot, thrombin also stimulates the release of t-PA from endothelial cells [18,19]. Tissue plasminogen activator can also be activated by complement, cytokines, and desamino-8-arginine-vasopressin [20]. Tissue plasminogen activator cleaves the circulating plasma protein plasminogen to plasmin. Plasmin cleaves fibrinogen, fibrin, and fibrin–fibrin dimers, thus dissolving the clot and leading to the formation of fibrin split products and D-dimers. These fibrin split products may themselves inhibit clotting by increasing vascular permeability and plasmin activity, inhibiting thrombin, and destroying factors V and VIII [21]. They also might activate factor XII, complement, and kallikrein [22]. There are 2 forms of plasmin. Plasmin bound to fibrinogen/fibrin is responsible for clot dissolution, whereas circulating free plasmin interacts with platelets, causing platelet dysfunction. Plasmin has been shown to proteolyze platelet surface GP Ib and impair platelet binding and aggregation [22, 23]. The fibrinolytic system is inhibited by plasminogen activator inhibitors (PAIs) such as PAI-1, and α-2 plasmin inhibitor.

The former prevents fibrinolysis by binding and deactivating t-PA and urokinase, whereas the latter inhibits plasmin [22, 24]. These actions and reactions allow hemostasis to occur locally, while systemic flow remains unaltered.

Cardiopulmonary Bypass-Induced Changes in Hemostasis

Exposure of blood to the artificial surfaces of the CPB circuit causes intense activation of the hemostatic and inflammatory systems. Although these processes are normal hemostatic reactions, the continuous ongoing exposure to a foreign surface results in an exaggerated response, leading to consumption of coagulation factors and platelets, as well as activation of the fibrinolytic system. The use of systemic heparinization does not fully prevent activation of the coagulation system [6]. Adding to the complexity of CPB-associated coagulopathies are patient comorbidities and procedural variables. Hemodilution, hypothermia, mechanical trauma to blood cells and components, and the hemostatic effects of a number of perioperative medications represent some of the variables involved in the development of a perioperative coagulation abnormality [6].

When blood comes into contact with a foreign surface, blood proteins rapidly become adsorbed onto the material [25-28]. Proteins shown to adhere to the foreign or injured surface include factors XII and VIII, vWF, fibrinogen, high-molecular-weight kininogen (HMWK), immunoglobulin G (IgG), albumin, fibronectin, and hemoglobin [6,25-28]. The intrinsic coagulation pathway is activated when factor XII is adsorbed onto the surface of the CPB circuit. Until recently, this was felt to be the major pathway for coagulation activation during CPB. Using a blood-primed simulated CPB circuit to assay for intrinsic pathway activation, Kappelmayer et al. [29] found very little intrinsic pathway activation, but extensive activation of the extrinsic system, resulting from induced expression of TF on the surface of activated monocytes. Bosclair et al. [30], using plasma-based enzyme-linked immunosorbent assays, showed that thrombin generation increased early in response to surgery and bypass. They observed a modest increase in factor XIIa levels and smaller increases in serum factor IX activation peptide (FIXAP) levels. The authors concluded that the main trigger to coagulation during CPB was from the TF/VIIa mechanism in response to surgical trauma, leading to subsequent activation of factor X and production of thrombin. The late activation of factor IX was probably due to the direct action of TF/VIIa or via a secondary feedback action of thrombin on the intrinsic system. The observation that thrombin was still formed during CPB in a patient with a congenital deficiency of factor XII lends further support to these conclusions [31]. Contact activation may still play an important role in the pathophysiologic response to CPB through the activation of kallikrein. Kallikrein, which is activated by factor XIIa, and mediates activation of neutrophils, the complement system, and the fibrinolytic system [32].

The major mechanism of coagulation activation during CPB is now felt to be via the TF pathway activated as a result of trauma and inflammation [33-38]. The endothelial cells and monocytes, activated during systemic inflammation, play a major role in the activation of the TF pathway during CPB[38]. In vitro studies have shown that the inflammatory mediators, such as tumor necrosis factor (TNF), interleukin-1, and lipopolysaccharide induce the expression of TF on endothelial cells and monocytes [34, 35].

Upon initiating CPB, there are reductions in plasma concentrations of coagulation factors II, V, VII, IX, X, and XIII [39]. Factor V levels decrease more than can be predicted by dilution alone, yet still remain above the level considered adequate for hemostasis (even in patients with excessive bleeding following CPB). By contrast, factor VIII levels remain within normal limits during and after CPB despite hemodilution [39]. All coagulation factor levels usually normalize within 12 hours after CPB39]. It is generally thought that only 20% to 25% of any particular clotting factor is necessary for coagulation, provided that the levels of other clotting factors are normal. In the setting of CPB, this teaching does not apply because most of the clotting factors and platelet are reduced together in number and function. In this particular setting, it is not readily discernible at what low serum level of any individual factor the risk for excessive bleeding is increased [6, 20].

Hemodilution alone does not account for the amount of protein depletion during CPB [6]. Denaturation of plasma proteins occurs at blood–air interfaces such as from the cardiotomy suction and the oxygenator, thus decreasing the availability of coagulation factors. Low-grade consumption of coagulation proteins is continuous and dependent upon the duration of CPB. Despite heparinization, there is a constant low-grade production of thrombin, as evidenced by the increasing concentration of thrombin–antithrombin complexes and thrombin fragment 1+2 levels throughout bypass [40].

This ongoing low-grade thrombin production leads to ongoing activation of the coagulation cascade, platelets, fibrinolysis, inflammation, and the endothelium [6].

Cardiopulmonary Bypass and Fibrinolysis

The fibrinolytic response to CPB is heterogeneous and multifactorial [41]. Diffuse microvascular coagulation and production of thrombin during CPB leads to activation of fibrinolysis resulting in increased production and conversion of plasminogen to plasmin. Fibrinolytic activity increases significantly during CPB and returns to normal shortly after termination of bypass [42]. Teufelsbauer et al. [43] showed that the activation of coagulation occurred before activation of fibrinolysis, suggesting that hyperfibrinolysis is directly or indirectly mediated by activation of coagulation. The pump, the oxygenator, the cardioplegia solution (high potassium-low temperature), and aspirated blood contribute to the activation of fibrinolysis.

This is evidenced by the production of fibrin split products during and after CPB [6,21,44-46]. Hypothermia may also play a role in the activation of plasminogen by activating prekallikrein and factor XII, which increases plasmin generation [42,45,46].

Fibrinolysis also results from endothelial cell activation and release of t-PA [47]. Tissue plasminogen activator levels rise on CPB, with the greatest increase seen during the first 30 minutes of bypass, then more slowly throughout the duration of bypass, followed by another large increase after protamine administration [41].

At the same time that t-PA levels rose, plasminogen activator inhibitor 1 (PAI-1) levels decreased, but then increased after surgery. The increase in PAI-1 seen postoperatively is associated with increased risk of arterial thrombosis, vascular graft occlusion, deep venous thrombosis, stroke, myocardial ischemia, and infarction [41].

Cardiopulmonary Bypass and Platelets

Cardiopulmonary bypass affects both platelet count and function. Thrombocytopenia during CPB is primarily due to hemodilution from the pump prime [39]. Shortly after initiating CPB, platelet counts fall to about 50% of preoperative levels [39, 48]. Holloway et al. [49] found that the degree of thrombocytopenia was greater than could be accounted for by hemodilution alone. Other possible causes of thrombocytopenia include mechanical disruption of the platelets, adhesion to the extracorporeal circuit, and organ sequestration [6,50]. The low platelet count persists for several days after surgery and is associated with an increased rate of platelet turnover until the count returns to normal [39].

Although several hemostatic abnormalities are induced by CPB, acquired platelet dysfunction is thought to be the major cause of nonsurgical bleeding after CPB. Bleeding time becomes prolonged shortly after commencement of CPB and increases further during the course of bypass. It decreases after protamine is administered and returns to normal within 4 hours [39,51].

Platelet dysfunction appears to result from contact with the synthetic surface of the extracorporeal circuit and subsequent activation, adhesion, and consumption [39,52,53]. Upon exposure of blood to artificial surfaces, there is a rapid adsorption and configurational changes of platelets and plasma proteins, including fibrinogen and vWF [32]. Platelet aggregation to adenosine diphosphate (ADP) or collagen is impaired [39,51]. Musial et al. [54] examined the effect of CPB on platelet fibrinogen receptors and found decreased fibrinogen-induced platelet aggregation and a diminished number of fibrinogen receptors on platelet surfaces.

Cardiopulmonary bypass is associated with several platelet receptor defects. After exposure to CPB, platelets undergo structural changes consistent with platelet aggregation and activation [52]. Upon activation, the platelets express glycoprotein binding sites on their membranes, which are involved in intercellular interactions [50]. Membrane surface expression of GP Ib, which binds vWF, is decreased by CPB, reaching a nadir 2 hours after the onset of CPB, followed by a gradual increase over the next 3 hours, until prebypass levels are reached [55,56]. The decrease in GP Ib correlates with the magnitude of platelet activation [56]. Glycoprotein IIb/IIIa, which binds fibrinogen, has also been reported to decrease during CPB [56,57]. Glycoprotein IV, which is involved in platelet aggregation and adhesion, is minimally decreased during hypothermic CPB but then increases significantly 2 to 4 hours after bypass [50]. This may be due to an influx of previously sequestered platelets from organs such as the spleen, rather than from production of new platelets [56].

Once platelets become activated, intracellular granules move to the cell surface and release a number of procoagulant substances important for platelet adhesion and aggregation. During CPB, the release and partial depletion of α granule constituents was observed [39, 48, 58]. Alpha granules release platelet factor-4 (PF4), β-thromboglobulin, and vWF [39]. A relationship between the increase in PF4, β-thromboglobulin, and bleeding time with the duration of bypass and/or the level of hypothermia has been demonstrated [39]. A decrease in

ADP secretion from platelets during CPB suggests that platelet dysfunction may be due to the persistence of activated degranulated platelets [59]. Activated platelets increase during CPB, peak before the termination of bypass, and continue to circulate after surgery. Cardiopulmonary bypass may be associated with platelet activation, release of α granules, prolonged circulation of activated, "spent" (degranulated) platelets, and impaired platelet aggregation [60].

Platelet dysfunction during CPB persists afterward for variable periods of time [6]. The peak platelet force development (PPFD) is a measure of the force generated by platelets during plasma clot retraction and of global clot strength. It depends upon the adhesion and aggregation properties of the platelets. It is abolished during bypass, recovers significantly after protamine administration, but remains abnormal after CPB [61]. The percent recovery of PPFD after CPB was shown to correlate inversely with nonsurgical (microvascular) blood loss in the first 24 hours [6].

Impact of Off-Pump Coronary Artery Bypass Grafting on Bleeding and Transfusion Requirements

In an attempt to avoid the deleterious effects of CPB, there has been a resurgence of interest in OPCAB [62]. OPCAB is fast becoming a safe alternative to conventional CABG. By avoiding CPB, OPCAB is a potentially more physiologic method to maintain the functional integrity of major organ systems with the possibility of reducing mortality and morbidity. In recent years, a large body of evidence has been presented in the medical literature on the safety and efficacy of off-pump coronary artery surgery [63]. Over the past decade several randomized controlled trials (RCTs) [64-66], systematic reviews[67,68], and meta-analyses[69-71] have consitently and clearly shown that there is less bleeding with off-pump procedures compared with CPB and there is less need for blood products.

Patients undergoing OPCAB do not show any impairing effect of CPB on hemostasis [72]. Because of the absence of the artificial surfaces of the heart-lung machine, the various platelet activation mechanisms and depletion caused by contact activation with extracorporeal surfaces, bubble oxygenator, cardiotomy suction, and filters are avoided [73,74] leading to reduced postoperative bleeding. In addition, excessive bleeding may be related to a coagulopathy resulting from greater heparin doses during CPB as guided by dosing protocols based on body weight and ACT values [75] or with maintenance of a defined heparin concentration [76]. In contrast, a low level of intraoperative heparinization in OPCAB patients preserves hemostasis [77,78]. Finally, markedly reduced systemic inflammatory response after OPCAB surgery [79] may also contribute to reduction in postoperative blood loss.

Casati et al. [80] were the first to provide an insight into the impact of OPCAB on coagulation and fibrinolysis. Their study was the first investigation directly comparing selected coagulation and fibrinolysis variables in CABG and OPCAB patients free of perioperative and postoperative complications. Because of the obvious difference in the degree of hemodilution occurring with the two surgical modalities, they chose to adjust the changes in hemostatic variables for those observed in total immunoglobulin G (IgG) concentrations. IgG concentrations have not been reported to be affected by surgery in the short term. They are not involved in metabolic pathways potentially altered by trauma, and, differently from erythrocytes, their plasma concentrations may account for the exchange of plasma proteins between intravascular and extravascular compartments. The results of this study showed that after correction for this variable, fibrinogen, antithrombin, and α_2-antiplasmin concentrations were not different in patients undergoing CABG or OPCAB and that both modalities of surgery involved a significant net consumption of antithrombin and fibrinogen. These findings are not surprising when considering the threefold higher dose of heparin infused in CABG patients and considering that thrombin generation during CPB does not result from exposure of blood to foreign surfaces (contact activation) but is triggered by the tissue factor–factor VIIa pathway, possibly in response to the cutting of blood vessels [31,81]. Earlier studies on CBP surgery reported conflicting results, with the additional bias represented by priming of the extracorporeal circuit with either blood or saline. Mammen et al. [82] found that the decreases in fibrinogen, antithrombin, plasminogen, and α_2-antiplasmin concentrations were consistent with the decrease in hematocrit. Plasminogen and antithrombin, but not α_2 antiplasmin, were found to decrease much more than dilution in another study [49]. In contrast, Konsgaard et al. [82] observed a decrease in α_2 antiplasmin, but not in plasminogen and antithrombin, when correcting for the hemoglobin concentration.

Casati et al. [80] further noticed that significant changes in platelet counts, D-dimer concentrations, and plasminogen concentrations were only associated with CPB surgery. When adjusted for the hematocrit, platelet counts were 24% lower than baseline in patients undergoing CABG. Plasma D-dimer concentrations were not significantly increased after surgery in OPCAB patients, but they were approximately fivefold higher in CABG patients. A 4% decrease in plasminogen concentrations was only observed after CABG surgery. These findings are consistent with increased plasminogen activation during CPB. Activation of fibrinolysis in CPB surgery has been reported in many studies, with both the intrinsic (factor XIIa- and kallikrein-dependent) and extrinsic (tissue plasminogen activator-dependent) mechanisms of plasminogen activation being involved [82]. Based on these findings the authors concluded that uncomplicated coronary artery bypass surgery involves a net consumption of antithrombin and fibrinogen. However, transient platelet consumption, plasminogen activation, and D-dimer formation are only observed with on-pump coronary surgery. Twenty-four hours after surgery, the hemostatic patterns of patients undergoing CABG and OPCAB are similar.

Ascione et al. [64] were the first to show in a randomized controlled setting the influence of beating-heart coronary operations on both blood loss and transfusion requirement. This study showed a significant decrease in postoperative blood loss measured as total chest tube drainage and transfusion requirement with beating-heart operations when compared with conventional CABG with CPB. In this study, 37% of the patients in the on-pump group and 35% in the off-pump group were unstable in-hospital referrals managed preoperatively with aspirin and low-molecular-weight heparin, which have been reported to increase perioperative blood loss [40]. The explanation for the reduced postoperative blood loss observed in the off-pump group is certainly multifactorial. Thrombocytopenia, platelet dysfunction, and clotting factor deficiencies all contributed to increased chest tube drainage in the on-pump group. Furthermore, as might be expected from the higher chest tube drainage, this study also showed a significantly greater transfusion requirement in the on-pump group. It is worth noting that less than one quarter of the patients in the off-pump group required transfusion compared with over half of the patients in the on-pump group.

Vedin et al. [83] in a small but sophisticated prospective, randomized study measured standard coagulation and fibrinolytic factors as well as platelet count and release of some markers of endothelial activation in low-risk patients undergoing elective coronary surgery with or without CPB. The measured parameters were: fibrin D dimer (D dimer), prothrombin fragment 1+2 (F1+2), α_2-macroglobulin, protein C1 esterase inhibitor (C1 inhibitor), fibronectin, and vWF. D dimer is a measure of fibrinolysis or increased coagulation; F1+2 is a degradation product from prothrombin indicating thrombin formation; α_2-macroglobulin is a protease inhibitor; C1 inhibitor is the only inhibitor of C1 esterase in the complement system, also inhibiting plasmin, kallikrein, and coagulation factors XI and XII; fibronectin is a marker of endothelial activation and involved in opsonization; and vWF, in addition to being carrier of factor VIII, is a platelet activating factor that is also suggested to be a marker of endothelial activation. This study demonstrated a tendency towards decreased activation of both coagulation and fibrinolysis in low risk patients during elective OPCAB compared with CABG on CPB. Similar findings have been reported by other researchers [64, 84-86].

Preservation of hemostasis after OPCAB on one hand is beneficial as it reduces postoperative bleeding and need for transfusion but on the other hand there is concern that OPCAB leads to a hypercoagulation, which may affect graft patency [72,83]. The issue of hypercoagulation after OPCAB is discussed in detail in a separate chapter in this book.

Conclusion

OPCAB reduces bleeding and need of allogeneic transfusion. This is perhaps due to less disturbed equilibrium between procoagulant and anticoagulant activity in patients operated with OPCAB technique. National blood shortages continue to surface periodically, new infectious sequelae of transfusion continue to threaten both the quality and the quantity of blood supply, and incompatibility and other immunologic reactions remain problems associated with allogeneic blood transfusion. In addition, cost and resource efficiency considerations now play a prominent role in mandating a reduction in blood transfusions. OPCAB can conserve blood during the perioperative period resulting in a concurrent decrease in the risk of transmitting blood-borne pathogens, blood transfusion reactions, and the associated risk of nonautologous transfusion as well as reduction of health care cost. Patients who are at a high risk of bleeding in the perioperative period as well as those who avoid transfusions such as Jehovah's Witnesses are likely to benefit from off-pump myocardial revascularization and must be offered the option of OPCAB surgery if expertise is available.

References

[1] Nader ND, Khadra WZ, Reich NT, *et al.* Blood product use in cardiac revascularization: Comparison of on- and off-pump techniques. *Ann. Thorac. Surg.*, 1999;68*:*1640-1643.

[2] Raja SG. Off-pump and on-pump coronary artery bypass surgery: Time to move on. *Chin. Med. J. (Engl)*, 2004;117*:* 959.

[3] Hein OV, Birnbaum J, Wernecke KD, et al. Three-year survival after four major post-cardiac operative complications. *Crit. Care. Med.,* 2006;34:2729-2737.

[4] Moulton MJ, Creswell LL, Mackey ME, et al. Reexploration for bleeding is a risk factor for adverse outcomes after cardiac operations. *J. Thorac. Cardiovasc. Surg.,* 1996;111:1037-1046.

[5] Christensen MC, Krapf S, Kempel A, von Heymann C. Costs of excessive postoperative hemorrhage in cardiac surgery. *J. Thorac. Cardiovasc. Surg.,* 2009;138:687-693.

[6] Maslow A, Schwartz C. Cardiopulmonary bypass-associated coagulopathies and prophylactic therapy. Int. Anesthesiol. Clin., 2004;42:103-33.

[7] Furie B, Furie BC. Molecular and cellular biology of blood coagulation. *N. Engl. J. Med.,* 1992;326:800-806.

[8] Mann KG. Biochemistry and physiology of blood coagulation. *Thromb. Haemost.,* 1999;82:165-174.

[9] Wiedmer T, Sims PJ. Participation of protein kinases in complement C5b-9-induced shedding of platelet plasma membrane vesicles. *Blood,* 1991;78:2880-2886.

[10] Luchtman-Jones L, Broze GJ Jr. The current status of coagulation. *Ann. Med.,* 1995;27:47-52.

[11] Esmon CT. The roles of protein C and thrombomodulin in the regulation of blood coagulation. *J. Biol. Chem.,* 1989;264:4743-4746.

[12] Boyle EM, Verrier ED, Spiess BD. Endothelial cell injury in cardiovascular surgery: the procoagulant response. *Ann. Thorac. Surg.,* 1996;62:1549-1557.

[13] Weitz JI, Hudoba M, Massel D, et al. Clot-bound thrombin is protected from inhibition by heparin-antithrombin III but is susceptible to inactivation by antithrombin III-independent inhibitors. *J. Clin. Invest.,* 1990;86:385-391.

[14] Weiss HJ. Platelet physiology and abnormalities of platelet function (Part 1). *N. Engl. J. Med.,* 1975;293:531-541.

[15] Weiss HJ. Platelet physiology and abnormalities of platelet function (Part 2). *N. Engl. J. Med.,* 1975;293:580-588.

[16] Ye J, Esmon NL, Esmon CT, et al. The active site of thrombin is altered upon binding to thrombomodulin. *J. Biol. Chem.,* 1991;266:23016-23021.

[17] Combes V, Simon AC, Grau GE, et al. In vitro generation of endothelial microparticles and possible prothrombotic activity in patients with lupus anticoagulant. *J. Clin. Invest.,* 1999;104:93-102.

[18] Vassalli JD, Sappino AP, Belin D. The plasminogen activator/plasmin system. *J. Clin. Invest.,* 1991;88:1067-1072.

[19] Levin EG, Marzec U, Anderson J, et al. Thrombin stimulates tissue plasminogen activator release from cultured human endothelial cells. *J. Clin. Invest.,* 1984;74:1988-1995.

[20] Spiess BD. Coagulation and cardiopulmonary bypass. In: Thys DM, Hillel Z, Schwartz AJ, eds. Textbook of Cardiothoracic Anesthesiology. New York, NY: McGraw Hill; 2001:378-403.

[21] Spiess BD. The contribution of fibrinolysis to postbypass bleeding. J Cardiothor Vasc Anesth 1991;5(suppl):13-17.

[22] Michelson AD, Barnard MR. Plasmin-induced redistribution of platelet glycoprotein Ib. *Blood,* 1990;76:2005-2010.

[23] Gouin I, Lecompte T, Morel MC, et al. In vitro effect of plasmin on human platelet function in plasma: Inhibition of aggregation caused by fibrinogenolysis. *Circulation*, 1992;85:935-941.

[24] Gelherter TD, Laszuk RS. Thrombin induction of plasminogen activator-inhibitor in cultured human endothelial cells. *J. Clin. Invest.*, 1986;77:165-169.

[25] Ziats NP, Pankowsky DA, Tierney BP, et al. Adsorption of Hageman factor (factor XII) and other human plasma proteins to biomedical polymers. *J. Lab. Clin. Med.*, 1990;116:687-696.

[26] 26.Vromen L, Adams AL, Fischer GC, et al. Interaction of high molecular weight kininogen, factor XII and fibrinogen in plasma at interfaces. *Blood*, 1980;55:156.

[27] Brash JL, Scott CF, Hove PT, et al. Mechanism of transient adsorption of fibrinogen from plasma to solid surfaces: role of the contact and fibrinolytic systems. *Blood*, 1988;71:932-939.

[28] Uniyal S, Brash JL. Patterns of adsorption of proteins from human plasma onto foreign surfaces. *Thromb. Haemost.*, 1982;47:285-290.

[29] Kappelmayer J, Bertiabei A, Edmunds LH Jr, et al. Tissue factor is expressed on monocytes during simulated extracorporeal circulation. *Circ. Res.*, 1993;72:1075-1081.

[30] Bosclair MD, Lane DA, Philippou H, et al. Mechanism of thrombin generation during surgery and cardiopulmonary bypass. *Blood*, 1993;82:3350-3357.

[31] Burman JF, Chung HI, Lane DA, et al. Role of factor XII in thrombin generation and fibrinolysis during cardiopulmonary bypass. *Lancet*, 1994;344:1192-1193.

[32] Edmunds LH Jr. Inflammatory response to cardiopulmonary bypass. *Ann. Thor. Surg.*, 1998;66:S12-S16.

[33] Chung JH, Gikakis N, Rao AK, et al. Pericardial blood activates the extrinsic coagulation pathway during clinical cardiopulmonary bypass. *Circulation*, 1996;93:2014-2018.

[34] Bevilacqua MP, Pober JS, Majeau GR, et al. Recombinant tumor necrosis factor induces procoagulant activity in cultured human vascular endothelium: characterization and comparison with the actions of interleukin 1. *Proc. Natl. Acad. Sci. US*, 1986;83:4533-4537.

[35] Mackman N, Brand K, Edgington T. Lipopolysaccharide-mediated transcriptional activation of the human tissue factor gene in THP-1 monocytic cells requires both activator protein 1 and nuclear factor kB binding sites. *J. Exp. Med.*, 1991;174:1517-1526.

[36] Bauer KA, Ten CH, Barzegar S, et al. Tumor necrosis factor infusions have a procoagulant effect on the hemostatic mechanism of humans. *Blood*, 1989;74:165-172.

[37] Altieri DC, Morrissey JH, Edgington T. Adhesive receptor Mac-1 coordinates the activation of factor X on stimulated cells of monocytic and myeloid differentiation: an alternative initiation of the coagulation protease cascade. *Proc. Natl. Acad. Sci. US*, 1988;85:7462-7466.

[38] Boyle EM, Verrier ED, Spiess BD. Endothelial cell injury in cardiovascular surgery: The procoagulant response. *Ann. Thorac. Surg.*, 1996;62:1549-1557.

[39] Harker LA, Malpass TW, Branson HE, et al. Mechanisms of abnormal bleeding in patients undergoing cardiopulmonary bypass: acquired transient platelet dysfunction associated with selective alpha-granule release. *Blood*, 1980;56:824-834.

[40] Despotis GJ, Filos KS, Zoys TN, et al. Factors associated with excessive postoperative blood loss and hemostatic transfusion requirements: a multivariate analysis in cardiac surgical patients. *Anesth. Analg.*, 1996;82:13-21.
[41] Chandler WL, Fitch JCK, Wall MH, et al. Individual variations in the fibrinolytic response during and after cardiopulmonary bypass. *Thromb. Haemost.*, 1995;74: 1293-1297.
[42] Kucuk O, Kwaan HC, Frederickson J, et al. Increased fibrinolytic activity in patients undergoing cardiopulmonary bypass operation. *Am. J. Hematol.*, 1986;23:223-229.
[43] Teufelsbauer H, Proidl S, Havel M, et al. Early activation of hemostasis during cardiopulmonary bypass: evidence for thrombin mediated hyperfibrinolysis. *Thromb. Haemost.*, 1992;68:250-252.
[44] Mammen E, Kocts MH, Washington B, et al. Hemostasis changes during cardiopulmonary bypass surgery. *Semin. Thromb. Hemost.*, 1985;11:281-292.
[45] Tanaka K, Takao M, Yada I, et al. Alterations in coagulation and fibrinolysis associated with cardiopulmonary bypass during open heart surgery. *J. Cardiothorac. Anesth.*, 1989;3:181-188.
[46] Pickering NJ, Brody JI, Fink GB, et al. The behaviour of antithrombin III, alpha2-macroglobulin and alpha-1-antitrypsin during cardiopulmonary bypass. *Am. J. Clin. Pathol.*, 1983;80:459.
[47] Stibbe J, Kluft C, Brommer EJP, et al. Enhanced fibrinolytic activity during cardiopulmonary bypass in open-heart surgery in man is caused by extrinsic (tissue-type) plasminogen activator. *Eur. J. Clin. Invest.*, 1984;14:375-382.
[48] Woodman RC, Harker LA. Bleeding complications associated with cardiopulmonary bypass. *Blood*, 1990;76:1680-1697.
[49] Holloway DS, Summaria L, Sanderasa J, et al. Decreased platelet number and function and increased fibrinolysis contribute to postoperative bleeding in cardiopulmonary bypass patients. *Thromb. Haemost.*, 1988;59:62-67.
[50] Weerasinghe A, Taylor KM. The platelet in cardiopulmonary bypass. *Ann. Thorac. Surg.*, 1998;66:2145-2152.
[51] Edmunds LH Jr, Ellison N, Colman RW, et al. Platelet function during cardiac operation: comparison of membrane and bubble oxygenators. *J. Thorac. Card. Surg.*, 1982;83:805-812.
[52] Zilla P, Fasol R, Groscurth P, et al. Blood platelets in cardiopulmonary bypass operations. *J. Thorac. Cardiovasc. Surg.*, 1989;97:379-388.
[53] Gemmell CH, Ramirez SM, Yeo EL, et al. Platelet activation in whole blood by artificial surfaces: identification of platelet-derived microparticles and activated platelet binding to leukocytes as material-induced activation events. *J. Lab. Clin. Med.*, 1995;125:276-287.
[54] Musial J, Niewiarowski S, Hershock D, et al. Loss of fibrinogen receptors from the platelet surface during simulated extracorporeal circulation. *J. Lab. Clin. Med.*, 1985;105:514-522.
[55] Kondo C, Tanaka K, Takagi K, et al. Platelet dysfunction during cardiopulmonary bypass surgery. With special reference to platelet membrane glycoproteins. *ASAIO J.*, 1993;39:M550-M553.
[56] Rinder CS, Mathew JP, Rinder HM, et al. Modulation of platelet surface adhesion receptors during cardiopulmonary bypass. *Anesthesiology*, 1991;75:563-570.

[57] Holada K, Simak J, Kucera V, et al. Platelet membrane receptors during short cardiopulmonary bypass—a flow cytometric study. *Perfusion*, 1996;11:401-406.
[58] Harker LA. Bleeding after cardiopulmonary bypass. *N. Engl. J. Med.,* 1986;314:1446-1447.
[59] Beurling-Harbury C, Galvan CA. Acquired decrease in platelet secretory ADP associated with increased postoperative bleeding in post-cardiopulmonary bypass patients and in patients with severe valvular heart disease. *Blood*, 1978;52:13-23.
[60] Rinder CS, Bohnert J, Rinder HM, et al. Platelet activation and aggregation during cardiopulmonary bypass. *Anesthesiology*, 1991;75:388-393.
[61] Greilich PE, Carr ME, Carr SL, et al. Reductions in platelet force development by cardiopulmonary bypass are associated with hemorrhage. *Anesth. Analg.,* 1995;80: 459-465.
[62] Raja SG. Decreased release of endothelin after OPCAB: Implications of the evidence. *J. Cardiothorac. Vasc. Anesth.,* 2004;18:680.
[63] Raja SG, Dreyfus GD. Off-pump coronary artery bypass surgery: To do or not to do? Current best available evidence. *J. Cardiothorac. Vasc. Anesth.,* 2004;18:486-505.
[64] Ascione R, Williams S, Lloyd CT, *et al.* Reduced postoperative blood loss and transfusion requirement after beating-heart coronary operations: A prospective randomized study. *J. Thorac. Cardiovasc. Surg.,* 2001;121:689-696.
[65] Puskas JD, Williams WH, Duke PG, *et al.* Off-pump coronary artery bypass grafting provides complete revascularization with reduced myocardial injury, transfusion requirements, and length of stay: A prospective randomized comparison of two hundred unselected patients undergoing off-pump versus conventional coronary artery bypass grafting. *J. Thorac. Cardiovasc. Surg.,* 2003;125:797-808.
[66] Angelini GD, Taylor FC, Reeves BC, *et al.* Early and midterm outcome after off-pump and on-pump surgery in Beating Heart against Cardioplegic Arrest Studies (BHACAS 1 and 2): A pooled analysis of two randomised controlled trials. *Lancet,* 2002;359:1194-1199.
[67] Raja SG, Dreyfus GD. Impact of off-pump coronary artery bypass surgery on postoperative bleeding: current best available evidence. J. Card. Surg., 2006;21:35-41.
[68] Bainbridge D, Martin J, Cheng D. Off pump coronary artery bypass graft surgery versus conventional coronary artery bypass graft surgery: a systematic review of the literature. *Semin. Cardiothorac. Vasc. Anesth.*, 2005;9:105-11.
[69] Reston JT, Tregear SJ, Turkelson CM. Meta-analysis of short-term and mid-term outcomes following off-pump coronary artery bypass grafting. *Ann. Thorac. Surg.*, 2003;76:1510-5.
[70] Parolari A, Alamanni F, Cannata A, et al. Off-pump versus on-pump coronary artery bypass: meta-analysis of currently available randomized trials. *Ann. Thorac. Surg.*, 2003;76:37-40.
[71] Kuss O, von Salviati B, Börgermann J. Off-pump versus on-pump coronary artery bypass grafting: a systematic review and meta-analysis of propensity score analyses. J. Thorac. Cardiovasc. Surg., 2010; 140:829-35.
[72] Mariani MA, Gu YJ, Boonstra PW, *et al.* Procoagulant activity after off-pump coronary operation: Is the current anticoagulation adequate? *Ann. Thorac. Surg.,* 1999;67:1370-1375.

[73] Gerrah R, Snir E, Brill A, *et al.* Platelet function changes as monitored by cone and plate(let) analyzer during beating heart surgery. *Heart Surg. Forum,* 2004*;7:* E191-E195.

[74] Bidstrup BP, Scarrott H, Luque M. Platelet function after off pump coronary surgery. *Heart. Surg. Forum,* 2003*;6:* 286-287.

[75] Boldt J, Schindler E, Osmer C, et al. Influence of different anticoagulation regimens on platelet function during cardiac surgery. *Br. J. Anaesth.,* 1994;73:639-644.

[76] Gravlee GP, Haddon WS, Rothberger HK, et al. Heparin dosing and monitoring for cardiopulmonary bypass. A comparison of techniques with measurement of subclinical plasma coagulation. *J. Thorac. Cardiovasc. Surg.,* 1990*;*99:518-527.

[77] Englberger L, Immer FF, Eckstein FS, et al. Off-pump coronary artery bypass operation does not increase procoagulant and fibrinolytic activity: Preliminary results. *Ann. Thorac. Surg.,* 2004;77:1560-1566.

[78] Donias HW, D'Ancona G, Pande RU, et al. Heparin dose, transfusion rates, and intraoperative graft patency in minimally invasive direct coronary artery bypass. *Heart. Surg. Forum.,* 2003*;*6*:*176-180.

[79] Larmann J, Theilmeier G. Inflammatory response to cardiac surgery: Cardiopulmonary bypass versus non-cardiopulmonary bypass surgery. *Best Pract. Res. Clin. Anaesthesiol.,* 2004*;*18*:* 425-438.

[80] Casati V, Gerli C, Franco A, et al. Activation of coagulation and fibrinolysis during coronary surgery: on-pump versus off-pump techniques. *Anesthesiology,* 2001;95: 1103-9.

[81] Boisclair MD, Lane DA, Philippou H, et al. Mechanisms of thrombin generation during surgery and cardiopulmonary bypass. *Blood,* 1993;82:3350-7.

[82] Kongsgaard UE, Smith-Erichsen N, Geiran O, Bjornskau L. Changes in the coagulation and fibrinolytic systems during and after cardiopulmonary bypass surgery. *Thorac. Cardiovasc. Surg.,* 1988;37:158-62.

[83] Vedin J, Antovic A, Ericsson A, Vaage J. Hemostasis in off-pump compared to on-pump coronary artery bypass grafting: a prospective, randomized study. *Ann. Thorac. Surg.,* 2005;80:586-93.

[84] Englberger L, Immer FF, Eckstein FS, et al. Off-pump coronary artery bypass operation does not increase procoagulant and fibrinolytic activity: preliminary results. *Ann. Thorac. Surg.*, 2004;77:1560-6.

[85] Vallely MP, Bannon PG, Bayfield MS, et al. Quantitative and temporal differences in coagulation, fibrinolysis and platelet activation after on-pump and off-pump coronary artery bypass surgery. *Heart. Lung. Circ.*, 2009;18:123-30.

[86] Paulitsch FS, Schneider D, Sobel BE, et al. Hemostatic changes and clinical sequelae after on-pump compared with off-pump coronary artery bypass surgery: a prospective randomized study. *Coron. Artery. Dis.*, 2009;20:100-5.

In: Off-Pump Coronary Artery Bypass Grafting
Editors: S.G. Raja and M. Amrani
ISBN 978-1-62081-575-5

Chapter 4

MYOCARDIAL OUTCOMES AFTER OFF-PUMP CORONARY ARTERY BYPASS GRAFTING

Ishtiaq A. Rahman and Raimondo Ascione
Cardiothoracic Surgery, Bristol Heart Institute,
University Hospitals Bristol NHS Trust Foundation, Bristol, UK

ABSTRACT

Current gold standard strategy of coronary artery bypass grafting (CABG) on cardiopulmonary bypass (CPB), despite being generally safe and efficient, is associated with numerous complications. Several of these complications such as bleeding diathesis, neurological deficits, tissue oedema and renal impairment are attributed to the use of CPB. Myocardial damage is known to occur following cross-clamping of the aorta and cardioplegic arrest. In the past two decades CABG without CPB on a beating heart has been increasingly performed. There is evidence to suggest that patients undergoing off-pump CABG have better preservation of left ventricular contraction than after cardioplegic arrest. Superior mitochondrial function, assessed using myocardial biopsy specimens, has also been reported after off-pump CABG. The avoidance of aortic cross-clamping may thus confer the potential advantage of minimizing the risks of global myocardial ischemia, myocardial stunning and the potentially damaging effects of cardioplegia administration.

This chapter provides a comprehensive and evidence-based discussion of the impact of off-pump CABG on myocardial outcomes.

INTRODUCTION

In conventional coronary artery bypass grafting (on-pump CABG) with cardiopulmonary bypass (CPB) and cardioplegic arrest (CA), adverse outcomes predominantly relate to the systemic impact of CPB and to cardiomyocyte injury due to myocardial protection failure. The advent of off-pump coronary surgery (off-pump CABG) with its potential to avoid CPB and CA has led to a prolonged debate on its efficacy in reducing myocardial injury compared to conventional technique. The adequacy of myocardial protection can be assessed using an array of measurements that are indicative of cardiomyocyte death, injury or dysfunction [1]. These include cardiac troponin (cTn) release, the incidence of post-operative low cardiac output episodes and ventricular arrhythmias, the need for inotropic support and functional assessment by hemodynamic monitoring and echocardiography. These measures contribute to an assessment of reversible and irreversible myocardial injury. In this chapter we will review the available evidence on the impact of off-pump CABG surgery on myocardial injury compared to on-pump CABG.

Impact of On-Pump and Off-Pump CABG Myocardial Injury at Biochemical Level

For assessment of perioperative myocardial injury a range of cardiac biochemical and inflammatory markers have been identified. The available evidence suggests that there is a significant release of markers of myocardial injury during on-pump CABG surgery and that this release appears to be reduced during off-pump [2-5].

Cardiac troponins are regarded as the most sensitive markers of myocardial injury [6]. There is debate regarding their site of origin and significance during coronary surgery. cTn release may be indicative of myofibrillar damage and myocyte necrosis or changes in sarcolemmal permeability with leakage from cytosolic pools [7,8]. CPB may itself affect sarcolemmal permeability.

The clinical relevance of cTn release is high given that it is regarded as an independent predictor of in-hospital death and that high concentrations are associated with a cardiac cause of death and major postoperative outcomes [9,10]. The magnitude of release has been shown to be related to the type of cardiac surgical procedure [11]. In one series perioperative elevation of cardiac Troponin I (cTnI) reliably predicted mortality in infants and children undergoing surgical repair of congenital heart defects [12].Since the advent of off-pump CABG a series of randomized and observational studies have utilised cTn as the primary endpoint to evaluate myocardial injury. Ascione et al reported in 1998, the first randomized controlled trial (RCT) in 80 elective patients undergoing coronary surgery, the serial release of cTnI to be minimal during off-pump CABG surgery (Figure 1) [13].

A similar trend in serial cTn release was confirmed later by others [14] and similar findings have also been seen in larger observational series [15]. Off-pump CABG has also demonstrated benefit in myocardial injury as assessed by postoperative creatine kinase MB (CK-MB). In the prospective, single centre, randomized PRAGUE-4 study (n=400) of unselected patients comparing non-emergent on- and off-pump surgery CK-MB levels where higher in the on-pump group (0.56 vs. 0.15 microkat/L; $p<0.01$).

In addition this study found the primary endpoint of any of death, myocardial infarction, stroke, or new renal failure requiring hemodialysis within 30 days to be similar between the groups (4.9% vs. 2.9%) as was mortality (1.1% vs. 2.0%) and preoperative crossover (5.4% in each group). However, intraoperative conversion was more common in the off-pump group (1.1% vs. 9.8%; $p<0.01$). On-pump patients received more distal anastomoses (2.7 vs. 2.3; $p<0.01$), suffered greater blood loss (680 vs. 560 mL; $p<0.01$) and higher total hospital costs (4387 vs. 3451; $p<0.01$) [16].

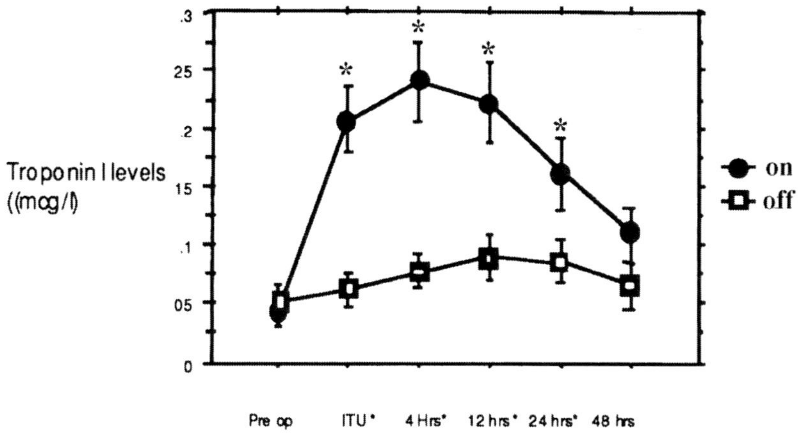

Figure 1. Perioperative Troponin I release. Data shown as mean±standard error of the mean.*p<0.05 on pump vs. off pump at 1, 4, 12 and 24h postoperatively. (Reproduced from reference 13 with permission from EACTS and Elsevier Inc.).

Puskas et al. in a prospective randomized comparison of two hundred unselected patients undergoing off-pump versus on-pump surgery by a single surgeon assessed myocardial injury with both CK-MB and cTnI markers. Once again the off-pump group demonstrated benefit with both markers. These patients were also found to have a shorter length of stay and reduced transfusion requirement. No difference in completeness of revascularisation, in-hospital and 30-day outcomes were observed however [17].

Debate remains over the most superior troponin measurement (12 hours; peak; area under the curve [AUC]). Khan et al. found on-pump surgery (n=50) to sustain the greater myocardial injury during the first 72 hours, as assessed by AUC cTnT (30.96 vs. 19.33 h.microg.l^{-1}; p=0.02), when compared to off-pump (n=50) in a prospective, randomized, controlled study. Other analyses found no difference in mean number of grafts (3.4 vs. 3.1; p=0.41) and median postoperative length of stay (seven days) between the groups. At three months on-pump graft patency, assessed by coronary angiography, was higher (127/130 (98%) vs. 114/130 (88%) patent grafts; p<0.01). and clearly this difference has implications with respect to long term outcomes. The patency rate was higher for all graft territories in the on-pump group than in the off-pump group [18].

Of interest, compared to a range of other surgical procedures off-pump CABG still appears to cause the smallest myocardial injury as determined by CK-MB and cTnI up to 18h postoperatively even for conditions with no coronary disease [19]. There appears to be an association between perioperative myocardial damage, as defined by cTnI and CK-MB and other clinical events. In a series of 261 patients those with cTnI>7.1 ng/ml (n=51) and CK-MB>36.3 ng/ml (n=48) were found to have longer mechanical ventilation and ICU length of stay and worse 3-year survival [20].

The sensitivity of cTn in measuring myocardial injury compared to other markers has been debated. In an RCT with 50 patients comparing on- pump vs. off-pump CABG the total amount of heart-type fatty acid-binding protein (hFABP), cTnI, and high-sensitivity C-reactive protein released was found to be higher in the on-pump group. Receiver operating characteristic curve analysis identified cTnI and hFABP to be the more superior diagnostic discriminators of myocardial injury, with optimal cut-off values >0.92 ng/mL and >6.8 ng/mL respectively. Logistic regression analysis revealed that patients with increased cTnI levels >0.92 ng/mL and hFABP levels >6.8 ng/mL were at 132 times and 54 times higher risk of myocardial injury after on-pump CABG [2]. Thus off-pump CABG was shown to provide better myocardial protection than on-pump CABG and high-sensitivity C-reactive protein did not prove to have superior diagnostic discriminator qualities. This has been confirmed by others [21-24].

The superiority of off-pump CABG in determining less release of cTn seems to persist also when excluding those patients suffering perioperative cardiac events. In one such study in 54 patients, to ensure no bias in results, those patients that had suffered perioperative myocardial infarctions, as defined as new Q wave on ECG, were excluded from the analysis. Yet, the off-pump CABG remained associated with less injury [25].

In addition, the purported increase in myocardial injury associated with on-pump CABG does not appear to depend on surgical priority and extension of coronary disease. In a large prospective cohort of 1511 coronary patients (on-pump n=778; off-pump n=733) mean cTnT levels were significantly higher in the on-pump group (0.9 vs. 0.2 ng/mL) consistently across urgent and elective surgeries and in those with 2- and 3-vessel disease [26].

Although the degree of myocardial injury measured by cTn is higher with on-pump CABG, it has been difficult over the years to determine the isolated contribution of CPB and CA to myocardial injury due to their concomitant use.

A study by Krejca et al. sought to differentiate three groups undergoing myocardial revascularization: those performed with intermittent cross-clamp (n=13); beating-heart on pump without CA (n=12); and off-pump CABG (n=13). cTnT levels were higher in those undergoing intermittent cross-clamp and significantly lower in the off-pump CABG [27].

Similar findings were observed in an RCT with 40 elective patients with normal left ventricular function and three vessels coronary artery disease assigned to off-pump CABG or on-pump beating heart surgery [28]. These studies suggest that CA itself might be the major determinant of myocardial injury. However, our group in a recent RCT with 80 elective patients allocated to on-pump CABG with CA vs. on-pump beating surgery showed no difference in serial cTnI release. The CA time in the on-pump CABG with CA group was only around 30 minutes and this might suggests that duration of CA is a key player in determining myocardial injury [29].

Although off-pump CABG is associated with less myocardial injury several factors, during this type of surgery, have been associated with an increased release of cTn and other markers.

These include the use of intracoronary shunts, anastomotic time and maintenance of appropriate hemodynamics during grafting. Yeatman et al. investigated the hemodynamic changes in patients undergoing multi-vessel beating heart coronary revascularization in the presence or absence of an intracoronary shunt.

Forty patients were randomized to off-pump with a shunt (n=20) or with the proximal coronary artery occluded by a soft snare (n=20). Hemodynamic measurements were recorded at base line, during construction, and after completion of each distal anastomosis. Stabilization of the left anterior descending coronary artery to perform the anastomosis resulted in temporary hemodynamic changes, which are prevented by the use of an intracoronary shunt.

The hemodynamic deterioration during the construction of the posterior descending coronary artery and circumflex coronary artery anastomoses were transient in the shunt group, whereas the snaring technique was associated with an impairment of early functional recovery [30]. Other determinants of myocardial cell injury during off-pump coronary artery bypass (OPCAB) grafting, assessed by serial release of cTn, are heart rate, blood pressure and anastomosis time [31-33].

Early after surgery OPCAB appears to result in better left ventricular function but does not reduce the incidence or extent of irreversible myocardial injury.

In a single-center randomized trial patients undergoing multivessel total arterial revascularization randomly assigned to OPCAB (n=30) and ONCAB (n=30) underwent preoperative and early postoperative cine MRI for assessment of global left ventricular function and contrast-enhanced CMRI for assessment of irreversible myocardial injury.

Serial troponin I measurements were obtained perioperatively and correlated with the CMRI findings. After surgery, the cardiac index was significantly higher in the OPCAB group compared to ONCAB (3.2±0.8 vs. 2.7±0.6; p=0.04). New irreversible myocardial injury was similar in incidence (44% vs. 36%; p=0.8) and magnitude (6.8±4.0 vs. 6.3±3.6 g; p=0.9) across the 2 groups. The median area-under-the-curve (AUC) troponin I values were significantly larger in ONCAB group (132 vs. 182 μg/L; p=0.02). There was a moderate correlation between the troponin I AUC values and mean mass of new myocardial hyperenhancement (r^2=0.4; p<0.01) [34].

In summary, it is evident, from a biochemical response perspective, that OPCAB surgery demonstrates advantage. However a greater understanding of the processes involved in myocardial injury is required and with it a refining of both the operative procedure and the development of novel techniques is necessary to further limit injurious factors.

Impact of On-Pump and Off-Pump CABG on the Incidence of Arrhythmias

Ischemic heart disease carries an increased risk of malignant ventricular fibrillation (VF), ventricular tachycardia (VT) and sudden death and post-CABG both VF and VT have been identified as potential life threatening complications [35-40].

The bulk of evidence in the literature relating to the anti-arrhythmic potential of off-pump CABG is focused on the incidence of atrial fibrillation (AF) rates. AF can impact on patient recovery post surgery, prolong hospital stay, and increase costs.

Ascione et al. reported the outcome of a large RCT in 200 patients (BHACAS trial) [41] which showed a reduced incidence of AF associated with off-pump CABG Thirty-nine patients in the on-pump group and 8 patients in the off-pump group had postoperative sustained AF (p<0.01). Univariate analysis showed that CPB inclusive of cardioplegic arrest, postoperative inotropic support, intubation time, chest infection, and hospital length of stay were predictors of AF (all p<0.05). However, stepwise multivariate regression analysis identified CPB inclusive of cardioplegic arrest as the only independent predictor of postoperative AF (OR 7.4; CI 3.4 to 17.9). This finding was confirmed in the pooled analysis of the BHACAS 1 and 2 trials by the same group in 401 patients [42].

In 2004 the ISMICS Conference conducted a systematic review and meta-analysis of the randomized and non-randomized evidence comparing off- and on-pump CABG and published evidence based consensus statements. Some but not all randomized trials showed significant reduction in AF with off-pump compared to on-pump surgery. In pooled analysis of randomized controlled trials evaluating outcomes in patient populations with mixed-risk factors, OPCAB reduced the incidence of atrial fibrillation (OR 0.58, 95% CI 0.44-0.77; $p<0.01$; n=2425 patients in 17 RCTs) [43].

In addition a meta-analysis of observational studies reported a comparison between on- and off-pump CABG in elderly patients (>70yrs) utilising postoperative AF incidence as the primary outcome of interest. The quality of each study included was evaluated by examining three items: patient selection, matching of the off-pump and CPB patient groups and assessment of outcome. Eight studies fulfilled inclusion criteria. In total the studies identified 3017 subjects of which 25% underwent off-pump (n=764) and 75% on-pump (n=2253) surgery. The meta-analysis showed that after off-pump surgery there was a significantly lower incidence of postoperative AF [44].

Perioperative protocols to reduce the incidence of AF post-cardiac surgery have been employed with varying success. In a multi-centre study comprising 2376 off-pump patients extubated immediately following surgery in the operating room there was found to be a reduced incidence of AF (10.6% vs. 18.5%; $p<0.01$), shorter length of stay (4.8±3.5 vs. 6.3±5.2 days; $p<0.01$) and reduced mortality (1.1% vs. 2.4%; p=0.04) [45]. However these protocols have not been adopted universally as the evidence for AF reduction with OPCAB has not been felt to be conclusive.

In an observational study of 670 patients that underwent revascularization by using in situ left internal mammary artery (LIMA) for single vessel disease (on-pump n=328; off-pump n=342) avoiding CPB did not alter incidence of AF. However, prophylactic beta-blocker usage was found to decrease the incidence of AF in both groups [46] and thus represents a useful management strategy.

Others have shown no evidence of reduced AF rate following off-pump surgery. Puskas et al. demonstrated in a prospective randomized comparison of 200 unselected patients undergoing off- vs. on-pump CABG that there was no significant difference in the incidence of postoperative AF between groups (n=16/98 for OPCAB vs. n=22/99 for on-pump CABG; p=0.367) [17]. In an observational study (off-pump n=99; on-pump n=100) the incidence of AF was also similar between the groups, (OPCAB 25% vs. on-pump CABG 18%; p=0.23) [47].

Impact of on-Pump and off-Pump CABG on Left and Right Ventricular Function

CABG is highly effective in improving life expectancy and quality of life in symptomatic patients with multivessel coronary artery disease [48]. Echocardiographic estimation of left ventricular ejection fraction (LVEF) has become the main method used in clinical practice to guide surgical management of patients with coronary artery disease [49,50].

While reduction in LVEF identifies those with most to benefit from revascularization, it is also a predictor both of in-hospital morbidity [51] and mortality [52]. Although LVEF above 40% is associated with reduced peri-operative complications [53], those with lower values suffer higher in-hospital mortality, longer cardiopulmonary bypass time, and longer hospital stays. In patients with impaired LV function and evidence of myocardial hibernation, CABG increases LVEF and improves regional LV function [54]. Furthermore, surgical revascularization of hibernating myocardium reduces mortality compared to medical therapy [55]. The improvement in LV systolic function following surgical revascularization of hibernating myocardium is greatest in those patients with the lowest preoperative LVEF [56].

Difference in surgical technique however, can affect post-operative LVEF, given that absolute difference has been observed in post-operative EF between off-pump and on-pump groups [34]. Off-pump CABG surgery has been shown to preserve LV systolic and diastolic function [57] and when compared with on-pump CABG surgery it has also been shown to improve more the indices of early diastolic filling and myocardial relaxation [58,59].

There appears to be evidence suggesting that the benefit of off-pump CABG may be more obvious in patients with impaired LV function. In a study of 142 patients undergoing off-pump CABG three groups defined by LVEF: <30% (n=48); 30-40% (n=48); >40% (n=46) were found to have similar late mortality [60]. The results of surgery were better than the preoperative predicted EuroSCORE and off-pump CABG was shown to be safe.

Similarly off-pump CABG (n=44) has been shown in another small study to be safe in the subset of patients with a severely decreased EF of ≤25% when compared to on-pump CABG (n=68) with fewer pulmonary complications, less postoperative pacing procedures and wound infections. However this was at expense of less number of grafts (2.5±0.9 vs. 3.±0.9; P=0.03) [61].

There is growing evidence that CABG may be associated with right ventricular (RV) dysfunction. RV function itself is a predictor of outcome and RV dysfunction has been associated with a high mortality [62]. RV function is markedly reduced following conventional on-pump CABG [63] and this persists up to 3 months with only partial recovery at 1 year [63-65].

Reduction in RV function does not appear to be related to the type of cardioplegia used during on-pump CABG [63,64,66,67]. Of interest, this appears to occur with both on- or off-pump surgical techniques. Pegg et al. showed a relative reduction of 12% in the off-pump and 7% in the on-pump groups respectively [33].

The study by Pegg et al. suggests that off-pump CABG surgery does not seem to provide superior functional protection of the RV over on-pump CABG surgery. This is confirmed by others. In a small RCT with a total of 50 patients right ventricular function was assessed by means of transthoracic echocardiographic analysis the day before the operation and 3 months later. Over the study period, RV myocardial performance index, a marker of global RV function, and right ventricular fractional area, a marker of overall RV systolic function change, did not change in comparison with the baseline values in both groups. Peak systolic velocity of the lateral tricuspid annulus was decreased significantly in both groups 3 months after the operation. There were no significant intergroup differences in any echocardiographic marker of right ventricular function [68, 69].

A difference in the impact on RV dysfunction does not appear to be influenced by the imaging technique used. Cardiac magnetic resonance imaging was performed in another study in 28 patients before and 3 months after elective coronary surgery. Both on-pump (47% vs. 62%; p<0.01) as well as off-pump CABG (47% vs. 55%; p<0.01) surgery resulted in an improvement in RV function in patients in a defined low RV ejection fraction group (below the median<53%) however there was no difference between the groups [70].

Hemodynamic Instability and Crossing over During off-Pump CABG

Off-pump CABG requires specific training and has a steep learning curve. Our group has shown that it can be taught to trainees both in elective and high-risk patients [71,72].

Adequate training allows preventing hemodynamic instability during off-pump CABG. In a series of 29 patients undergoing OPCAB using the 'Bristol Technique' patients were assessed for hemodynamic changes with the beating heart positioned for grafting. Three different surgical settings of exposure and stabilization were used according to the site of anastomosis: left anterior descending (LAD), posterior descending (PDA), and circumflex (Cx) coronary arteries. Reassuringly the technique produced no marked changes in heart rate (HR) and systemic mean arterial pressure during the construction of the anastomoses for any of the three surgical settings. LAD showed a decrease of 15.5% in stroke volume (SV) and an increase of 9% in pulmonary capillary wedge pressure (PCWP) compared to baseline. PDA showed a marked decrease in SV and cardiac index (CI), and an increase in central venous pressure (CVP) when compared to baseline.

The most extensive changes were observed in Cx with a considerable reduction in SV and CI, and an increase in CVP, PCWP, pulmonary arterial pressure, and systemic vascular resistance index. These hemodynamic changes were transient and totally recovered after the heart was returned to its anatomical position [73] and no adverse clinical events were encountered. Similar results were obtained by others in a study in 26 patients using a 'no compression' technique which involves enucleation of the heart without any compression on the cavities, and stabilization of the target area with a suction device [74]. In addition, in a study of 99 off-pump CABG patients matched and compared with 99 on-pump CABG patients no significant difference among the groups was found regarding early hemodynamics in terms of cardiac index (CI), systemic vascular resistance index (SVRI), left ventricular stroke work index (LVSWI), and inotropic support [75]. However, lack of appropriate training or specific clinical conditions might trigger hemodynamic instability during off-pump CABG leading to crossing over with emergency cardiopulmonary bypass and/or intra-aortic balloon pump (IABP) support.

The reported incidence of hemodynamic instability requiring crossing over differs markedly in the literature possibly as result of difference in learning curve. In a prospective study of 500 patients undergoing off-pump CABG hemodynamic instability was found in 24 (4.8%) patients, IABP support was instituted in 16 (3.2%) patients, and 8 (1.6%) required crossing over to CPB. A stepwise logistic regression identified ejection fraction <25%, myocardial infarction of <1-month, congestive heart failure and preoperative hemodynamic instability as predictors of crossing over [76]. Our group assessed the incidence of acute crossing over in relation to learning curve and associated clinical outcome in a large series of patients. The risk of acute conversion between 1996 and 2004 was 1.1% (27/2492): 5.1% in the first 2 years, 2.2% in the third year and 0.8% subsequently. Odds ratios for death in hospital compared to unconverted OPCAB and CABG-CPB were 4.4 (95% confidence interval (CI) 0.67-29.1) and 4.7 (95% CI 1.03-21.1), respectively, and ranged from 0 to 4.5 for serious complications. Converted patients had an increased hazard of death for 3 years after surgery compared to unconverted OPCAB (hazard ratio 3.21, 95% CI 1.20-8.59) and CABG-CPB patients (hazard ratio 3.23, 95% CI 1.41-7.39) [77]. Other research has concluded the cause of haemodynamic instability during elective OPCAB to be ischaemic, mechanical, or a combination of both [78].

Finally, the recent ROOBY trial in 2203 patients, randomized to on-pump and off-pump CABG, reported no significant difference between groups in the 30-day composite outcome (7.0% and 5.6%, respectively; p=0.19). The rate of the 1-year composite outcome was higher for off-pump than for on-pump CABG (9.9% vs. 7.4%, p=0.04). Of interest, the incidence of acute crossing over for this trial was very high (12.4% vs. 3.7% in the off- vs. on-pump groups). Of note, more than 55% of off-pump procedures were performed by residents with limited experience confirming the importance of the learning curve to minimise crossing over [79]. This was a major reason for concern when the outcome of this trial was published [80].

IMPACT OF ON-PUMP AND OFF-PUMP CABG ON MORTALITY

A review of the literature for mortality benefit attributed to on-pump over off-pump CABG has proved ambiguous ranging from advantage to similar to disadvantage.

Analysis comparing on- and off-pump CABG data from The Society of Thoracic Surgeons National Adult Cardiac Surgery Database included 126 centres having performed 118,140 total CABG procedures (off-pump: n=11717; 9.9% of total cases). Mortality and major complications were examined, both as unadjusted rates and after adjusting for known base line patient risk factors.

The use of an off-pump procedure decreased risk-adjusted operative mortality when compared to on-pump (2.3% vs. 2.9%; p<0.01) and decreased the risk-adjusted major complication rate (10.62% vs. 14.15%; p<0.01). Patients receiving off-pump procedures were less likely to die (adjusted odds ratio 0.81, 95% CI 0.70 to 0.91) and less likely to have major complications (adjusted odds ratio 0.77, 95% CI 0.72 to 0.82) [81].

In a study of 12812 patients over a 10 year follow up period comparing in-hospital major adverse cardiac events (MACE) and long-term survival after off-pump vs. on-pump CABG, off-pump CABG was associated with a significant reduction in operative mortality, stroke and MACE [82]. Female gender was associated with higher rates of death, stroke, myocardial infarction and MACE and women, but not men, disproportionately benefited from OPCAB in operative mortality. The male gender was associated with longer-term survival but surgery type (OPCAB vs. On-pump CABG) was not. Thus OPCAB itself provided significant early mortality and morbidity advantages, especially for women.

In 2004 the ISMICS Conference conducted a systematic review and meta-analysis of the randomized and non-randomized evidence comparing off- and on-pump CABG and published evidence based consensus statement[43]. For mixed-risk patient populations comparing off- and on-pump CABG a meta-analysis of 37 randomized clinical trials reported across 53 papers (3369 patients, level A) and two meta-analyses of non-randomized trials (Level B) were identified. For high-risk patient populations a meta-analysis of 3 randomized and 42 non-randomized trials (26349 patients, Level B) was conducted. Thus in patients undergoing surgical myocardial revascularization the following consensus statements were published:

1) OPCAB should be considered a safe alternative to CCAB with respect to mortality [Class I, Level A];
2) With appropriate use of modern stabilizers, heart positioning devices, and adequate surgeon experience, similar completeness of revascularization and graft patency can be achieved [Class IIa,Level A];
3) OPCAB is recommended to reduce perioperative morbidity [Class I, Level A];
4) OPCAB may be recommended to minimize mid-term cognitive dysfunction [Class IIa, Level A];
5) OPCAB should be considered as an equivalent alternative to CCAB in regard to quality of life [Class I, Level A];
6) OPCAB is recommended to reduce the duration of ventilation, ICU and hospital stay and resource utilization [Class I, Level A];
7) OPCAB should be considered in high-risk patients to reduce perioperative mortality, morbidity and resource utilization [Class IIa, Level B]

Equivocally a meta-analysis comparing the two techniques of 10 randomized trials (n=2018 patients) showed similar results in 1-year mortality, stroke, myocardial infarction, and need for repeat revascularization [83]. This finding was corroborated by a prospective observational study comparing mortality and morbidity between OPCAB (n=254) and conventional CABG (n=347) in three major preoperative groups as assessed by EuroSCORE. No difference in mortality, stroke, renal dysfunction, atrial fibrillation, re-exploration for bleeding, deep sternal wound infection, or pulmonary complications in any of the three groups after risk adjustment was elicited. However, inotropic requirement and requirements of blood products were less in OPCAB group [84].

In the Veterans Affairs Randomized On/Off Bypass (ROOBY) study (n=2203) patients underwent both urgent and elective CABG. No significant difference between off- and on-pump CABG in the primary short-term composite end point of death or complications (reoperation, new mechanical support, cardiac arrest, coma, stroke, or renal failure) within 30 days after surgery (7.0% vs. 5.6%; p=0.19) was found. The rate of the 1-year composite outcome of death from any cause, a repeat revascularization procedure, or a nonfatal myocardial infarction after surgery was higher for off-pump (9.9% vs. 7.4%; p=0.04). The proportion of patients with fewer grafts completed than originally planned was higher with off-pump CABG than with on-pump CABG (17.8% vs. 11.1%; p<0.01). Follow-up angiograms in 1371 patients who underwent 4093 grafts revealed that the overall rate of graft patency was lower in the off-pump group than in the on-pump group (82.6% vs. 87.8%; p<0.01). There were no treatment-based differences in neuropsychological outcomes or short-term use of major resources [79].

In a series of 200 patients randomly assigned to undergo off-pump vs. on-pump CABG with patients and nonoperative care providers blinded to surgical group, number of grafts performed per patient, index of completeness of revascularization (number of grafts performed/number of grafts intended), combined hospital and 30-day mortalities and stroke rates were again similar between groups [17].

The data for benefit of off-pump surgery is not universal. In a RCT with 341 stable patients, with triple vessel disease, EF>30% and a EuroSCORE ≥5 the primary outcome measure of a composite of major adverse cardiac and cerebrovascular events (MACCE) was found to be more common in off-pump CABG patients (69(40%) vs. 54(33%); p=0.26). All-cause mortality was increased in the off-pump CABG group (24% vs. 15%; p=0.04) but cardiac-related death was not different (10% vs. 7%; p=0.47) [85].

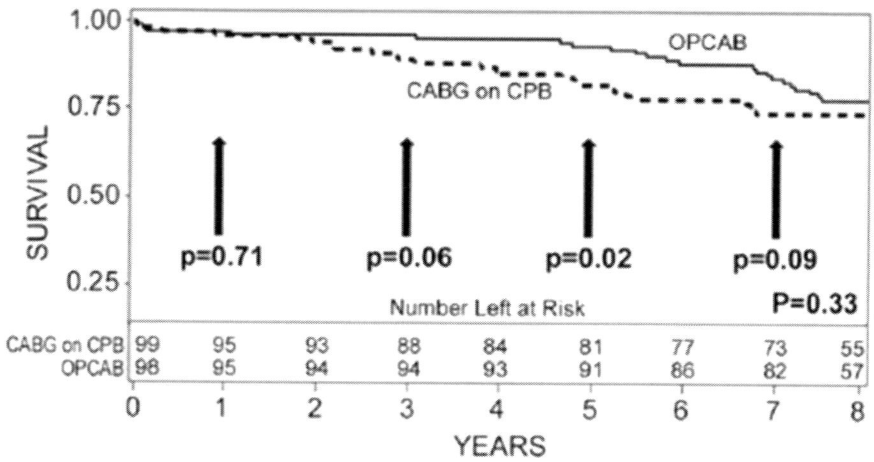

Figure 2. Late survival outcome of SMART trial. (Reproduced from reference 87 with permission from STS and Elsevier Inc.).

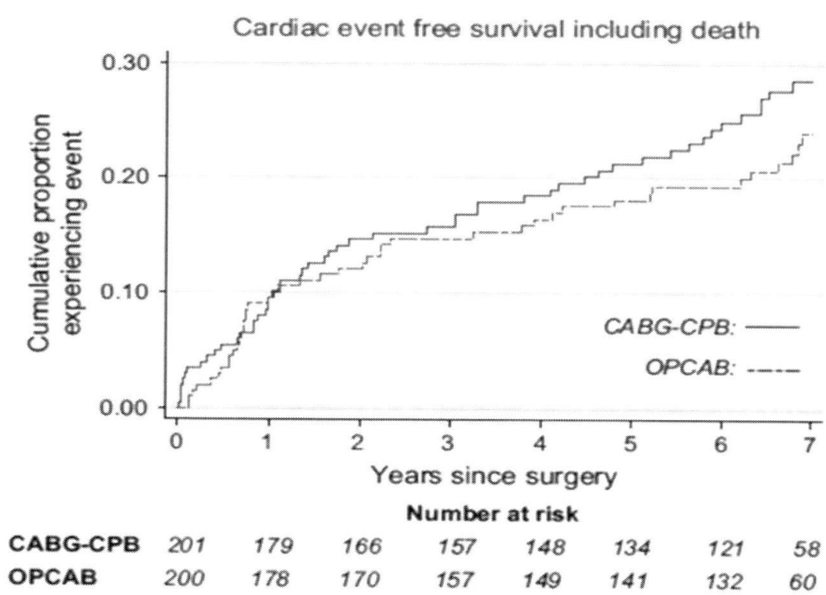

Figure 3. 7-year cardiac event free survival from BHACAS trials (Reproduced from reference 88 with permission from AATS and Elsevier Inc.).

A meta-analysis of randomized controlled trials comparing off-pump with on-pump CABG for (≥1yr) all-cause mortality with a total pool of 4326 patients suggested a statistically significant increase in midterm all-cause mortality by a factor of 1.37 with off-pump CABG. Exclusion of any single result, except for the largest (>2,000 patients) trial, from the analysis did not substantively alter the overall result. Eliminating the largest trial demonstrated a nonsignificant benefit of on-pump over off-pump CABG for midterm all-cause mortality [86]. The results suggest that off-pump CABG may increase late all-cause mortality by a factor of 1.37 over on-pump CABG. These findings however contrast with the late survival outcome of the SMART trial published recently which reported no difference between on- vs. off-pump CABG [Figure 2][87]. Similar late 7-year cardiac event free survival between groups was also observed in the BHACAS trials [Figure 3] [88].

Impact of On-Pump and Off-Pump Coronary Surgery on Late Graft Patency Rate and Need for Repeat Revascularization

Early matched sample data from New York databases of off-pump (n=13889) or on-pump CABG (n=35941) demonstrated off-pump CABG patients had lower rates of freedom from subsequent revascularization (89.9% vs. 93.6%; p<0.01) which favoured on-pump CABG [89]. In a later study with 503 on-pump patients matched to 503 off-pump patients twice as many off-pump patients (n=24) required repeat revascularization and Cox regression analysis confirmed off-pump surgery to be an independent predictor of poorer freedom from revascularization (95±3% vs. 92±2%; p=0.02) and cardiac event-free survival (76±5% vs. 62±8%; p=0.05) [90].

More recently a study by our group reported the 6-8 years follow-up of the BHACAS 1and2 trials. Patency was assessed in 199 of 349 survivors by using multidetector computed tomographic coronary angiographic analysis with a 16-slice scanner. The graft patency rate was 89.6% vs. 89% in the off-pump and on-pump group respectively. There was no difference between groups in cardiac event free survival including death [Figure 3] [88].

In a randomised trial by Puskas et al. of 200 unselected patients with multivessel coronary artery disease assigned to OPCAB or CABG with CPB 140 patients survived of which 87 returned for follow up after a minimum of 6.8 years. Early and late graft patency, assessed by computed tomographic angiography, was similar between OPCAB and CABG with CPB groups before hospital discharge (622 grafts assessed: 99% vs. 97.7%), at 1 year follow up (511 grafts assessed: 93.6% vs. 95.8%), and at late follow up (190 grafts assessed: 76% vs. 83.5%). The incidence of recurrent and residual myocardial ischaemia assessed by cardiac positron emission tomography and 12-lead electrocardiogram was also similar as was the need for reinterventions and long-term survival [87].

The ROOBY trial was published in 2009 reporting also 1 year patency rate. Follow-up angiograms in 1371 patients who underwent 4093 grafts revealed that the overall rate of graft patency was lower in the off-pump group than in the on-pump group (82.6% vs. 87.8%; p<0.01). Of interest, there was no difference in patency rate for LIMA-LAD graft between groups (95.3% vs. 96.2%; p=0.4), while a large difference in patency rate was observed for vein grafts (76.6% vs. 83.8%; p<0.01) [79].

Very recently the late follow-up of the SMART trial has been published [87]. This is in keeping with the late outcome analyses of the BHACAS trials which corroborate no difference between groups in terms of graft patency, myocardial ischemia, and freedom from repeat revascularization.

Off-Pump Surgery in High Risk Patients

Over the years there has been suggestion that off-pump coronary surgery might be particularly beneficial for high-risk patients. Our group reported the impact of on- vs. off-pump CABG in 1570 consecutive high-risk patients (defined as the presence of one or more of ten adverse prognostic factors), 332 (21.1%) of whom underwent an off-pump operation. Intensive care unit or high-dependency unit stay, total length of stay, blood loss of more than 1000 mL, postoperative hemoglobin and transfusion requirement all showed a highly significant benefit for the off-pump group ($p \leq 0.005$; odds ratios, 0.33 to 0.65) [91]. In a further study focussing on 2844 overweight patients (on-pump CABG n=2170 (76.3%)) Ascione et al. compared the clinical outcome of overweight patients undergoing coronary surgery with or without CPB. After adjustment for confounding prognostic factors, the benefits of off-pump surgery were still significant for death in hospital, transfusion requirement, neurological complications, intensive care unit and hospital stay (ORs 0.35 to 0.79; $p<0.05$) [92].Reoperative coronary artery bypass surgery is associated with increased surgical risk. A recent study compared the outcome of two surgical cohorts undergoing either off-pump or on-pump CABG. The early mortality was 3.3% vs. 5.5% for off-pump vs. on-pump CABG ($p<0.01$) [93].

Those who had undergone off-pump reoperations were found to have suffered less postoperative complications. Evidence suggests that off-pump CABG can also be performed safely in octogenarians, with excellent early and late outcomes. In a larger series of octogenarians (n=1993; 1589 on-pump vs. 404 off-pump). Patients undergoing off-pump CABG were older, had higher rates of preoperative AF ($p=0.01$) and New York Heart Association class IV heart failure ($p<0.01$). The use of on-pump surgery was associated with higher incidence of blood transfusion rates, (2.0±1.7 vs. 1.6±1.9units; $p=0.05$), AF (28.4% vs. 21.5%; $p<0.01$), prolonged ventilation (14.7% vs. 11.4%; $p=0.05$), and major complications (20.1% vs. 15.6%; $p=0.04$) [94]. Similar results were observed by others [95]. Of note recently Puskas et al. have reported that off-pump CABG disproportionately benefits high-risk patients undergoing coronary surgery [96]. Isolated, primary coronary artery bypass graft patients, over a 10 year period, were derived from the Society of Thoracic Surgeons (STS) database (14766 patients: OPCAB n=7083 (48%); on-pump CABG n=7683 (52%)). STS Predicted Risk of Mortality (PROM) was calculated by a formula based on 30 preoperative risk factors and 30-day operative mortality was compared between the two groups. Comparison of quartiles derived from PROM demonstrated no difference in operative mortality for those in the lower two risk quartiles. However in the higher risk quartiles there was a mortality benefit for OPCAB (odds ratio, 0.62 and 0.45 for OPCAB in the third and fourth risk quartiles). Logistic regression analysis, testing for an interaction between surgery type and PROM, confirmed a significant interaction ($p<0.01$) meaning that OPCAB is especially beneficial to patients with higher PROM.

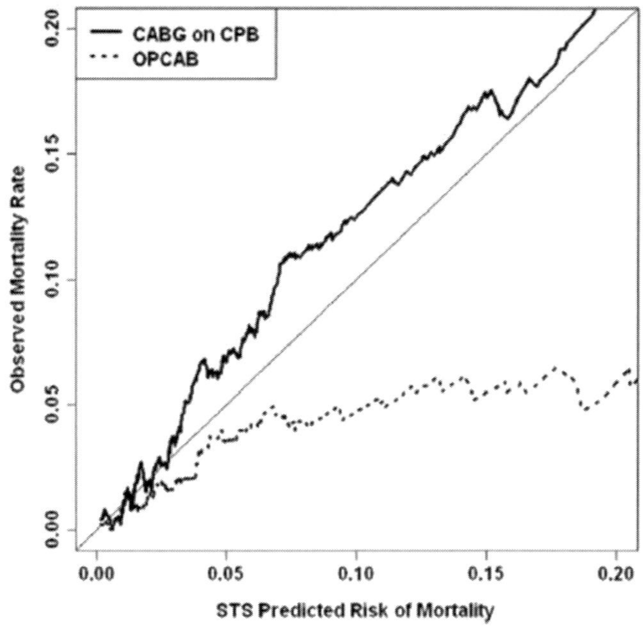

Figure 4. Regression curve comparison of observed mortality rates for off-pump coronary artery bypass grafting (OPCAB) and coronary artery bypass grafting (CABG) on cardiopulmonary bypass (CPB) across all levels of predicted risk. (Reproduced from reference 96 with permission from the Society of Thoracic Surgeons [STS] and Elsevier Inc.).

Locally smoothed kernel regression curves used to visually estimate a threshold PROM point at which mortality rates diverge found the benefit to be most significant for patients with PROM values above 2.5% to 3%. Thus OPCAB disproportionately benefits high-risk patients [Figure 4] [96].

Conclusion

A comprehensive review of the literature has shown off-pump surgery to reduce myocardial injury as defined by release of biochemical markers. Evidence suggests an anti-arrhythmic potential as well as functional benefit that can be quantified using a range of cardiac imaging techniques. With careful manipulation of the heart hemodynamic stability can be maintained with no compromise of precision of coronary anastomosis with comparable patency rates as on-pump surgery. Overall late mortality rates may appear controversial however there appears to be benefit associated with the use of off-pump CABG in high-risk patients.

References

[1] Hearse DJ, Braimbridge MV, Jynge P. Protection of ischaemic myocardium. New York: Raven Press, 1989.

[2] Chowdhury UK, Malik V, Yadav R, et al. Myocardial injury in coronary artery bypass grafting: on-pump versus off-pump comparison by measuring high-sensitivity C-reactive protein, cardiac troponin I, heart-type fatty acid-binding protein, creatine kinase-MB, and myoglobin release. *J. Thorac. Cardiovasc. Surg.,* 2008;135:1110-9, 1119.e1-10.

[3] Piacenza AE, Cacheda JH, Badaracco JR, Benetti FJ. Troponin as a marker of myocardial damage during coronary surgery with and without cardiopulmonary bypass. *J. Cardiovasc. Surg.,* (Torino) 2001;42:709-12.

[4] Koh TW, Carr-White GS, DeSouza AC, et al. Intraoperative cardiac troponin T release and lactate metabolism during coronary artery surgery: comparison of beating heart with conventional coronary artery surgery with cardiopulmonary bypass. *Heart,* 1999;81:495-500.

[5] Hammer S, Loeff M, Reichenspurner H, et al. Effect of cardiopulmonary bypass on myocardial function, damage and inflammation after cardiac surgery in newborns and children. *Thorac. Cardiovasc. Surg.,* 2001;49:349-54.

[6] Daubert MA, Jeremias A. The utility of troponin measurement to detect myocardial infarction: review of the current findings. *Vasc. Health Risk Manag.,* 2010;6:691-9.

[7] Remppis A, Scheffold T, Greten J, et al. Intracellular compartmentation of troponin T: release kinetics after global ischemia and calcium paradox in the isolated perfused rat heart. *J. Mol. Cell Cardiol.,* 1995;27:793-803.

[8] Fredericks S, Merton GK, Lerena MJ, Heining P, Carter ND, Holt DW. Cardiac troponins and creatine kinase content of striated muscle in common laboratory animals. *Clinica. Chimica. Acta.,* 2001;304:65-74.

[9] Hashemzadeh K, Dehdilani M. Postoperative cardiac troponin I is an independent predictor of in-hospital death after coronary artery bypass grafting. *J. Cardiovasc. Surg.,* (Torino) 2009;50:403-9.

[10] Lasocki S, Provenchère S, Bénessiano J, et al. Cardiac troponin I is an independent predictor of in-hospital death after adult cardiac surgery. *Anesthesiology,* 2002;97: 405-11.

[11] Fellahi JL, Hedoire F, Le Manach Y, Monier E, Guillou L, Riou B. Determination of the threshold of cardiac troponin I associated with an adverse postoperative outcome after cardiac surgery: a comparative study between coronary artery bypass graft, valve surgery, and combined cardiac surgery. *Crit. Care,* 2007;11:R106.

[12] Montgomery VL, Sullivan JE, Buchino JJ. Prognostic value of pre- and postoperative cardiac troponin I measurement in children having cardiac surgery. *Pediatr. Dev. Pathol.,* 2000;3:53-60.

[13] Ascione R, Lloyd CT, Gomes WJ, Caputo M, Bryan AJ, Angelini GD. Beating versus arrested heart revascularization: evaluation of myocardial function in a prospective randomized study.*Eur. J. Cardiothorac. Surg.,* 1999;15:685-90.

[14] Alwan K, Falcoz PE, Alwan J, et al. Beating versus arrested heart coronary revascularization: evaluation by cardiac troponin I release. *Ann. Thorac. Surg.,* 2004;77:2051-5.

[15] Badruzzaman M, Hossain A, Adhikary AB, et al. Evaluation of myocardial protection in off-pump vs. on-pump coronary bypass surgery by troponin I estimation. *Bangladesh Med. Res. Counc. Bull.,* 2010;36:93-6.

[16] Straka Z, Widimsky P, Jirasek K, Stros P, Votava J, Vanek T, Brucek P, Kolesar M, Spacek R. Off-pump versus on-pump coronary surgery: final results from a prospective randomized study PRAGUE-4. *Ann. Thorac. Surg.,* 2004;77:789-93.
[17] Puskas JD, Williams WH, Duke PG, et al. Off-pump coronary artery bypass grafting provides complete revascularization with reduced myocardial injury, transfusion requirements, and length of stay: A prospective randomized comparison of two hundred unselected patients undergoing off-pump versus conventional coronary artery bypass grafting. *J. Thorac. Cardiovasc. Surg.,* 2003;125:797-808.
[18] Khan NE, De Souza A, Mister R, et al. A randomized comparison of off-pump and on-pump multivessel coronary-artery bypass surgery. *N. Engl. J. Med.,* 2004;350:21-8.
[19] Landoni G, Pappalardo F, Calabrò MG, et al. Myocardial necrosis biomarkers after different cardiac surgical operations. *Minerva. Anestesiol.,* 2007;73:49-56.
[20] Paparella D, Cappabianca G, Malvindi P, et al. Myocardial injury after off-pump coronary artery bypass grafting operation. *Eur. J. Cardiothorac. Surg.,* 2007;32:481-7.
[21] Malik V, Kale SC, Chowdhury UK, et al. Myocardial injury in coronary artery bypass grafting: On-pump versus off-pump comparison by measuring heart-type fatty-acid-binding protein release. *Tex. Heart Inst. J.,* 2006;33:321-7.
[22] Tzimas PG, Milionis HJ, Arnaoutoglou HM, et al. Cardiac troponin I versus creatine kinase-MB in the detection of postoperative cardiac events after coronary artery bypass grafting surgery. *J. Cardiovasc. Surg.,* (Torino) 2008;49:95-101.
[23] Benoit MO, Paris M, Silleran J, Fiemeyer A, Moatti N. Cardiac troponin I: its contribution to the diagnosis of perioperative myocardial infarction and various complications of cardiac surgery. *Crit. Care Med.,* 2001;29:1880-6.
[24] Bonnefoy E, Filley S, Kirkorian G, et al. Troponin I, troponin T, or creatine kinase-MB to detect perioperative myocardial damage after coronary artery bypass surgery. *Chest,* 1998;114:482-6.
[25] Bennetts JS, Baker RA, Ross IK, Knight JL. Assessment of myocardial injury by troponin T in off-pump coronary artery grafting and conventional coronary artery graft surgery. *ANZ J. Surg.,* 2002;72:105-9.
[26] Brown JR, Hernandez F Jr, Klemperer JD, et al. Cardiac troponin T levels in on- and off-pump coronary artery bypass surgery. *Heart Surg. Forum,* 2007;10:E42-6.
[27] Krejca M, Skiba J, Szmagala P, Gburek T, Bochenek A. Cardiac troponin T release during coronary surgery using intermittent cross-clamp with fibrillation, on-pump and off-pump beating heart. *Eur. J. Cardiothorac. Surg.,* 1999;16:337-41.
[28] Rastan AJ, Bittner HB, Gummert JF, et al. On-pump beating heart versus off-pump coronary artery bypass surgery-evidence of pump-induced myocardial injury. *Eur. J. Cardiothorac. Surg.,* 2005;27:1057-64.
[29] Narayan P, Rogers CA, Bayliss KM, et al. On-pump coronary surgery with and without cardioplegic arrest: comparison of inflammation, myocardial, cerebral and renal injury and early and late health outcome in a single-centre randomised controlled trial. *Eur. J. Cardiothorac. Surg.,* 2011;39:675-83.
[30] Yeatman M, Caputo M, Narayan P, et al. Intracoronary shunts reduce transient intraoperative myocardial dysfunction during off-pump coronary operations. *Ann. Thorac. Surg.,* 2002;73:1411-7.
[31] Ketenci B, Enc Y, Ozay B, et al. Myocardial injury during off-pump surgery. The effect of intraoperative risk factors. *Saudi Med. J.,* 2008;29:203-8.

[32] Kurita A, Shintani H. Risk factors for myocardial injury during off-pump coronary artery bypass grafting. *Heart Surg. Forum,* 2005;8:E401-5.
[33] Pegg TJ, Selvanayagam JB, Karamitsos TD, et al. Effects of off-pump versus on-pump coronary artery bypass grafting on early and late right ventricular function. *Circulation,* 2008;117:2202-10.
[34] Selvanayagam JB, Petersen SE, Francis JM, et al. Effects of off-pump versus on-pump coronary surgery on reversible and irreversible myocardial injury: a randomized trial using cardiovascular magnetic resonance imaging and biochemical markers. *Circulation,* 2004;109:345-50.
[35] Ducceschi V, D'Andrea A, Liccardo B, et al. Ventricular tachyarrhythmia's following coronary surgery: predisposing factors. *Int. J. Cardiol.,* 2000;73:43-48.
[36] Steinberg JS, Gaur A, Sciacca R, et al. New-onset sustained ventricular tachycardia after cardiac surgery. *Circulation,* 1999;99:903-908.
[37] Holman WL, Spruell RD, Vicente WV, et al. Electrophysiological mechanisms for postcardioplegia reperfusion ventricular fibrillation. *Circulation,* 1994;90(suppl II):II-293–II-298.
[38] Pinto RP, Romerill DB, Nasser WK, et al. Prognosis of patients with frequent premature ventricular complexes and nonsustained ventricular tachycardia after coronary artery bypass graft surgery. *Clin. Cardio.,* 11996;19:321-324.
[39] Pires LA, Wagshal AB, Lancey R, et al. Arrhythmias and conduction disturbances after coronary artery bypass graft surgery: epidemiology, management, and prognosis. *Am. Heart J.,* 1995;129:799-808.
[40] Azar RR, Berns E, Seecharran B, et al. De novo monomorphic and polymorphic ventricular tachycardia following coronary artery bypass grafting. *Am. J. Cardiol.,* 1997;80:76-78.
[41] Ascione R, Caputo M, Calori G, Lloyd CT, Underwood MJ, Angelini GD. Predictors of atrial fibrillation after conventional and beating heart coronary surgery: A prospective, randomized study. *Circulation,* 2000;102:1530-5.
[42] Angelini GD, Taylor FC, Reeves BC, Ascione R. Early and midterm outcome after off-pump and on-pump surgery in Beating Heart Against Cardioplegic Arrest Studies (BHACAS 1 and 2): a pooled analysis of two randomised controlled trials. *Lancet,* 2002;359:1194-9.
[43] Puskas J, Cheng D, Knight J, et al. Off-pump versus conventional coronary artery bypass grafting: a meta-analysis and consensus statement from The 2004 ISMICS Consensus Conference. Innovations: *Technology and Techniques in Cardiothoracic and Vascular Surgery,* 2005:1:3-27.
[44] Athanasiou T, Aziz O, Mangoush O, et al. Do off-pump techniques reduce the incidence of postoperative atrial fibrillation in elderly patients undergoing coronary artery bypass grafting? *Ann. Thorac. Surg.,* 2004;77:1567-74.
[45] Edgerton JR, Herbert MA, Prince SL, et al. Reduced atrial fibrillation in patients immediately extubated after off-pump coronary artery bypass grafting. *Ann. Thorac. Surg.,* 2006;81:2121-6.
[46] Enc Y, Ketenci B, Ozsoy D, Camur G, Kayacioglu I, Terzi S, Cicek S. Atrial fibrillation after surgical revascularization: is there any difference between on-pump and off-pump? *Eur. J. Cardiothorac. Surg.,* 2004;26:1129-33.

[47] Place DG, Peragallo RA, Carroll J, Cusimano RJ, Cheng DC. Postoperative atrial fibrillation: a comparison of off-pump coronary artery bypass surgery and conventional coronary artery bypass graft surgery. *J. Cardiothorac. Vasc. Anesth.,* 2002;16:144-8.

[48] Yusuf S, Zucker D, Charles TC. Ten-year results of the randomized controlled trials of coronary artery bypass graft surgery: tabular data compiled by the collaborative effort of the original trial investigators. *Online J. Curr. Clin. Trials.* 1994;Doc No 145.

[49] Shiran A, Adawi S, Dobrecky-Mery I, Halon DA, Lewis BS. Echocardiographic predictors of late mortality in elderly patients with acute coronary syndromes. *Isr. Med. Assoc. J.,* 2007;9:247-51.

[50] Bierig SM, Ryan A, Ziaee A, et al. Serial changes in systolic and diastolic echocardiographic indices as predictors of outcome in patients with decreased left ventricular ejection fraction. *Eur. J. Echocardiogr.,* 2007;8:369-74.

[51] Vavlukis M, Georgievska-Ismail LJ, Bosevski M, Borozanov V. Predictors of in-hospital morbidity and mortality in patients with coronary artery disease treated with coronary artery bypass surgery. *Prilozi,* 2006;27:97-113.

[52] Del Rizzo DF, Fremes SE, Christakis GT, Sever J, Goldman BS. The current status of myocardial revascularization: changing trends and risk factor analysis. *J. Card. Surg.,* 1996;11:18-29.

[53] Wang J, Xiao F, Ren J, Li Y, Zhang ML. Risk factors for mortality after coronary artery bypass grafting in patients with low left ventricular ejection fraction. *Chin. Med. J. (Engl),* 2007;120:317-22.

[54] Erentürk S, Yildiz CE, Gulbaran M. Revascularization in patients with severe left ventricular impairment who have ischemic heart disease. *Saudi Med. J.,* 2007;28:54-9.

[55] Allman KC, Shaw LJ, Hachamovitch R, Udelson JE. Myocardial viability testing and impact of revascularization on prognosis in patients with coronary artery disease and left ventricular dysfunction: a meta-analysis. *J. Am. Coll. Cardiol.,* 2002;39:1151-8.

[56] Gasior Z, Krejca M, Szmagala P, Bochenek A. Long term left ventricular systolic function assessment following CABG. A prospective, randomised study. Blood versus crystalloid cardioplegia. *J. Cardiovasc. Surg.,* (Torino) 2000;41:695-702.

[57] Royse CF, Royse AG, Wong CT. Assessment of left ventricular function during off-pump coronary artery bypass surgery. *Ann. Thorac. Cardiovasc. Surg.,* 2003;9:371-7.

[58] Ng KK, Popovic ZB, Troughton RW, et al. Comparison of left ventricular diastolic function after on-pump versus off-pump coronary artery bypass grafting. *Am. J. Cardiol.,* 2005;95:647-50.

[59] Diller GP, Wasan BS, Kyriacou A, Mayet J, et al. Effect of coronary artery bypass surgery on myocardial function as assessed by tissue Doppler echocardiography. *Eur. J. Cardiothorac. Surg.,* 2008;34:995-9.

[60] Darwazah AK, Snaineh YA, Kiswani MO, Yassin IH, Abu Sham'a RA. Off-pump coronary artery bypass in multi-vessel disease: effect of ejection fraction on early and midterm mortality and morbidity. *J. Cardiovasc. Surg.,* (Torino) 2008;49:519-26.

[61] Emmert MY, Emmert LS, Martinez EC, Lee CN, Kofidis T. Off-pump coronary bypass surgery is safe in patients with a low ejection fraction (< or =25%). *Heart Surg., Forum,* 2010;13:E136-42.

[62] Davila-Roman VG, Waggoner AD, Hopkins WE, Barzilai B. Right ventricular dysfunction in low output syndrome after cardiac operations: assessment by transoesophageal echocardiography. *Ann. Thorac. Surg.,* 1995;60:1081-1086.

[63] Hedman A, Alam M, Zuber E, Nordlander R, Samad BA. Decreased right ventricular function after coronary artery bypass grafting and its relation to exercise capacity: a tricuspid annular motion-based study. *J. Am. Soc. Echocardiogr.,* 2004;17:126-31.

[64] Alam M, Hedman A, Nordlander R, Samad B. Right ventricular function before and after an uncomplicated coronary artery bypass graft as assessed by pulsed wave Doppler tissue imaging of the tricuspid annulus. *Am. Heart J.,* 2003;146:520-6.

[65] Schirmer U, Calzia E, Lindner KH, Hemmer W, Georgieff M. Right ventricular function after coronary artery bypass grafting in patients with and without revascularization of the right coronary artery. *J. Cardiothorac Vasc. Anesth.,* 1995;9:659-64.

[66] Roshanali F, Yousefnia MA, Mandegar MH, Rayatzadeh H, Alinejad S. Decreased right ventricular function after coronary artery bypass grafting. *Tex. Heart Inst. J.,* 2008;35:250-5.

[67] Diller GP, Wasan BS, Kyriacou A, et al. Effect of coronary artery bypass surgery on myocardial function as assessed by tissue Doppler echocardiography. *Eur. J. Cardiothorac. Surg.,* 2008;34:995-999.

[68] Michaux I, Filipovic M, Skarvan K, et al . A randomized comparison of right ventricular function after on-pump versus off-pump coronary artery bypass graft surgery. *J. Thorac. Cardiovasc. Surg.,* 2011;141:361-7.

[69] Michaux I, Filipovic M, Skarvan K, et al. Effects of on-pump versus off-pump coronary artery bypass graft surgery on right ventricular function. *J. Thorac. Cardiovasc. Surg.,* 2006;131:1281-8.

[70] Joshi SB, Roswell RO, Salah AK, et al. Right ventricular function after coronary artery bypass graft surgery--a magnetic resonance imaging study. *Cardiovasc. Revasc. Med.,* 2010;11:98-100.

[71] Caputo M, Reeves BC, Rogers CA, Ascione R, Angelini GD. Monitoring the performance of residents during training in off-pump coronary surgery. *J. Thorac. Cardiovasc. Surg.,* 2004;128:907-15.

[72] Ascione R, Reeves BC, Pano M, Angelini GD. Trainees operating on high-risk patients without cardiopulmonary bypass: a high-risk strategy? *Ann. Thorac. Surg.,* 2004;78: 26-33.

[73] Watters MP, Ascione R, Ryder IG, et al. Haemodynamic changes during beating heart coronary surgery with the 'Bristol Technique'. *Eur. J. Cardiothorac. Surg.,* 2001;19: 34-40.

[74] Mueller XM, Chassot PG, Zhou J, et al. Hemodynamics optimization during off-pump coronary artery bypass: the 'no compression' technique. *Eur. J. Cardiothorac. Surg.,* 2002;22:249-54.

[75] Thielmann M, Massoudy P, Marggraf G, et al. Impact of intraoperative myocardial cellular damage on early hemodynamics after off-pump versus on-pump coronary artery bypass surgery. *Eur. J. Med. Res.,* 2005;10:218-26.

[76] Mishra M, Shrivastava S, Dhar A, et al. A prospective evaluation of hemodynamic instability during off-pump coronary artery bypass surgery. J. *Cardiothorac. Vasc. Anesth.,* 2003;17:452-8.

[77] Reeves BC, Ascione R, Caputo M, Angelini GD. Morbidity and mortality following acute conversion from off-pump to on-pump coronary surgery. *Eur. J. Cardiothorac. Surg.,* 2006;29:941-7.

[78] Vassiliades TA Jr, Nielsen JL, Lonquist JL. Hemodynamic collapse during off-pump coronary artery bypass grafting. *Ann. Thorac. Surg.*, 2002;73:1874-9.

[79] Shroyer AL, Grover FL, Hattler B, et al for the Veterans Affairs Randomized On/Off Bypass (ROOBY) Study Group. On-Pump versus Off-Pump Coronary-Artery Bypass Surgery. *N. Engl. J. Med.*, 2009; 361:1827-1837.

[80] Puskas JD, Mack MJ, Smith CR. On-pump versus off-pump CABG. *N. Engl. J. Med.*, 2010;362:851.

[81] Cleveland JC Jr, Shroyer AL, Chen AY, Peterson E, Grover FL. Off-pump coronary artery bypass grafting decreases risk-adjusted mortality and morbidity. *Ann. Thorac. Surg.*, 2001;72:1282-8.

[82] Puskas JD, Kilgo PD, Lattouf OM, et al. Off-pump coronary bypass provides reduced mortality and morbidity and equivalent 10-year survival. *Ann. Thorac. Surg.*, 2008;86:1139-46.

[83] Feng ZZ, Shi J, Zhao XW, Xu ZF. Meta-analysis of on-pump and off-pump coronary arterial revascularization. *Ann. Thorac. Surg.*, 2009;87:757-65.

[84] Singhal P, Mahon B, Riordan J. A prospective observational study to compare conventional coronary artery bypass grafting surgery with off-pump coronary artery bypass grafting on basis of EuroSCORE. *J. Card. Surg.*, 2010;25:495-500.

[85] Møller CH, Perko MJ, Lund JT, et al. Three-year follow-up in a subset of high-risk patients randomly assigned to off-pump versus on-pump coronary artery bypass surgery: the Best Bypass Surgery trial. *Heart,* 2011;97:907-13.

[86] Takagi H, Matsui M, Umemoto T. Off-pump coronary artery bypass may increase late mortality: a meta-analysis of randomized trials. *Ann. Thorac. Surg.*, 2010;89:1881-8.

[87] Puskas JD, Williams WH, O'Donnell R, Patterson RE, Sigman SR, Smith AS, Baio KT, Kilgo PD, Guyton RA. Off-pump and on-pump coronary artery bypass grafting are associated with similar graft patency, myocardial ischemia, and freedom from reintervention: long-term follow-up of a randomized trial. *Ann. Thorac. Surg.*, 2011;91:1836-42.

[88] Angelini GD, Culliford L, Smith DK, et al. Effects of on- and off-pump coronary artery surgery on graft patency, survival, and health-related quality of life: Long-term follow-up of 2 randomized controlled trials. *J. Thorac. Cardiovasc. Surg.*, 2009;137:295-303.

[89] Hannan EL, Wu C, Smith CR, et al. Off-pump versus on-pump coronary artery bypass graft surgery: differences in short-term outcomes and in long-term mortality and need for subsequent revascularization. *Circulation*, 2007;116:1145-52.

[90] Ivanov J, Borger MA, Tu JV, Rao V, David TE. Mid-term outcomes of off-pump versus on-pump coronary artery bypass graft surgery. *Can. J. Cardiol.,* 2008;24:279-84.

[91] Chamberlain MH, Ascione R, Reeves BC, Angelini GD. Evaluation of the effectiveness of off-pump coronary artery bypass grafting in high-risk patients: an observational study. *Ann. Thorac. Surg.*, 2002;73:1866-73.

[92] Ascione R, Reeves BC, Rees K, Angelini GD. Effectiveness of coronary artery bypass grafting with or without cardiopulmonary bypass in overweight patients. *Circulation,* 2002;106:1764-70.

[93] Mishra YK, Collison SP, Malhotra R, Kohli V, Mehta Y, Trehan N. Ten-year experience with single-vessel and multivessel reoperative off-pump coronary artery bypass grafting. *J. Thorac. Cardiovasc. Surg.*, 2008;135:527-32.

[94] LaPar DJ, Bhamidipati CM, Reece TB, Cleveland JC, Kron IL, Ailawadi G. Is off-pump coronary artery bypass grafting superior to conventional bypass in octogenarians? *J. Thorac. Cardiovasc. Surg.*, 2011;141:81-90.
[95] Takase S, Yokoyama H, Satokawa H, et al. Short-term and long-term outcomes of octogenarians after off-pump coronary artery bypass surgery. *Gen. Thorac. Cardiovasc. Surg.*, 2010;58:561-7.
[96] Puskas JD, Thourani VH, Kilgo P, et al. Off-pump coronary artery bypass disproportionately benefits high-risk patients. *Ann. Thorac. Surg.*, 2009;88:1142-7.

In: Off-Pump Coronary Artery Bypass Grafting
Editors: S.G. Raja and M. Amrani
ISBN 978-1-62081-575-5

Chapter 5

PULMONARY OUTCOMES AFTER OFF-PUMP CORONARY ARTERY BYPASS GRAFTING

Ana Maria Rocha Pinto e Silva and Luíz Antônio Rivetti
Faculty of Medical Sciences of Santa Casa de São Paulo,
Hospital Samaritano, São Paulo, Brazil

ABSTRACT

Pulmonary function following surgery for myocardial revascularization with cardiopulmonary bypass (CPB) has been extensively studied by several authors. Disturbance of pulmonary function after cardiac surgery remains an important issue because it increases postoperative morbidity and mortality. The disturbance may range from subclinical functional changes that occur in most patients, to full-blown adult respiratory distress syndrome in < 2% after CPB.

With growing interest in minimally invasive techniques, there has been an upsurge in off-pump coronary artery bypass (OPCAB) grafting. Resurgence of interest in OPCAB is associated with the expectation that avoiding deleterious effects of the CPB pump leads to better outcomes and possibly decreased costs and resource utilization.

Recently several researchers have compared impact of off-pump and on-pump coronary artery bypass surgery on pulmonary function and the results are controversial. This chapter discusses in detail the impact of on-pump and off-pump coronary artery bypass grafting on pulmonary function.

INTRODUCTION

The concern about pulmonary function after heart surgery started in the 1950s and1960s [1, 2] with the advent of cardiopulmonary bypass (CPB). Schramel et al.[1] studying diffusion of carbon monoxide in patients operated on CPB, suggested that there were alterations of alveolar-capillary membrane. Osborn and associates [2] discussed the effect of CPB in the formation of microatelectasis, secondary to the collapse of the lungs during the procedure.

Surgery for myocardial revascularization with CPB through sternotomy was standardized by Favaloro [3] and since that time pulmonary function has been extensively studied by several researchers who found it to be quite compromised [4-8] Many factors have been analyzed as the causes of pulmonary changes after heart surgery including sternotomy, anesthesia, pleurotomy, hypothermia, transfusion, fluid balance, cardiopulmonary bypass and systemic inflammatory response.

Surgery without CPB reported by Ankeney [9], Benetti [10], Buffolo [11] and Rivetti [12, 13] are currently being performed in large series. With the growing interest in minimally invasive techniques, there has been an increase in myocardial revascularization without CPB.

In 1984 Rivetti [12] started to perform revascularization without CPB with the aid of a temporary intraluminal coronary device (shunt). The behavior of patients submitted to this technique was found to involve better postoperative clinical recovery, and their pulmonary function was also studied [14].

The initial results showed that all the pulmonary function tests were significantly decreased on the 4th postoperative day when compared with the preoperative value. An improvement of all tests was observed on the 10th postoperative day, despite persistent significant changes.

After this preliminary investigation another prospective study was carried out, comparing two groups of patients submitted to coronary artery revascularization with and without CPB[15] and it was concluded that measures of pulmonary function deteriorate significantly after coronary revascularization with and without CPB, but the deterioration was more pronounced after on-pump coronary artery bypass grafting (CABG). Furthermore, even though pulmonary function did not return to baseline after 10 days postoperatively for both the groups, the off-pump patients showed significant great improvement compared to those who had surgery on CPB.

Buffolo [16] reported pulmonary complications in 3.2% of patients without CPB and in 9.7% of patients with CPB, but no pulmonary function tests were applied to these patients. Later at the same institution Guizilini [17, 18] evaluated and compared the pulmonary function in patients undergoing on- and off-pump surgeries and the influence of pleurotomy on pulmonary function after off-pump CABG using the left internal thoracic artery.

This study demonstrated that an evident impairment of pulmonary function occurs in the early postoperative period after off-pump CABG, regardless of the pleurotomy, and the spirometry showed significant reduction of parameters until the 5th postoperative day.

Impact on Pulmonary Function Tests

Many studies have shown important changes in lung function tests after CABG. The beneficial impact of off-pump surgery on pulmonary function remains controversial. In order to analyze the effect of different surgical myocardial revascularization strategies on pulmonary function, authors have performed several studies. The tests consist of two parts: spirometry and arterial blood gas measurements [19].

Spirometry

We prospectively compared pulmonary function tests for two well-matched groups of patients undergoing off-pump (Group I) and on-pump CABG (Group II). All patients had normal pulmonary function preoperatively. Pulmonary function tests were repeated at the 4th (PO_4) and 10th (PO_{10}) day postoperative. On PO_4 all spirometry indices were reduced, although the percentages of alteration differed significantly between Group I and Group II. On PO_{10}, the parameters of spirometry improved in both groups but all indices remained below preoperative values, with significant differences between groups and better performance in the off-pump group [15].

Vital capapcity (VC) was reduced on average by 39.62% in Group I and by 51.08% in Group II (p = 0.018) on PO_4. It continued to be reduced on average by 24.46% in Group I and by 39.39% in Group II (p = 0.005) on PO_{10}. It is known that VC can be reduced by limitation of thoracic movements because of postoperative changes in the chest, impaired diaphragm excursion due to changes in the phrenic nerve, and limitations of lung expansibility owing to the presence of pleural effusion or parenchymatous changes. VC has been studied by several authors after the use of CPB.

Shapira et al.[6] have reported an average 46.42% rate of VC alteration on PO_{10}. Cimen and associates[20] referred that VC dropped from 3.25 ± 0.78 to 1.01 ± 0.45L (31% of preoperative value) in on-pump and dropped from 2.8 ± 0.77 to 1.11 ± 0.23L (39% of preoperative value) in off-pump patients on the first postoperative day. Thereafter, although the values of VC improved in both groups until the day of discharge, they did not differ from each other significantly.

In our study [15], forced vital capacity (FVC) was reduced in all patients of Groups I and II in a similar fashion as described above for VC. FVC requires a greater effort on the part of the patient, who must execute maximum inspiration followed by maximum expiration. On PO_4, FVC was reduced on average by 38.85% in Group I and by 46.94% in Group II (p = 0.012). On PO_{10}, FVC continued to be reduced, on average, by 24.23% in Group I and by 39.22% in Group II (p = 0.005). Several investigators have reported changes in FVC after surgery with the use of CPB [8, 21-24]. Vargas and colleagues [8] performed daily FVC measurements after CABG on CPB and observed a persistent mean decrease of 30% on PO_{10}. Montes et al.[25] found that during the postoperative period FVC dropped from 92% of predicted value to 50% and from 94% to 52% in the on-pump and off-pump groups, respectively.

Tests showed a significant reduction in both groups, but with no statistical differences between the 2 groups. They reported that off-pump does not confer major protection from postoperative pulmonary dysfunction compared with on-pump, but the authors observed the patients for only 72 hours postoperatively. They suggested that the general strategies used to decrease postoperative pulmonary dysfunction in on-pump CABG patients should also be used in OPCAB patients.

We found that forced expiratory volume in the first second (FEV_1) was reduced in both groups[15]. By representing the initial part of the FVC curve, this index reflects the same behavior and suffers the same postoperative influences as described for FVC and is considered to be a parameter of high specificity. The changes in FEV_1 reported in the literature for cardiac surgeries with CPB are similar to those of our Group II, while the values obtained for our Group I are significantly lower. Some investigators have reported similar changes in FEV_1 in patients operated with the aid of extracorporeal circulation [7, 21, 23]. Guizilini [17] reported significant falls in the FVC and FEV_1 up to the fifth postoperative day, comparing 2 groups of patients operated on- or off-pump. The decreases of FVC and FEV_1 were higher in the on-pump group ($p < 0.050$). Staton and associates [26] in a prospective randomized trial found that the FVC and FEV_1 were significantly reduced at 4 to 6 weeks postoperatively in the off-pump and on-pump groups.

Forced expiratory flow between 25%-75% of FVC (FEF_{25-75}) showed a mean decrease of 30.01% in Group I, and of 44.46% in Group II, on PO_4. Group I patients already presented a lower mean FEF_{25-75} value than group II during the preoperative period ($p = 0.043$). However, on PO_4 the reduction of FEF_{25-75}, despite the alterations already existing in Group I, was even greater in Group II ($p = 0.014$). On PO_{10} there was a mean 8.93% decrease in Group I, and a mean 37.84% decrease in Group II ($p < 0.001$). Analysis of the factors that alter FEF_{25-75} shows that this parameter indicates the earlier changes that occur in the airways, which are directly affected by pulmonary expansibility.

The decreases in FEF_{25-75} observed in our patients may be explained by the presence of atelectasis, interstitial edema and general anesthesia itself. There was a marked improvement on PO_{10} in Group I patients, indicating that the pulmonary changes were more noticeable in patients submitted to CPB, and that these patients, despite physiotherapy, continued to have more intense and longer lasting changes in FEF_{25-75}.

The decreases in FEF_{25-75} reported in the literature on revascularization surgeries with CPB are 40% and 51.3% [7, 22]. Cimen et al.[20] reported that FEF_{25-75} dropped on the first postoperative day in the off-pump and on-pump groups and increased thereafter steadily but no significant difference occurred between them, until the 6th day. They concluded that pulmonary function was not improved in off-pump patients when compared with on-pump patients. The extubation times were similar between groups. They commented that early discharge of patients with off-pump surgery cannot be related merely to better preservation of respiratory functions.

Maximum voluntary ventilation (MVV) was the last index evaluated by spirometry in our study [15]. MVV is the most difficult test to be performed by the patients during the postoperative period and this may be the reason why few reports are available in the literature about the execution of this test after surgery [23,24].

MVV depends on good patient orientation, on neuromuscular coordination and on the degree of fatigue, since it is under the influence of muscle strength, the expansibility of chest and lungs, the resistance of the airway and of the tissues, and on the presence or absence of pain. Analysis of our results showed that Group I patients presented lower percentages of alterations on PO_4 and PO_{10}, and their recovery on PO_{10} was better than that of Group II. Considering that both groups were submitted to sternotomy, the conditions concerning to the properties of the chest were identical for all patients [15]. Cimen et al.[20] found decrease of MVV on the first postoperative day with no statistically significant difference between groups. On the fifth day mean values of each group were approximately the same.

In our study, five patients in on-pump group were not in a stable enough condition for execution of the tests on the 4th postoperative day. Despite this occurrence, differences between groups were statistically significant.

Arterial Blood Gas Measurements

The arterial blood gases are measured from a blood sample obtained from the radial or brachial artery of the patient. The analysis consist of partial oxygen pressures (PaO_2), considering the normal range to be 80 to 90 mmHg, and of partial carbon dioxide pressures ($PaCO_2$), considering the normal range to be from 30 to 40 mmHg. The alveolar-arterial gradient ($A\text{-}aDO_2$) is used to diagnose the source of hypoxemia and it can be calculated at 21% or 100% of O_2. The patient is asked to breathe for 15 minutes in a closed circuit into a rubber balloon with 100% oxygen and with a valve at the end, so that expired air would exit into the environment. After wards, a new arterial blood sample is collected and blood gases are measured. $A\text{-}aDO_2$ at 100% is calculated by subtracting PaO_2 from alveolar oxygen pressure to determine if there are changes in pulmonary gas exchange. $A\text{-}aDO_2 = PAO_2 - PaO_2$, with PAO_2 being calculated by the following formula:

$$PAO_2 = (BP - PH_2O) \times FiO_2 - PACO_2/RQ$$

where: BP = barometric pressure, PH_2O = water vapor pressure, FiO_2 = inspired oxygen fraction, $PaCO_2$ = arterial carbonic gas pressure, and RQ = respiratory quotient (0.8 to 1.0)

Finally the clinical shunt measurement can be calculated whenever both systemic arterial and pulmonary arterial blood gas samples are available[19]. The end-pulmonary capillary oxygen content is calculated by assuming that the end-pulmonary capillary hemoglobin content is the same as arterial and by calculating the alveolar PO_2 by the alveolar gas equation. Determination of blood gases and calculation of $A\text{-}aDO_2$ were part of our study[15].

Partial Oxygen Pressure

Several authors have studied the decrease in PaO_2 during the postoperative period of surgeries in which CPB was used [4,24,27,28]. A drop of 15.17 ± 2.36% in off-pump group and 16.41 ± 2.35% in the on-pump group on the 4th postoperative day was found. The mean values of the changes observed in our study were slightly lower than those reported in the literature, and that both groups studied here had a decrease in PaO_2 up to the 10th postoperative day, although no significant difference was observed between groups[15].

Partial Carbon Dioxide Pressure

We observed that $PaCO_2$ had small changes, less significant than those observed for PaO_2. On the 4th day we had a decrease of 3.68 ± 2.10% in off-pump and 10.49 ± 2.40% in on-pump, which was not significant [15]. This reduction in $PaCO_2$ can be explained by the hyperventilation performed by the patient in an attempt to improve PaO_2, while struggling against the changes in the thorax caused by the surgical incision, such as tissue edema, restriction of expansion, and pain [28, 29].

Cimen and colleagues [20] referred in their experience that preoperative PaO_2 levels were 80.92 ± 10.13 mmHg in on-pump group and 89.44 ± 6.24 mmHg in off-pump group. Maximal drop was on the second postoperative day in both groups that was 17% less than preoperative value. Preoperative $PaCO_2$ levels of on-pump and off-pump groups were 38.1 ± 4.5 and 39.17 ± 3.1 mmHg respectively. No disparity occurred during postoperative course in both groups. It was concluded that elective off-pump surgery offers no major advantage compared to on-pump surgery with respect to postoperative pulmonary function tests and blood gases [15].

Kochamba et al. [30] in their study comparing early pulmonary function after on-pump and off-pump surgery have mentioned that there was no statistical difference in gas exchange. In this study pulmonary dysfunction in off-pump group was attributed to pulmonary congestion resulting from cardiac manipulation, cardiac immobilization, coronary vessel occlusion, drugs used during operation, and Trendelenburg position.

Alveolar-Arterial Gradient

The alveolar-arterial gradient ($A\text{-}aDO_2$), is a measure of the difference between the alveolar concentration and the arterial concentration of oxygen. $A\text{-}aDO_2$ has been studied by many authors [28, 29, 31]. The changes observed in our patients were similar to those reported in the literature. The gradient increased on the 4th day in both groups and a significant difference persisted on 10th day when the off-pump group showed greater recovery [15].

Factors Responsible for Alterations of Pulmonary Function

Pulmonary Factors

The complications we observe during the postoperative period, which might influence pulmonary function, are: atelectasis, pleural effusions, pneumothorax, paralysis of the phrenic nerve, pulmonary edema, bronchopneumonia, acute respiratory distress syndrome and pulmonary embolism, all of them detected by a thoracic X-ray, that is taken immediately after surgery in the intensive care unit and daily until the drains are removed and the patients are discharged from unit.

The high incidence of pulmonary complications is partly due to the alteration of normal ventilatory function, which is inherent to surgery carried out in the thoracic region, moreover, the development of minimally invasive surgery and no bypass techniques are further evidences of the attempts to reduce the homeostatic disruptions of cardiac surgery [32].

Off-pump CABG compared to on-pump CABG can reduces pulmonary complications in high-risk subgroups [33]. In a group of 87 elderly patients submitted to off-pump revascularization in our institution, we found a mean extubation time of 18.50 ± 19.09 hours, range from 2 to 120 hours. None was extubated in operating room. This prolonged time of intubation is reflective of less muscular mass and preexisting pulmonary comorbidities present in these patients. Related to this fact there was a significant postoperative incidence of pneumonia (10.3%) in this group [34].

Inflammatory Syndrome and Extracorporeal Circulation (CPB)

There is accumulation of interstitial fluid in the lungs after CPB [27]. This fluid accumulation is due to the fluid manipulation occurring in CPB itself and to the systemic inflammatory syndrome [35], caused by blood contact with the CPB circuit with the resultant reperfusion damage in the lungs.

Studies looking at impact of extracorporeal circulation on lungs have shown high circulating C3a and C5a complement levels in the lungs[36], migration and aggregation of polymorphonuclear leukocytes causing damage to endothelial cells [37], activation of the kallikrein cascade, presence of circulating endotoxins, synthesis of various oxytocins by activated leukocytes, and release of oxygen free radicals[38,39]. Despite the technological advances in the production of oxygenators [40], there still are histologically confirmed changes characterized by endothelial edema and leukocyte and platelet clusters in the pulmonary capillaries in patients submitted to CPB with membrane oxygenators [41]. These alterations in the pulmonary capillaries may to contribute to the increased alveolar-arterial difference in oxygen detected in the patients [42].

The impact of OPCAB technology on systemic inflammation has been studied in detail. Raja et al. in a review article analyzed 19 randomized clinical trials with low-risk patients [43]. Evidence was evaluated for impact of OPCAB on: neutrophils, endothelial cells, platelets, complement, cytokines, endotoxemia and oxidative stress and other mediators of inflammation.

They concluded that plenty of evidence from these studies is available to validate that the magnitude of inflammatory response is significantly less with OPCAB than CPB, yet very few trials have actually correlated the biochemical findings with the clinical outcomes.

Finally they remark that it would be incorrect to expect that OPCAB would abolish the systemic inflammatory response completely, taking into account the response to surgical trauma, manipulation of the heart, heparin and protamine use, other drugs and anesthesia, all of them producing an increase in the markers of acute inflammation. Analysis of current best available evidence from randomized controlled trials indicates that OPCAB reduces the systemic inflammatory response but does not prevent it. There is a limitation of these trials in not recruiting high-risk population with an adequate sample size correlating inflammatory response and clinical outcome.

Fluid Balance

Off-pump surgery usually requires increasing fluid volume in order to maintain hemodynamic stability particularly during grafting on the lateral and inferior aspects. According to Staton and associates [26] this creates a higher intraoperative fluid balance and reduces the postoperative pulmonary compliance. This is a very important point to be elucidated in future studies. Techniques to reduce the necessity of extra intravenous fluids during surgery should be examined as methods to reduce the compliance changes. We believe that the use of an intra-coronary shunt during off-pump surgery, which causes better hemodynamic stability by avoiding regional ischemia [44], allows us to use less fluid volume intraoperatively. There is need for a new study to measure the fluid volume given during off-pump revascularization and its impact on pulmonary compliance and function.

Anesthesia and Sternotomy

General anesthesia causes pulmonary changes itself [45-47] such as hypoxemia, formation of atelectasis, interstitial pulmonary edema, changes in compliance, effects of inhibitory drugs on the central nervous system and of muscle relaxants, changes in cardiac output, increased dead space, and changes in the hemoglobin dissociation curve. All of these factors should be taken into consideration for the patients undergoing on- and off-pump CABG, since all are submitted to the same anesthesia protocol.

Another factor to be analyzed is the access route used in CABG patients. Sternotomy causes changes in pulmonary function from the very first moment when the chest is opened. When the movement of the chest wall is measured after sternotomy, reduced and uncoordinated wall expansion is observed, contributing to the restrictive ventilatory alterations observed after heart surgeries performed through this access route [48]. In our study the two patient groups were submitted to median sternotomy and equally suffered, permitting us to state that the significant differences in pulmonary function between groups were not simply due to the sternotomy [15].

Pleurotomy

A great decrease in postoperative pulmonary function has been attributed to pleurotomy that often occurs during internal thoracic artery harvesting [6, 22]. The role of pleural opening has been debated by many authors.

Rolla and associates [49] demonstrated that on-pump revascularization using internal thoracic artery and maintaining pleural integrity has beneficial effects on pulmonary function, which could reduce respiratory morbidity. Guizilini et al. [22] studied the influence of pleurotomy on pulmonary function after OPCAB grafting using the left internal thoracic artery. They compared two groups: with an opened left pleural cavity and with an intact pleural cavity, performing pulmonary function tests and arterial blood gas analyses. Both groups had a significant reduction in early postoperative pulmonary function until the 5th day, and they concluded that the patients undergoing pleurotomy demonstrated more pronounced pulmonary dysfunction.

Role of Physiotherapy

All patients should be submitted to respiratory physiotherapy. Preoperative physiotherapy on the chest, including deep-breathing exercises, improves spirometry values, compared to a regime without breathing instructions, following CABG surgery [50]. It must be used during the postoperative period, after extubation. A CPAP mask placed for 20 minutes, with increased PEEP if necessary, according to O_2 saturation measured with a pulse-oximeter, repeated each 2 hours for 12 hours, is effective in avoiding atelectasis.

CONCLUSION

Recently several authors [15, 18, 20, 25, 26, 33] have studied pulmonary function, comparing off-pump versus on-pump coronary artery bypass surgery and the results are controversial.

In our experience at the Department of Surgery of Santa Casa São Paulo Medical School, we found that pulmonary function deteriorates significantly after coronary artery revascularization with or without CPB, but to a greater degree in patients undergoing on-pump CABG. Furthermore, off-pump patients showed significantly greater improvement at 10 days postoperatively despite pulmonary function failing to return to baseline in both groups.

REFERENCES

[1] Schramel RJ, Cameron R, Ziskind MM, Adam M, Creech O. Studies of pulmonary diffusion after open-heart surgery. *J. Thorac. Cardiovasc. Surg.*, 1959;38:281-91.

[2] Osborn JJ, Popper RW, Kerth WJ, Gerbode F. Respiratory insufficiency following open-heart surgery. *Ann. Surg.*, 1962;156:638-47.

[3] Favaloro RG. Saphenous vein graft in the surgical treatment of coronary artery disease. Operative technique. *J. Thorac. Cardiovasc. Surg.*, 1969;58:178-85.

[4] Braun SR, Birnbaum ML, Chopra PS. Pre and postoperative pulmonary function abnormalities in coronary artery revascularization surgery. *Chest*, 1978;73:316-20.

[5] Rea HH, Harris EA, Seelye ER, Whitlock RM, Withy SJ. The effects of cardiopulmonary bypass upon pulmonary gas exchange. *J. Thorac. Cardiovasc. Surg.*, 1978;75:104-20.

[6] Shapira N, Zabatino SM, Ahmed S, et al. Determinants of pulmonary function in patients undergoing coronary bypass operations. *Ann. Thorac. Surg.*, 1990;50:268-73.

[7] Vargas FS, Cukier A, Terra-Filho M, et al. Influence of atelectasis on pulmonary function after coronary artery bypass grafting. *Chest*, 1993;104:434-7.

[8] Vargas FS, Terra-Filho M, Hueb W, et al. Pulmonary function after coronary artery bypass surgery. *Respir. Med.*, 1997;91:629-33.

[9] Ankeney JL. To use or not use the pump oxygenator in coronary bypass operations. [Editorial] *Ann. Thorac. Surg.*, 1975;19:108-9.

[10] Benetti FJ. Cirurgia coronaria directa con bypass de vena safena sin circulatión extracorpórea o parada cardíaca. Comunicación previa. *Rev. Fed. Argent. Cardiol.*, 1980;8:3-5.

[11] Buffolo E, Andrade JC, Succi JE, et al. Revascularização direta do miocárdio sem circulação extracorpórea: descrição da técnica de resultados iniciais. *Arq. Bras. Cardiol.*, 1982;38:365-73.

[12] Rivetti LA, Gandra SMA. Initial experience using an intraluminal shunt during revascularization of the beating heart. *Ann. Thorac. Surg.*, 1997;63:1742-7.

[13] Rivetti LA, Gandra SMA. Intraluminal shunt for off-pump coronary artery by-pass grafting. Report of 501 consecutive cases and review of the technique. *Heart Surg. Forum*, 1998;1:30-6.

[14] Pinto AMR, Stirbulov R, Rivetti, LA, Saad Junior R. Estudo da função pulmonar em pacientes submetidos a revascularização do miocárdio sem circulação extracorpórea com derivação intraluminal. *Rev. Col. Bras. Cir.*, 1998;25:363-8.

[15] e Silva, AMRP, Saad Junior R, Stirbulov R, Rivetti LA. Off-pump versus on-pump coronary artery revascularization:effects on pulmonar function. *Interact. Cardiovasc. Thorac. Surg.*, 2010;11:42-45.

[16] Buffolo E, de Andrade CS, Branco JN, et al. Coronary artery bypass grafting without cardiopulmonary bypass. *Ann. Thorac. Surg.*, 1996;61:63-6.

[17] Guizilini S, Gomes WJ, Faresin SM, et al. Influence of pleurotomy on pulmonary function after off-pump coronary artery bypass grafting. *Ann. Thorac. Surg.*, 2007;84:817-22.

[18] Guizilini S, Gomes WJ, Faresin SM, et al. Evaluation of pulmonary function in patients following on- and off-pump coronary artery bypass grafting. *Rev. Bras. Cir. Cardiovasc.*, 2005;20:310-316.

[19] Shapiro BA, Harrison RA, Trout CA. Clinical assessment of intrapulmonary shunt, oxygenation, and cardiac output. In: Shapiro BA, Harrison RA, Trout CA. Clinical application of respiratory care. 2nd ed. Chicago: *Year Book Medical Publishers,* 1982:419-27.

[20] Cimen S, Ozkul V, Ketenci B, et al. Daily comparison of respiratory functions between on-pump and off-pump patients undergoing CABG. *Eur. J. Cardiothorac. Surg.*, 2003;23:589-594.

[21] Ferdinande P, Lauwers P, Van Buyten L, Van de Walle J. Pulmonary function tests before and after open heart surgery. *Acta. Anesthesiol. Belg.*, 1980;31(suppl.):127-36.

[22] Berrizbeitia LD, Tessler S, Jacobowitz IJ, et al. Effect of sternotomy and coronary bypass surgery on postoperative pulmonary mechanics. Comparison of internal mammary and saphenous vein bypass grafts. *Chest,* 1989;96:873-6.

[23] Petelenz T, Gaszewska I, Elertowicz M. Effect of long-term physical training on the parameters of pulmonary ventilation after cardiac operations. *Mater. Med. Pol.*, 1987;19:267-70.

[24] Turnbull KW, Miyagishima RT, Gerein AN. Pulmonary complications and cardiopulmonary bypass: a clinical study in adults. *Can. Anaesth. Soc. J.*, 1974;21: 181-94.

[25] Montes FR, Maldonado JD, Paez S, Ariza F. Off-pump versus on-pump coronary artery bypass surgery and postoperative pulmonary dysfunction. *J. Cardiothorac. Vasc. Anesth.*, 2004;18:698-703.

[26] Staton GW, Willians WH, Mahoney EM, Hu J, Chu H, Duke PG, Puskas JD. Pulmonary outcomes of off-pump versus on-pump coronary artery bypass surgery in a randomized trial. *Chest,* 2005;127:892-901.

[27] Korsten HH, Leusink JA, Spierdijk J, et al. Pulmonary shunting after cardiopulmonary bypass. *Eur. Heart J.*, 1989;10(suppl. H):17-21.

[28] Singh NP, Vargas FS, Cukier A, et al. Arterial blood gases after coronary artery bypass surgery. *Chest,* 1992;102:1337-41.

[29] Geha AS, Sessler AD, Kirklin JW. Alveolar-arterial oxygen gradients after open intracardiac surgery. *J. Thorac. Surg.*, 1966;51:609-15.

[30] Kochamba GS, Yun KL, Pfeffer TA, Sintek CF, Khonsari S. Pulmonary abnormalities after coronary arterial bypass grafting operation: cardiopulmonary bypass versus mechanical stabilization. *Ann. Thorac. Surg.*, 2000:69:1466-70.
[31] Kanber GJ, King FW, Eshchar YR, Sharp JT. The alveolar-arterial oxygen gradient in young and elderly men during air and oxygen breathing. *Am. Rev. Respir. Dis.*, 1968;97:376-81.
[32] Weissman C Pulmonary complications after cardiac surgery Semin Cardiothorac Vasc Anesth 2004,8:185-211.
[33] Yokoyama T, Baumgartner FJ, Gheissari A, et al. Off-pump versus on-pump coronary bypass in high-risk subgroups. *Ann. Thorac. Surg.*, 2000;70:1546-15.
[34] Silva AMRP, Campagnucci VP, Pereira WL, et al. Off-pump myocardial revascularization in the elderly: analysis of morbidity and mortality. *Rev. Bras. Cir. Cardiovasc.*, 2008;23:40-45.
[35] Kirklin JK, Westaby S, Blackstone EH, et al. Complement and the damaging effects of cardiopulmonary bypass. *J. Thorac. Cardiovasc. Surg.*, 1983;86:845-57.
[36] Chenoweth DE, Cooper SW, Hugli TE, et al. Complement activation during cardiopulmonary bypass: evidence for generation of C3a and C5a anaphylatoxins. *N. Engl. J. Med.*, 1981;304:497-503.
[37] Ratliff NB, Young WG Jr, Hackel DB, Mikat E, Wilson JW. Pulmonary injury secondary to extracorporeal circulation - an ultrastructural study. *J. Thorac. Cardiovasc. Surg.*, 1973;65:425-32.
[38] Cremer J, Martin M, Redl H, et al. Systemic inflammatory response syndrome after cardiac operations. *Ann. Thorac. Surg.*, 1996;61:1714-20.
[39] Brasil LA, Gomes WJ, Salomão R, Buffolo E. Inflammatory response after myocardial revascularization with or without cardiopulmonary bypass. *Ann. Thorac. Surg.*, 1998;66:56-9.
[40] Gaylor JD. Membrane oxygenators: current developments in design and application. *J. Biomed. Eng.*, 1988;10:541-7.
[41] Nilsson L, Tydén H, Johansson O, et al. Bubble and membrane oxygenators: comparison of postoperative organ dysfunction with special reference to inflammatory activity. *Scand. J. Thorac. Cardiovasc. Surg.*, 1990; 24:59-64.
[42] Tönz M, Mihaljevic T, von Segesser LK, et al. Acute lung injury during cardiopulmonary bypass. Are the neutrophils responsible? *Chest*, 1995; 108:1551-6.
[43] Raja SG, Berg GA. Impact of off-pump coronary artery bypass on systemic inflammation: current best available evidence. *J. Card. Surg.*, 2007;22:445-455.
[44] Gandra S, Rivetti LA. Experimental evidence of regional ischemia during beating heart bypass: Prevention with temporary intraluminal shunt, *Heart Surg. Forum.*, 2003;6: 10-17.
[45] Magnusson L, Zemgulis V, Wicky S, Tydén H, Thelin S, Hedenstierna G. Atelectasis is a major cause of hypoxemia and shunt after cardiopulmonary bypass: an experimental study. *Anesthesiology*, 1997;87:1153-63.
[46] Marshall BE, Wyche Junior MQ. Hypoxemia during and after anesthesia. *Anesthesiology*, 1972;37:178-209.
[47] Rehder K, Sessler AD, Marsh HM. General anesthesia and the lung. *Am. Rev. Respir. Dis.*, 1975;112:541-63.

[48] Locke TJ, Griffiths TL, Mould H, Gibson GJ. Rib cage mechanics after median sternotomy. *Thorax,* 1990;45:465-8.

[49] Rolla G, Fogliati P, Bucca C, et al. Effect of pleurotomyon pulmonary function after coronary artery bypass grafting with internal mammary artery. *Respir. Med.,* 1994;88:417-20.

[50] Westerdahl E, Lindmark B, Eriksson T, et al. Deep-breathing exercises reduce atelectasis and improve pulmonary function after coronary artery bypass surgery. *Chest,* 2005;128:3482-3488.

In: Off-Pump Coronary Artery Bypass Grafting
Editors: S.G. Raja and M. Amrani
ISBN 978-1-62081-575-5

Chapter 6

Renal Outcomes after Off-Pump Coronary Artery Bypass Grafting

Sagar U. Nigwekar, Praveen Kandula, Charuhas V. Thakar and John K. Hix
Clinical and Research Fellow, Division of Nephrology,
Massachusetts General Hospital, Scholars in Clinical Science Program,
Harvard Medical School, Boston, MA, US

Abstract

Acute kidney injury (AKI) is a serious post coronary artery bypass grafting complication associated with significant morbidity and mortality. The origin of this condition is multifactorial and includes factors relating to the conduct and management of cardiopulmonary bypass, such as the systemic inflammatory response, emboli, hypoperfusion, and loss of pulsatile perfusion. Furthermore, the use of aortic cross-clamping and cardioplegic arrest can result in myocardial dysfunction, which can lead to renal hypoperfusion and subsequent renal impairment. In an attempt to avoid these deleterious effects of cardiopulmonary bypass, off-pump coronary artery bypass surgery has been rediscovered. Resurgence of interest in off-pump coronary artery bypass surgery is associated with the expectation that avoiding deleterious effects of cardiopulmonary bypass leads to better outcomes including prevention of AKI. This chapter summarizes the existing literature on this approach to prevent AKI and provides expert guidelines for clinicians and for future research. Issues related to off pump coronary artery bypass surgery in end stage renal disease and renal transplant population are also discussed.

Introduction

Coronary artery disease remains responsible for over 1/3rd causes of death [1]. Options for treatment include medical management, percutaneous coronary intervention and coronary artery bypass grafting (CABG). Over the past several decades, the effectiveness of non-surgical interventions has been debated, and surgical revascularization continues to remain a cornerstone of treatment in symptomatic coronary artery disease. Over 400,000 CABG surgeries are performed annually in the United States [2].

Post-operative acute kidney injury (AKI) is one of the most serious complications after CABG and it has been reported in the setting of cardiac surgery for over five decades now [3]. Its reported incidence has varied in the literature from 0.3%-30% [4-8] and AKI severe enough to require renal replacement therapy is reported to occur in 1-3% of the patients[5, 9]. Thakar et al. in a recent database analysis of 33,217 patients identified an increase in AKI from 5.1 to 6.6% and an increase in AKI requiring dialysis from 1.5% to 2% over a 10 year period. The changing definitions and increased awareness of AKI have been reported as possible reasons for increasing trend for acute kidney injury. To tackle the problem of inconsistent definitions, Acute Kidney Injury Network (AKIN) has recently proposed a 3 stage classification of AKI (Table 1) [10]. This classification has been validated in multiple studies [11-13].

It is also possible that the rise in AKI is a true phenomenon given that older and sicker patients are being operated on as well as introduction of potentially nephrotoxic agents like aprotinin. There is unequivocal evidence that AKI in this post-surgery setting is associated with significant increase in length of hospital stay, healthcare resource utilization, morbidity, and mortality [14-18]. Patients who develop moderate-to-severe AKI after CABG surgery have mortality rates of 19% during hospitalization [17], and may rise to almost 80% within 30 days of surgery [19]; this reflects more than 5–10 fold increase in mortality as compared to those without AKI, who experience a mortality rate of 0.9% -6.4%[9,] [17]. Even small increments of creatinine post CABG surgery adversely impact survival [15]. AKI has been reported to be associated with 1.6 fold increase in the intensive care unit length of stay as well as 1.6 fold increase in post-operative costs [18].

Table 1. Acute Kidney Injury Network (AKIN) criteria

Stage*	Serum creatinine criteria±	Urine output criteria
1	Increase in serum creatinine of more than or equal to 0.3 mg/dl or increase to more than or equal to 150% to 200% from baseline	Less than 0.5 ml/kg per hour for more than 6 hours
2	Increase in serum creatinine to more than 200% to 300% from baseline	Less than 0.5 ml/kg per hour for more than 12 hours
3	Increase in serum creatinine to more than 300% from baseline or serum creatinine of more than or equal to 4.0 mg/dl with an acute increase of at least 0.5 mg/dl	Less than 0.3 ml/kg per hour for 24 hours or anuria for 12 hours

*Only one of the criteria (either creatinine based or urine output based) is needed to assign stage.
± Change in serum creatinine is calculated over 48 hour period.
Patients who develop acute kidney injury requiring renal replacement therapy are assigned to stage 3.

Clearly, given the magnitude of the problem that we face, prevention of AKI, amelioration of ongoing injury, and treatment of established injury are all necessary targets of intervention to improve the outcomes. Several therapeutic agents have been tested in the setting of post-operative AKI, without promising results [20-21]. Use of vasodilators like dopamine [22-23], ionoptropic agents like dobutamine [24], diuretics like, mannitol, furosemide [23, 25-26], anti -inflammatory agents like N-acetylcysteine [27-29], and steroids [30] have not been effective in improving the outcomes. A small study evaluating prophylactic dialysis found reduction in operative morbidity and mortality but it may not be practical to subject all patients undergoing CABG to dialysis [31]. Other therapies like fenoldopam [32-33] and natriuretic peptides [21, 34-36] were found to be variably effective. Suboptimal timing of application of therapy, inappropriate risk stratification, small sample sizes, and difficulties in translating a therapy that targets single-hit paradigm to a multi-factorial injury in clinical settings are all likely contributors to the lack of success in treatment of AKI.

Although not insurmountable, planning new clinical trials with the advent of early biomarkers will be costly, and remains a challenging frontier [37]. Thus, prevention of AKI remains one of the key cornerstones in improving patient outcomes.

Operative techniques have also been reported to alter the development of AKI. Several studies have been conducted to evaluate renal outcomes following off-pump technique compared to on-pump technique [38]. This chapter summarizes rationale for this approach, critically appraises the current available evidence and provides guidelines for clinicians and for future research. We also address issues related to off- pump bypass surgery in end stage renal disease (ESRD) and renal transplant population.

Mechanisms of Renal Injury from Cardiopulmonary Bypass

Patients undergoing CABG have several risk factors that predispose them to develop AKI. These include but are not limited to advanced age, presence of multiple co-morbid illnesses like diabetes, hypertension, congestive heart failure, peripheral vascular disease and most importantly preexisting renal insufficiency [8, 39-41].

However, the risk of developing AKI is related to the surgical procedure itself. One of the major causes is the application of cardio pulmonary bypass circuit that requires placement of aortic cross clamp and the inevitable reduction in blood supply, albeit for a short time, and loss of pulsatile blood flow to the kidney [42].

In addition, exposure of blood to circuit membranes stimulates release of inflammatory mediators like catecholamines and free hemoglobin that may be involved in the development of AKI [43-47]. The length of the use of the bypass circuit further dictates likelihood of development of AKI. At a pathological level, although no biopsy based studies have been done, based on the pathophysiology of developing AKI, acute tubular necrosis is suspected to be the most likely cause [8].

This constellation of changes described above provides a reasonable explanation for cardiopulmonary bypass associated AKI and it can be hypothesized that avoiding cardiopulmonary bypass may reduce the AKI risk. On the other hand, off-pump technique is technically difficult and can impair renal perfusion from low cardiac output caused by ventricular compression during manipulation of the heart [48-49]. In effect, both approaches entail AKI risk. Results from clinical studies evaluating these 2 approaches are outlined below.

Evidence for Renal Injury Prevention by Applying off-Pump Technique

Observational Studies

Despite potential pathophysiological mechanisms that link AKI and cardiopulmonary bypass, early clinical data were conflicting. Weinstein et al. conducted a study of 18 adult patients undergoing cardiopulmonary bypass for CABG or valve procedures [50]. They evaluated urine output and creatinine clearance in peri-operative period and reported improvements in urine output and creatinine clearance during the cardiopulmonary bypass. At the end of the bypass, urine output and creatinine clearance were at baseline at 8 hour follow up. They concluded that the modern bypass techniques are not nephrotoxic. On the other hand, Abel et al. reported that as the duration of cardiopulmonary bypass pump increased, the risk for AKI also increased [51]. Multiple observational studies since then have identified cardiopulmonary bypass time as an independent risk factor for the development of AKI after cardiac surgery [6, 39].

Early observational studies and randomized controlled clinical trials comparing off-pump bypass technique with on-pump bypass technique were focused primarily on evaluating its impact on mortality and stroke and did not adequately assess the renal outcomes [52-54]. Gamoso et al. reported one of the earliest observational studies comparing renal outcomes from off pump and on pump techniques [55]. They evaluated perioperative changes in creatinine clearance using the Cockroft-Gault equation. In this retrospective study involving 690 primary coronary artery bypass graft surgeries (55 off-pump, 635 on-pump), pre-surgery creatinine level was defined as the level closest to cardiac surgery and post-surgery creatinine was defined as the highest of the daily in-hospital post-surgery levels. In multivariate analysis, authors did not identify off- pump CABG as an independent predictor of changes in creatinine clearance. In addition to the methodological limitations inherent to any observational study, this study was also limited by the fact that the off-pump surgeries included in these analyses were the first 55 off-pump surgeries performed at the participating institution. Relative inexperience of surgeons performing off-pump surgeries in this study may have contributed to the lack of renal benefits.

Hix et al. reported one of the largest observational studies on this topic [56]. Their single center observational cohort study involved 10,061 patients (8,696 patients in on-pump group and 1,365 were in off-pump group) who underwent isolated first time CABG between 1998 and 2002 at the Cleveland Clinic, Cleveland, OH. Patients who were on dialysis therapy prior to surgery were excluded from the analysis. Based on propensity score matching, authors selected a subgroup of 1,365 patients from 8,696 patients who underwent coronary artery bypass surgery using a bypass pump and analyses regarding the outcomes were conducted using this propensity score matched cohort (1,365 patients in on pump group and 1,365 patients in off pump group). Patients included in this study had relatively preserved pre-operative renal function with mean estimated glomerular filtration rate of 76.6 mL/min/1.73 m^2 in the off pump cohort and 76.8 mL/min/1.73 m^2 in the on pump cohort.

Table 2. Summary of observational studies addressing renal outcomes comparing off-pump to on-pump coronary artery bypass grafting. (Reproduced with permission[38])

Study, year [Reference]	Country	Population	Patients included (N per group)		Baseline renal function∞		Study definition of AKI	Propensity Score Matching
			OPCAB	CABP	OPCAB	CABP		
Ascione, 2001[57]	UK	Elective primary CABG patients with creatinine >1.7 mg/dl	51	202	2.1 ±0.6	2.0 ±0.4	*Renal replacement therapy requirement*	Yes
Beauford, 2004[58]	USA	Isolated CABG patients with creatinine >1.5 mg/dl	188	103	45 ±16*	47 ±17*	*Doubling of the preoperative creatinine level or renal replacement therapy requirement*	No
Bucerius, 2004[59]	Germany	Isolated CABG patients	761	8870	Not available		*Renal replacement therapy requirement*	No
Chukwuemeka, 2005[60]	Canada	Isolated CABG patients with creatinine clearance <60 mL/min	146	438	1.6 ± 1.3	1.5 ±1.3	Decrease in post-operative creatinine clearance ≥ 25% or renal replacement therapy requirement	Yes
Di Mauro, 2007[44] Analysis A	Italy	Isolated CABG patients with multivessel coronary disease with normal pre-operative renal function	862	862	1.0 ±0.2	1.0 ±0.2	Postoperative creatinine ≥2.0 mg/dl	Yes
Di Mauro, 2007[44] Analysis B	Italy	Isolated CABG patients with multivessel coronary disease with creatinine ≥1.5 mg/dl	80	80	2.4 ±1.6	2.4 ±1.9	Increase of ≥1 mg/dl in postoperative creatinine	Yes
Fischer, 2006[61]	USA	Elective aortocoronary operative patients with multivessel disease	313	2863	83 ±36*	86 ±36*	Not available	No
Gamoso, 2000[55]	USA	Primary elective CABG operative patients	55	635	1.1 ±0.4	1.1 ±0.7	Postoperative creatinine increase ≥ 0.7 mg/dl	No
Hayashida, 2002[62]	Japan	CABG patients	52	53	1.3 ± 0.2	1.4 ± 0.1	Postoperative creatinine increase >1.5 mg/dl or oliguria (<0.5ml/kg/min) or RRT requirement	No

Table 2. (Continued)

Study, year [Reference]	Country	Population	Patients included (N per group)		Baseline renal function∞		Study definition of AKI	Propensity Score Matching
			OPCAB	CABP	OPCAB	CABP		
Hirose, 2001[63]	Japan	Isolated CABG patients with creatinine >2.0 mg/dl	16	43	2.6 ±0.6	2.7 ±0.9	Postoperative creatinine increase > 2.0 mg/dl or ≥ 50% increase in creatinine or renal replacement therapy requirement	No
Hix, 2006[56]	USA	Low risk isolated first CABG	1365	1365	1.0	1.0	≥50% decline in glomerular filtration rate or renal replacement therapy requirement	Yes
Landoni, 2007[64]	Italy	First CABG patients	848	2255	Not available		Doubling of the pre-operative creatinine level	No
Loef, 2002[65]	Netherlands	Elective CABG patients with a normal pre-operative renal function	10	12	0.9 ± 0.1	1.0 ± 0.1	Not available	No
Massoudy, 2008[66]	Germany	Isolated CABG patients	100	101	1.16 ± 0.3	1.2 ±0.2	Post-operative creatinine increase ≥50% or ≥0.3 mg/dl	No
Schwann, 2004[49]	USA	Primary, isolated, elective CABG patients	220	119	1.4 ±0.4	1.2 ± 0.3	Post-operative creatinine increase ≥ 50% or postoperative creatinine increase ≥2 mg/dl	No
Stallwood, 2004[67]	UK	Isolated CABG patients with normal pre-operative renal function	716	1483	1.1 ± not available	1.1± not available	Postoperative creatinine > 2.25 mg/dl or RRT requirement	No
Weerasinghe, 2005[68]	UK	First CABG patients with multivessel disease and normal pre-operative renal function	817	1224	Not available		Post-operative creatinine increase >20% or composite end point of postoperative creatinine > 2.25 mg/dl and RRT requirement	Yes

∞ Renal function reported as mean serum creatinine ± standard deviation (mg/dl) except in studies with * where mean creatinine clearance± standard deviation (ml/minute) is reported.

Abbreviations: CABG = coronary artery bypass graft; CABP = coronary artery bypass pump; OPCAB = off pump coronary artery bypass; RRT = renal replacement therapy.

Incidence of dialysis requiring acute kidney injury was significantly lower in the off-pump group (1.2% vs. 2.6%). There was also significant reduction in the incidence of non-dialysis requiring AKI defined as >50% decline in postoperative glomerular filtration rate (2.5% vs. 5.0%). AKI among matched patients was associated with significantly increased risk of mortality when compared to patients who did not develop AKI; relative risk for mortality of 13.14 (95% CI, 8.43–30.50) in patients with AKI requiring dialysis and 9.33 (95% CI, 4.83–19.00) in those with >50% decline in glomerular filtration rate but not requiring dialysis.

Characteristics of the observational studies performed to date comparing off-pump to on-pump CABG for renal outcomes are summarized in Table 2 [44' 55-68]. Nigwekar et al. previously conducted a systematic review and meta-analysis of these studies [38]. In this analysis, in the observational cohort, both overall AKI (OR, 0.61; 95% CI, 0.45 to 0.81) and requirement of renal replacement therapy (OR, 0.54; 95% CI, 0.40 to 0.73) were significantly less in the off-pump surgery group. As is common in medical literature, AKI definition varied widely in these observational studies. Adequate information regarding serum creatinine, creatinine clearance, estimated glomerular filtration rate and urine output were not available in most studies. Nigwekar et al. observed a significant statistical heterogeneity in the analysis of outcome of overall AKI which was eliminated in the sensitivity analysis restricted to studies involving patients with pre-existing kidney disease, a major risk factor for development of post cardiac surgery AKI. Inability to control for known and unknown covariates limits the internal validity of observational studies when compared to the randomized controlled trials. Statistical method of propensity score matching may be able to control for known covariates [69].

A recent review summarizing propensity score analyses comparing off pump to on pump surgeries reported reduction in AKI (17 studies, 38, 866 patients, OR 0.60 [0.51–0.70]) [70]. However, definition of AKI was not provided in this review. Five of 16 observational studies included in the analysis by Nigwekar et al. had applied propensity score matching [38]. When analyses were restricted to studies that applied propensity score matching, similar reductions in overall AKI and requirement of renal replacement therapy were observed. Well conducted observational studies, despite their inherent limitations of inability to adequately address confounders, have advantages over the randomized controlled trials. First of all, findings from observational studies are more generalizable since unlike randomized controlled trials the enrollment is frequently not restricted to relatively "healthier" patients. Secondly, for studying outcomes such as requirement of renal replacement therapy which is relatively rare in cardiac surgery setting, sample size requirement for a well powered randomized controlled trial is large and often not feasible.

Randomized Controlled Trials

Compared to the number of observational studies, limited numbers of randomized controlled trials have evaluated the outcome of AKI in the setting of off-pump CABG. One of the earliest randomized trials that reported renal outcomes on this topic was conducted by Ascione et al in 1999 [71]. This trial enrolled 50 patients with normal pre-surgery renal function and assessed glomerular and tubular function at 48 hours post-surgery.

Table 3. Summary of randomized controlled trials addressing renal outcomes comparing off-pump to on-pump coronary artery bypass grafting. (Reproduced and modified with permission[38])

Study, year [Reference]	Country	Population	Patients randomized (N per group)		Baseline renal function∞		Assessment of renal function	Study definition of AKI
			OPCAB	CABP	OPCAB	CABP		
Ascione, 1999[71]	UK	Low risk first elective CABG patients with normal pre-operative renal function	25	25	93 ± 25*	88 ± 27*	Creatinine clearance, urine albumin to creatinine ratio, N-acetyl glucosaminidase	Not available
Carrier, 2003[113]	Canada	High risk CABG patients (creatinine > 1.5 mg/dl was one of the high risk defining criterion)	28	37	Not available		Serum creatinine	Increase of > 1.13 mg/dl of the postoperative creatinine value from baseline or renal replacement requirement
Celik, 2005[114]	Turkey	Low risk CABG patients with normal pre-operative renal function	30	30	1.4 ± 0.2	1.3 ± 0.4	Creatinine clearance, serum creatinine, free water clearance	Not available
Kobayashi, 2005[115]	Japan	Elective primary multiple arterial grafts CABG patients with	81	86	Not available		Not available	Renal replacement therapy requirement
		normal pre-operative renal function						
Sajja, 2007[116]	India	Non-dialysis dependent elective primary CABG patients with estimated glomerular filtration rate<60 ml/min/1.73m^2	59	60	1.4 ± 0.6	1.5 ± 0 .6	Serum creatinine, estimated glomerular filtration rate	Post-operative creatinine > 20% or post-operative estimated glomerular filtration rate by < 20 % with respect to baseline
Shroyer, 2009[72]	USA	Non-dialysis dependent elective and urgent CABG patients	1104	1099	Not available		Not available	Renal replacement therapy requirement
Tang, 2002[117]	UK	Elective CABG patients with normal pre-operative renal function	20	20	1.6 ± 0.2	1.2 ± 0.2	Serum creatinine, urine microalbumin:creatinine ratio, urine retinol binding protein:creatinine ratio	Not available

∞ Renal function reported as mean serum creatinine ± standard deviation (mg/dl) except in studies with * where mean creatinine clearance± standard deviation (ml/minute) is reported.

Abbreviations: CABG = coronary artery bypass graft; CABP = coronary artery bypass pump; OPCAB = off pump coronary artery bypass

The authors reported that the glomerular filtration rate, urinary micro albumin-creatinine ratio as well as N-acetylglucosaminidase activity (marker of renal tubular function) were much better in the off-pump group. None of the study patients developed hard end points such as AKI requiring renal replacement therapy or death during the study period. Subsequent randomized trials over the last two decades have continued to demonstrate a general bias towards enrolling low risk patients and have also been largely underpowered to definitively address the renal outcomes. These trials are summarized in Table 3. Recently published Randomized Off/On Bypass (ROOBY) study (N=2,203) analyzed AKI requiring dialysis as a component of composite end point and did not demonstrate any difference in the incidence of AKI requiring dialysis between the off pump and on pump groups [72].

This study despite its large sample size was not powered to detect difference in AKI requiring dialysis and authors did not report the incidence of AKI or any other measures of renal function which is not an uncommon problem amongst the studies on this topic. Studies continue to either not report renal outcomes or they may not be reported in a consistent manner making any conclusions difficult. The AKIN criteria as mentioned earlier in this chapter will hopefully make this issue less common. In the absence of conclusive data from randomized studies, we are left with the data from observational studies, especially those with propensity score matching, to make clinical decisions regarding which approach to use for patients at risk for AKI post-surgery.

Evidence for off Pump Surgery in ESRD and Renal Transplant Population

It is well known that patients suffering from chronic kidney disease are more likely to die from cardiac disease than to reach ESRD, and that among dialysis patients who suffer an acute myocardial infarction, the majority die within 2 years of the event [73]. Cardiovascular disease is the most common cause of death in the dialysis population, and survival is demonstrably better with intervention compared to medical therapy [74-75]. Despite improvements in availability and techniques of angioplasty, surgical coronary revascularization remains the gold standard for treatment of advanced coronary artery disease in patients on dialysis [76-85]. A large retrospective review found that the proportion of patients with ESRD undergoing CABG has increased significantly from 1988 to 2003 with simultaneous decline in the annual in-hospital mortality rate despite increasing co-morbidities in this population [84, 86]. It is worth noting however that some studies have shown comparable mortality between angioplasty and CABG in patients with ESRD although a trend towards better outcomes in non-hemodialysis chronic kidney disease was noted [86]. A recent systematic review of studies comparing angioplasty and CABG noted little definitive difference in mortality although existing data properly comparing the two approaches was sparse and lacking in completeness [87].

Patients with advanced renal disease including those on dialysis who undergo CABG have higher mortality rates than comparable cohorts [79, 88-93]. Attempts to compare CABG outcomes in dialysis dependent patients versus those with chronic kidney disease not requiring dialysis are limited and retrospective in nature and it is difficult to draw conclusions beyond the fact that both groups are high risk surgical patients. Complication rates are high in dialysis patients and this finding is pronounced in centers with relatively less experience with surgical revascularization of ESRD patients [94-98]. After undergoing CABG, patients with chronic kidney disease tend to experience less improvement in physical function than other cohorts, impacting adversely upon quality of life [99]. Some researchers have theorized that higher complication rates in dialysis patients relate to the potential for atheroemboli, inflammation, and chemotaxis attributed to exposure to the cardiopulmonary bypass process, while others suggest that dialysis patients may fall victim to fluctuations in fluid volume and electrolytes that are difficult to control precisely with cardi [94, 100]. Another study suggested both 30 day and late (>48 month) mortality in ESRD patients undergoing CABG was significantly related to age, pulmonary complications and blood product transfusion, suggesting that measures to limit the latter two should be emphasized in this population [97]. Rehabilitation after CABG is delayed short term in the ESRD population, most likely because of the time burden imposed by dialysis, but is an important and modifiable factor in improving long term survival [101-102].

The high incidence of coronary artery disease in the ESRD population and the potential adverse effects of cardiopulmonary bypass have led to interest in the use of off-pump techniques in this high risk population. Whether avoiding bypass pump can improve these parameters is uncertain; it does appear that ESRD increases the likelihood of prolonged ventilation post-CABG and one small retrospective study of patients on dialysis did show off-pump technique was associated with improved pulmonary function and reduced right atrial volume compared to on pump technique, although no difference in short term mortality was noted [82, 103]. In patients suffering myocardial infarction prior to CABG there is increased risk for adverse outcomes particularly if ESRD is present. Enhanced vulnerability to fluctuations in volume is one likely reason and off-pump technique would be one mechanism to address this, however a large retrospective study in this population found no difference in hospital mortality between the two techniques [73]. One interesting area of research has linked long term memory deficits in ESRD patients to exposure to cardiopulmonary bypass, although that study was not designed to demonstrate whether the use of off-pump technique would reduce this morbidity [104].

Others have found higher operative mortality in patients with advanced chronic kidney disease not on dialysis compared to those on dialysis, suggesting off pump technique might have less benefit in the dialysis population compared to the pre-dialysis chronic kidney disease group [90]. Efforts to directly compare off-pump against on-pump in the dialysis patient population are hampered by differences in surgical approaches, technical competency, degree of revascularization, differences in dialysis prescription, difference in length of follow-up, and lack of powered direct randomized trials. Data is generally retrospective in nature and predominantly influenced by one large retrospective review of a national database [78, 100] (Table 4).

As a result it is difficult to draw definitive conclusions. It does seem that in centers with good experience with the technique, off-pump CABG has been shows to be safe in patients on dialysis without significant differences in hospital or short term mortality, adequacy or revascularization, or number of bypass grafts utilized [83, 105-107]. Direct mortality comparisons between on-pump and off-pump techniques in this population are difficult outside of short term or hospital mortality. In a large retrospective review, off-pump technique was associated with a significant 8% reduction in all cause mortality compared to on pump technique in dialysis patients, an effect most prominent in the first year after surgery [100].

Table 4. Comparison of off-pump versus on-pump technique in ESRD*

Study, year [Reference]	Country	Population	Number of patients		Study Outcomes
			OPCAB	CABP	
Ariyoshi, 2006[76]	Japan	ESRD patients on dialysis undergoing CABG	12	23	No difference in mortality Significantly lower atrial fibrillation, duration of mechanical ventilation, and heart failure in the OPCAB group
Beckerman n, 2006[78]	USA	Dialysis requiring patients undergoing CABG	21	16	*Lower incidence of atrial fibrillation in the off pump group* *No difference in other outcomes including mortality*
Beckerman n, 2006[78]	USA	ESRD patients on dialysis undergoing CABG	540	3382	*No difference in mortality*
Bruschi, 2010[94]	Italy	ESRD patients on dialysis undergoing isolated CABG	17	23	*No difference in mortality* Significantly lower requirement of blood transfusions, inotropic support, ventilation support, atrial fibrillation, and days of intensive care unit stay in the OPCAB group
Dewey 2006[75]	USA	Dialysis requiring patients undergoing CABG	59	99	Lower in-hospital and 1 year mortality in OPCAB group Significantly lower requirement of blood transfusions, ventilation support, and days of intensive care unit stay in the OPCAB group
Kan 2004[79]	Taiwan	ESRD patients undergoing isolated CABG	6	17	*No difference in mortality* Significantly lower requirement of ventilation support, intensive care unit stay, and length of hospital stay in the OPCAB group
Manabe 2006[81]	Japan	ESRD patients on dialysis undergoing CABG	15	10	*No difference in major post surgery complications*
Nishimura 2004[106]	Japan	ESRD patients on dialysis undergoing elective CABG	19	34	*No significant difference in mortality* OPCAB significantly decreased blood loss, blood transfusion, intensive care unit stay, and major perioperative morbidity
Shroff 2010[100]	USA	ESRD patients on dialysis undergoing CABG	2335	10750	Significant reduction in in-hospital and one-year mortality

* All studies listed in this table have observational design.

Abbreviations: CABG = coronary artery bypass graft; CABP = coronary artery bypass pump; ESRD = end stage renal disease; OPCAB = off-pump coronary artery bypass.

In one study, off-pump technique was associated with strikingly lower short term mortality in ESRD patients, yet subsequently was associated with significantly worse long term mortality rates compared with the on-pump technique survivors or even unselected ESRD patients with coronary artery disease and not undergoing any intervention, suggesting that comparisons between off-pump and on-pump in this patient population must be evaluated in the context of the duration of follow-up [75]. This discordant short versus long term survival in the ESRD population may relate to inadequate revascularization, which is more common in off pump compared with on pump and is a critical determinant of mortality [75, 80, 108]. Conversely, others have shown complete revascularization is attainable without short term mortality[83, 109]. In fact, one center's experience with off-pump technique demonstrated that completely revascularized ESRD patients enjoyed greater than 91% freedom from cardiac death at 3 years [83, 109]. These data indicate that off-pump technique may have a beneficial role in the ESRD population. This cohort should not only be denied this technique as there can be significant non-renal benefits but also should be the focus of future randomized controlled trials.Data regarding safety and efficacy of off-pump technique in renal transplant population have largely been limited to case reports [110-111]. To our knowledge, there is one retrospective study that compared off-pump vs. on-pump technique in 43 renal transplant patients [112]. This study did not find any difference between mortality and renal allograft function between the two groups. Although, there was no clinical benefit from off-pump technique in this study, off-pump surgery was performed safely in the included patients (n=22).

Clinical Practice and Future Research Implications

The pathophysiological aspects of cardiopulmonary bypass on renal function and abundant observational cohort literature support the efficacy of off-pump technique to improve renal outcomes. Especially the observational studies with better methodology such the ones with propensity score analysis are very useful in deciding whether the off-pump technique is the appropriate one for a patient scheduled to undergo CABG. Surgical team's experience must however be taken into account. Data from randomized trials have been inadequate and are likely to remain so since the sample size needed to adequately address outcomes such as AKI requiring renal replacement therapy is quite large and may not be achievable. Current observational data suggest that off-pump technique is a reasonable approach for patients at high risk for AKI provided the surgical team is experienced with this technique. Identification of high risk patients should be performed using validated scoring systems as the one proposed by Thakar et al. [39]. Renal biomarker literature suffers from imprecise diagnostic performance due to imperfect gold standard [37] and thus risk stratification with renal biomarkers is not clinically indicated at this time.

Conclusion

Off-pump bypass surgery is likely to be an effective approach to prevent AKI post-surgery. Based upon the high quality observational data, we recommend this approach in patients identified as high risk for post-CABG AKI. Risk stratification should be based upon the validated scoring systems (such as the one by Thakar et al. [39]). Surgical team's experience in performing off-pump CABG needs to be taken into account while offering this technique to the patients.

Future trials in this field need to be powered for specific renal outcomes and should define AKI as per the standard AKI criteria such as the AKIN criteria.

Further studies on renal biomarkers may help in effective risk stratification; however, the present biomarker literature has limitations. Off-pump CABG is safe in ESRD and renal transplant population and these populations should also be a focus of future studies.

REFERENCES

[1] Lloyd-Jones D, Adams RJ, Brown TM, et al. Executive summary: heart disease and stroke statistics--2010 update: a report from the American Heart Association. *Circulation*, 2010;121:948-54.

[2] Epstein AJ, Polsky D, Yang F, Yang L, Groeneveld PW. Coronary revascularization trends in the United States, 2001-2008. *JAMA*, 2011;305:1769-76.

[3] Doberneck RC, Reiser MP, Lillehei CW. Acute renal failure after open-heart surgery utilizing extracorporeal circulation and total body perfusion. Analysis of 1000 patients. *J. Thorac. Cardiovasc. Surg.*, 1962;43:441-52.

[4] Leacche M, Rawn JD, Mihaljevic T, et al. Outcomes in patients with normal serum creatinine and with artificial renal support for acute renal failure developing after coronary artery bypass grafting. *Am. J. Cardiol.*, 2004;93:353-6.

[5] Thakar CV, Worley S, Arrigain S, Yared JP, Paganini EP. Improved survival in acute kidney injury after cardiac surgery. *Am. J. Kidney. Dis.*, 2007;50:703-11.

[6] Conlon PJ, Stafford-Smith M, White WD, et al. Acute renal failure following cardiac surgery. *Nephrol. Dial.Transplant.*, 1999;14:1158-62.

[7] Chertow GM, Levy EM, Hammermeister KE, Grover F, Daley J. Independent association between acute renal failure and mortality following cardiac surgery. *Am. J. Med.*, 1998;104:343-8.

[8] Rosner MH, Okusa MD. Acute kidney injury associated with cardiac surgery. *CJASN*, 2006;1:19-32.

[9] Gaudino M, Luciani N, Giungi S, et al. Different profiles of patients who require dialysis after cardiac surgery. *Ann. Thorac.Surg.*, 2005;79:825-9.

[10] Mehta RL, Kellum JA, Shah SV, et al. Acute Kidney Injury Network: report of an initiative to improve outcomes in acute kidney injury. *Crit. Care*, 2007;11:R31.

[11] Haase M, Bellomo R, Matalanis G, Calzavacca P, Dragun D, Haase-Fielitz A. A comparison of the RIFLE and Acute Kidney Injury Network classifications for cardiac surgery-associated acute kidney injury: a prospective cohort study. *J.Thorac. Cardiovasc. Surg.*,2009;138:1370-6.

[12] Ricci Z, Cruz DN, Ronco C. Classification and staging of acute kidney injury: beyond the RIFLE and AKIN criteria. *Nat. Rev. Nephrol.*, 2011;7:201-8.

[13] Cruz DN, Ricci Z, Ronco C. Clinical review: RIFLE and AKIN--time for reappraisal. *Crit. Care*, 2009;13:211.

[14] Chertow GM, Burdick E, Honour M, Bonventre JV, Bates DW. Acute kidney injury, mortality, length of stay, and costs in hospitalized patients. *J. Am. Soc. Nephrol.,* 2005;16:3365-70.

[15] Lassnigg A, Schmidlin D, Mouhieddine M, et al. Minimal changes of serum creatinine predict prognosis in patients after cardiothoracic surgery: a prospective cohort study. *J. Am. Soc. Nephrol.,* 2004;15:1597-605.

[16] Swaminathan M, Shaw AD, Phillips-Bute BG, et al. Trends in acute renal failure associated with coronary artery bypass graft surgery in the United States. *Crit. Care. Med,* 2007;35:2286-91.

[17] Mangano CM, Diamondstone LS, Ramsay JG, Aggarwal A, Herskowitz A, Mangano DT. Renal dysfunction after myocardial revascularization: risk factors, adverse outcomes, and hospital resource utilization. The Multicenter Study of Perioperative Ischemia Research Group. *Ann. Intern. Med.,* 1998;128:194-203.

[18] Dasta JF, Kane-Gill SL, Durtschi AJ, Pathak DS, Kellum JA. Costs and outcomes of acute kidney injury (AKI) following cardiac surgery. *Nephrol. Dial. Transplant.,* 2008;23:1970-4.

[19] Bahar I, Akgul A, Ozatik MA, et al. Acute renal failure following open heart surgery: risk factors and prognosis. *Perfusion,* 2005;20:317-22.

[20] Park M, Coca SG, Nigwekar SU, Garg AX, Garwood S, Parikh CR. Prevention and treatment of acute kidney injury in patients undergoing cardiac surgery: a systematic review. *Am. J. Nephrol.,* 2010;31:408-18.

[21] Nigwekar SU, Navaneethan SD, Parikh CR, Hix JK. Atrial natriuretic peptide for preventing and treating acute kidney injury. *Cochrane Database Syst. Rev.,* 2009:CD006028.

[22] Woo EB, Tang AT, el-Gamel A, et al. Dopamine therapy for patients at risk of renal dysfunction following cardiac surgery: science or fiction? *Eur. J. Cardiothorac. Surg.,* 2002;22:106-11.

[23] Lassnigg A, Donner E, Grubhofer G, Presterl E, Druml W, Hiesmayr M. Lack of renoprotective effects of dopamine and furosemide during cardiac surgery. *J. Am. Soc. Nephrol.,* 2000;11:97-104.

[24] Duke GJ, Briedis JH, Weaver RA. Renal support in critically ill patients: low-dose dopamine or low-dose dobutamine? *Crit. Care. Med .,*1994;22:1919-25.

[25] Mahesh B, Yim B, Robson D, Pillai R, Ratnatunga C, Pigott D. Does furosemide prevent renal dysfunction in high-risk cardiac surgical patients? Results of a double-blinded prospective randomised trial. *Eur. J. Cardiothorac. Surg.,* 2008;33:370-6.

[26] Smith MN, Best D, Sheppard SV, Smith DC. The effect of mannitol on renal function after cardiopulmonary bypass in patients with established renal dysfunction. *Anaesthesia,* 2008;63:701-4.

[27] Adabag AS, Ishani A, Koneswaran S, et al. Utility of N-acetylcysteine to prevent acute kidney injury after cardiac surgery: a randomized controlled trial. *Am. Heart J.,* 2008;155:1143-9.

[28] Wijeysundera DN, Beattie WS, Rao V, Granton JT, Chan CT. N-acetylcysteine for preventing acute kidney injury in cardiac surgery patients with pre-existing moderate renal insufficiency. *Can. J. Anaesth.,* 2007;54:872-81.

[29] Nigwekar SU, Kandula P. N-acetylcysteine in cardiovascular-surgery-associated renal failure: a meta-analysis. *Ann. Thorac. Surg.,* 2009;87:139-47.

[30] Loef BG, Henning RH, Epema AH, et al. Effect of dexamethasone on perioperative renal function impairment during cardiac surgery with cardiopulmonary bypass. *Br. J. Anaesth.,* 2004;93:793-8.

[31] Durmaz I, Yagdi T, Calkavur T, et al. Prophylactic dialysis in patients with renal dysfunction undergoing on-pump coronary artery bypass surgery. *Ann. Thorac. Surg.,* 2003;75:859-64.

[32] Cogliati AA, Vellutini R, Nardini A, et al. Fenoldopam infusion for renal protection in high-risk cardiac surgery patients: a randomized clinical study. *J. Cardiothorac. Vasc. Anesth.,* 2007;21:847-50.

[33] Caimmi PP, Pagani L, Micalizzi E, et al. Fenoldopam for renal protection in patients undergoing cardiopulmonary bypass. *J. Cardiothorac. Vasc. Anesth.,* 2003;17:491-4.

[34] Sezai A, Hata M, Wakui S, et al. Efficacy of continuous low-dose hANP administration in patients undergoing emergent coronary artery bypass grafting for acute coronary syndrome. *Circ. J.,* 2007;71:1401-7.

[35] Hayashida N, Chihara S, Kashikie H, et al. Effects of intraoperative administration of atrial natriuretic peptide. *Ann. Thorac. Surg.*, 2000;70:1319-26.

[36] Nigwekar SU, Hix JK. The role of natriuretic peptide administration in cardiovascular surgery-associated renal dysfunction: a systematic review and meta-analysis of randomized controlled trials. *Cardiothoracic. Vasc. Anesth.,* 2009;23:151-60.

[37] Waikar SS, Betensky RA, Emerson SC, Bonventre JV. Imperfect Gold Standards for Kidney Injury Biomarker Evaluation. *J. Am. Soc. Nephrol.,* 2011.

[38] Nigwekar SU, Kandula P, Hix JK, Thakar CV. Off-pump coronary artery bypass surgery and acute kidney injury: a meta-analysis of randomized and observational studies. *Am. J. Kidney. Dis.,* 2009;54:413-23.

[39] Thakar CV, Arrigain S, Worley S, Yared JP, Paganini EP. A clinical score to predict acute renal failure after cardiac surgery. Journal of the American Society of Nephrology : *JASN,* 2005;16:162-8.

[40] Chertow GM, Lazarus JM, Christiansen CL, et al. Preoperative renal risk stratification. *Circulation*, 1997;95:878-84.

[41] Karkouti K, Wijeysundera DN, Yau TM, et al. Acute kidney injury after cardiac surgery: focus on modifiable risk factors. *Circulation,* 2009;119:495-502.

[42] Hickey PR, Buckley MJ, Philbin DM. Pulsatile and nonpulsatile cardiopulmonary bypass: review of a counterproductive controversy. *Ann. Thorac. Surg.,* 1983;36:720-37.

[43] Zhou W, Farrar CA, Abe K, et al. Predominant role for C5b-9 in renal ischemia/reperfusion injury. *J. Clin. Invest.,* 2000;105:1363-71.

[44] Di Mauro M, Gagliardi M, Iaco AL, et al. Does off-pump coronary surgery reduce postoperative acute renal failure? The importance of preoperative renal function. *Ann. Thorac. Surg.,* 2007;84:1496-502.

[45] Fransen E, Maessen J, Dentener M, Senden N, Geskes G, Buurman W. Systemic inflammation present in patients undergoing CABG without extracorporeal circulation. *Chest,* 1998;113:1290-5.

[46] Dybdahl B, Wahba A, Haaverstad R, et al. On-pump versus off-pump coronary artery bypass grafting: more heat-shock protein 70 is released after on-pump surgery. *Eur. J. Cardiothorac. Surg.,* 2004;25:985-92.

[47] Karkouti K, Beattie WS, Wijeysundera DN, et al. Hemodilution during cardiopulmonary bypass is an independent risk factor for acute renal failure in adult cardiac surgery. *J. Thorac. Cardiovasc. Surg.,* 2005;129:391-400.

[48] Patel NC, Grayson AD, Jackson M, et al. The effect off-pump coronary artery bypass surgery on in-hospital mortality and morbidity. *Eur. J. Cardiothorac. Surg.,* 2002;22:255-60.

[49] Schwann NM, Horrow JC, Strong MD, 3rd, Chamchad D, Guerraty A, Wechsler AS. Does off-pump coronary artery bypass reduce the incidence of clinically evident renal dysfunction after multivessel myocardial revascularization? *Anesth. Analg.,* 2004;99:959-64.

[50] Weinstein GS, Rao PS, Vretakis G, Tyras DH. Serial changes in renal function in cardiac surgical patients. *Ann. Thorac. Surg.,* 1989;48:72-6.

[51] Abel RM, Buckley MJ, Austen WG, Barnett GO, Beck CH, Jr., Fischer JE. Etiology, incidence, and prognosis of renal failure following cardiac operations. Results of a prospective analysis of 500 consecutive patients. *J. Thorac. Cardiovasc. Surg.,* 1976;71:323-33.

[52] van der Heijden GJ, Nathoe HM, Jansen EW, Grobbee DE. Meta-analysis on the effect of off-pump coronary bypass surgery. *Eur. J. Cardiothorac. Surg.,* 2004;26:81-4.

[53] Tasdemir O, Vural KM, Karagoz H, Bayazit K. Coronary artery bypass grafting on the beating heart without the use of extracorporeal circulation: review of 2052 cases. *J. Thorac. Cardiovasc. Surg.,* 1998;116:68-73.

[54] Vural KM, Tasdemir O, Karagoz H, Emir M, Tarcan O, Bayazit K. Comparison of the early results of coronary artery bypass grafting with and without extracorporeal circulation. *Thorac. Cardiovasc. Surg.,* 1995;43:320-5.

[55] Gamoso MG, Phillips-Bute B, Landolfo KP, Newman MF, Stafford-Smith M. Off-pump versus on-pump coronary artery bypass surgery and postoperative renal dysfunction. *Anesth. Analg.,* 2000;91:1080-4.

[56] Hix JK, Thakar CV, Katz EM, Yared JP, Sabik J, Paganini EP. Effect of off-pump coronary artery bypass graft surgery on postoperative acute kidney injury and mortality. *Crit. Care. Med.,* 2006;34:2979-83.

[57] Ascione R, Nason G, Al-Ruzzeh S, Ko C, Ciulli F, Angelini GD. Coronary revascularization with or without cardiopulmonary bypass in patients with preoperative nondialysis-dependent renal insufficiency. *Ann. Thoracic. Surg.,* 2001;72:2020-5.

[58] Beauford RB, Saunders CR, Niemeier LA, et al. Is off-pump revascularization better for patients with non-dialysis-dependent renal insufficiency? *Heart Surg. Forum.,* 2004;7:E141-6.

[59] Bucerius J, Gummert JF, Walther T, et al. On-pump versus off-pump coronary artery bypass grafting: impact on postoperative renal failure requiring renal replacement therapy. *Ann.Thorac. Surg.,* 2004;77:1250-6.

[60] Chukwuemeka A, Weisel A, Maganti M, et al. Renal dysfunction in high-risk patients after on-pump and off-pump coronary artery bypass surgery: a propensity score analysis. *Ann. Thorac. Surg.,* 2005;80:2148-53.

[61] Fischer SS, Phillips-Bute B, Swaminathan M, Milano C, Stafford-Smith M. Symmetry aortic connector devices and acute renal injury: a comparison of renal dysfunction after three different aortocoronary bypass surgery techniques. *Anesth. Analg.,* 2006;102:25-31.

[62] Hayashida N, Teshima H, Chihara S, et al. Does off-pump coronary artery bypass grafting really preserve renal function? *Circ. J.*, 2002;66:921-5.

[63] Hirose H, Amano A, Takahashi A, Nagano N. Coronary artery bypass grafting for patients with non-dialysis-dependent renal dysfunction (serum creatinine > or =2.0 mg/dl). *Eur. J. Cardiothorac. Surg.*, 2001;20:565-72.

[64] Landoni G, Bove T, Crivellari M, et al. Acute renal failure after isolated CABG surgery: six years of experience. *Minerva. Anestesiol.*, 2007;73:559-65.

[65] Loef BG, Epema AH, Navis G, Ebels T, van Oeveren W, Henning RH. Off-pump coronary revascularization attenuates transient renal damage compared with on-pump coronary revascularization. *Chest,* 2002;121:1190-4.

[66] Massoudy P, Wagner S, Thielmann M, et al. Coronary artery bypass surgery and acute kidney injury--impact of the off-pump technique. *Nephrol. Dial. Transplant.*, 2008;23:2853-60.

[67] Stallwood MI, Grayson AD, Mills K, Scawn ND. Acute renal failure in coronary artery bypass surgery: independent effect of cardiopulmonary bypass. *Ann. Thorac. Surg.*, 2004;77:968-72.

[68] Weerasinghe A, Athanasiou T, Al-Ruzzeh S, et al. Functional renal outcome in on-pump and off-pump coronary revascularization: a propensity-based analysis. *Ann. Thorac. Surg.*, 2005;79:1577-83.

[69] Joffe MM, Rosenbaum PR. Invited commentary: propensity scores. *Am. J. Epidemiol.*, 1999;150:327-33.

[70] Kuss O, von Salviati B, Borgermann J. Off-pump versus on-pump coronary artery bypass grafting: a systematic review and meta-analysis of propensity score analyses. *J. Thorac. Cardiovasc. Surg.*, 2010;140:829-35, 835 e1-13.

[71] Ascione R, Lloyd CT, Underwood MJ, Gomes WJ, Angelini GD. On-pump versus off-pump coronary revascularization: evaluation of renal function. *Ann. Thorac. Surg.*, 1999;68:493-8.

[72] Shroyer AL, Grover FL, Hattler B, et al. On-pump versus off-pump coronary-artery bypass surgery. *N. Engl. J. Med.*, 2009;361:1827-37.

[73] Moore GJ, Trachiotis GD. Outcomes of off-pump versus on-pump coronary artery bypass surgery in end-stage renal disease patients with a history of myocardial infarction. *Heart Surg. Forum,* 2006;9:E774-8.

[74] De Lima JJ, Gowdak LH, de Paula FJ, et al. Treatment of coronary artery disease in hemodialysis patients evaluated for transplant-a registry study. *Transplant,* 2010;89:845-50.

[75] Dewey TM, Herbert MA, Prince SL, et al. Does coronary artery bypass graft surgery improve survival among patients with end-stage renal disease? *Ann. Thorac. Surg.*, 2006;81:591-8; discussion 8.

[76] Ariyoshi T, Eishi K, Yamachika S, et al. Perioperative and mid-term results of coronary bypass surgery in patients undergoing chronic dialysis. *Ann. Thorac. Cardiovasc. Surg.*, 2006;12:257-64.

[77] Bechtel JF, Detter C, Fischlein T, et al. Cardiac surgery in patients on dialysis: decreased 30-day mortality, unchanged overall survival. *Ann. Thorac. Surg.*, 2008;85:147-53.

[78] Beckermann J, Van Camp J, Li S, Wahl SK, Collins A, Herzog CA. On-pump versus off-pump coronary surgery outcomes in patients requiring dialysis: perspectives from a

single center and the United States experience. *J. Thorac. Cardiovasc. Surg.*, 2006;131:1261-6.

[79] Kan CD, Yang YJ. Coronary artery bypass grafting in patients with dialysis-dependent renal failure. *Tex. Heart Inst. J.*, 2004;31:224-30.

[80] Liu JF, Lin CH, Chua CH, et al. Outcome of off-pump coronary artery bypass in renal dialysis patients. *Thorac. Cardiovasc. Surg.*, 2008;56:412-7.

[81] Manabe S, Arai H, Tanaka H, Tabuchi N, Sunamori M. Physiological comparison of off-pump and on-pump coronary artery bypass grafting in patients on chronic hemodialysis. *Jpn. J. Thorac. Cardiovasc. Surg.*, 2006;54:3-10.

[82] Manabe S, Shimokawa T, Fukui T, et al. Coronary artery bypass surgery versus percutaneous coronary artery intervention in patients on chronic hemodialysis: does a drug-eluting stent have an impact on clinical outcome? *J. Card. Surg*., 2009;24:234-9.

[83] Milani R, Brofman PR, Souza JA, et al. OPCAB in patients on hemodialysis. *Rev. Bras. Cir. Cardiovasc.*, 2007;22:104-8.

[84] Parikh DS, Swaminathan M, Archer LE, et al. Perioperative outcomes among patients with end-stage renal disease following coronary artery bypass surgery in the USA. *Nephrol. Dial. Transplant.*, 2010;25:2275-83.

[85] Sunagawa G, Komiya T, Tamura N, Sakaguchi G, Kobayashi T, Murashita T. Coronary artery bypass surgery is superior to percutaneous coronary intervention with drug-eluting stents for patients with chronic renal failure on hemodialysis. *Ann. Thorac. Surg.*, 2010;89:1896-900; discussion 900.

[86] Ashrith G, Lee VV, Elayda MA, Reul RM, Wilson JM. Short- and long-term outcomes of coronary artery bypass grafting or drug-eluting stent implantation for multivessel coronary artery disease in patients with chronic kidney disease. *Am. J. Cardiol.*, 2010;106:348-53.

[87] Nevis IF, Mathew A, Novick RJ, et al. Optimal method of coronary revascularization in patients receiving dialysis: systematic review. *Clin. J. Am. Soc. Nephrol.*, 2009;4:369-78.

[88] Akman B, Bilgic A, Sasak G, et al. Mortality risk factors in chronic renal failure patients after coronary artery bypass grafting. *Ren. Fail*, 2007;29:823-8.

[89] Charytan DM, Kuntz RE. Risks of coronary artery bypass surgery in dialysis-dependent patients--analysis of the 2001 National Inpatient Sample. *Nephrol. Dial. Transplant.*, 2007;22:1665-71.

[90] Chikwe J, Castillo JG, Rahmanian PB, Akujuo A, Adams DH, Filsoufi F. The impact of moderate-to-end-stage renal failure on outcomes after coronary artery bypass graft surgery. *J. Cardiothorac. Vasc. Anesth.*, 2010;24:574-9.

[91] Hedley AJ, Roberts MA, Hayward PA, et al. Impact of chronic kidney disease on patient outcome following cardiac surgery. *Heart Lung. Circ.*, 2010;19:453-9.

[92] Herzog CA, Strief JW, Collins AJ, Gilbertson DT. Cause-specific mortality of dialysis patients after coronary revascularization: why don't dialysis patients have better survival after coronary intervention? *Nephrol. Dial. Transplant.*, 2008;23:2629-33.

[93] Moore GJ, Pfister A, Trachiotis GD. Outcomes for off-pump coronary artery bypass grafting in high-risk groups: a historical perspective. *Heart Surg. Forum,* 2005;8:E19-22.

[94] Bruschi G, Colombo T, Botta L, et al. Off-pump coronary revascularization in chronic dialysis-dependent patients: early outcomes at a single institution. *J. Cardiovasc. Med.,* (Hagerstown) 2010;11:481-7.

[95] Gharsallah H, Trabelsi W, Hajjej Z, et al. Cardiac surgery in patients on hemodialysis: eight years experience of the Tunisian military hospital. *Saudi. J. Kidney. Dis. Transpl.,* 2010;21:1157-64.

[96] Imamaki M, Ishida A, Shimura H, Miyazaki M. Steal phenomenon with kinked graft caused a loss of viability in a dialysis patient. *J. Card. Surg.,* 2005;20:377-9.

[97] Jayasekera H, Pinto N, Mundy J, et al. Cardiac surgery in the presence of dialysis: effect on mid-term outcomes and quality of life. *Heart Lung. Circ.,* 2011;20:105-10.

[98] Nyawo B, Pawale A, Pardeshi L, Talbot D, Forty J. The effect of a large proximal haemodialysis arterio-venous fistula on weaning off cardiopulmonary bypass: case report. *J. Cardiothorac. Surg.,* 2008;3:44.

[99] Parikh CR, Coca SG, Smith GL, Vaccarino V, Krumholz HM. Impact of chronic kidney disease on health-related quality-of-life improvement after coronary artery bypass surg. *Arch. Intern. Med.,*2006;166:2014-9.

[100] Shroff GR, Li S, Herzog CA. Survival of patients on dialysis having off-pump versus on-pump coronary artery bypass surgery in the United States. *J. Thorac. Cardiovasc. Surg.,* 2010;139:1333-8.

[101] Kobayashi J, Ikebuchi M, Fujita Y, Irie H. Early postoperative recovery by chronic dialysis patients after coronary artery bypass grafting. *Ann. Thorac. Cardiovasc. Surg.,* 2009;15:243-6.

[102] Kutner NG, Zhang R, Huang Y, Herzog CA. Cardiac rehabilitation and survival of dialysis patients after coronary bypass. *J. Am. Soc. Nephrol.,* 2006;17:1175-80.

[103] Nakasuji M, Nishi S, Nakasuji K, Hamaoka N, Ikeshita K, Asada A. Duration of dialysis is a significant predictor of prolonged postoperative mechanical ventilation in dialysis-dependent patients undergoing cardiac surgery. *Anesth. Analg.,*2006;102:2-7.

[104] Harciarek M, Williamson JB, Biedunkiewicz B, Lichodziejewska-Niemierko M, Debska-Slizien A, Rutkowski B. Memory performance in adequately dialyzed patients with end-stage renal disease: is there an association with coronary artery bypass grafting? *J. Clin. Exp. Neuropsychol.,*2010;32:881-9.

[105] Fukushima S, Kobayashi J, Tagusari O, et al. Early results of off-pump coronary artery bypass grafting for patients on chronic renal dialysis. Jpn *J. Thorac. Cardiovasc. Surg.,* 2005;53:186-92.

[106] Nishimura J, Akagi H, Sawa Y, et al. Advantages of off-pump coronary artery bypass grafting in long-term hemodialysis patients: multicenter analysis. *Heart Surg. Forum,* 2004;7:E370-3.

[107] Oyamada S, Kobayashi J, Tagusari O, et al. Is diabetic nephropathy a predicted risk factor?--Kaplan-Meier and multivariate analysis of confounding risk factors in off-pump coronary artery bypass grafting for chronic dialysis patients. *Circ. J.,* 2009;73:2056-60.

[108] Murai N, Kodera K, Sasaki A, et al. Prognosis after off-pump coronary artery bypass in patients receiving hemodialysis. *Ann. Thorac. Cardiovasc. Surg.,* 2007;13:396-9.

[109] Horai T, Fukui T, Tabata M, Takanashi S. Early and mid-term results of off-pump coronary artery bypass grafting in patients with end stage renal disease: surgical

outcomes after achievement of complete revascularization. *Interact. Cardiovasc. Thorac. Surg.,* 2008;7:218-21.

[110] Sakao T, Kashu Y, Nakagawa H, Kajiwara S. Off-pump coronary artery bypass grafting in two renal transplant patients. *Jpn. J. Thorac. Cardiovasc. Surg.,* 2003;51:678-80.

[111] Hattori K, Hoshino R, Tochii M, Sato M, Yamashita M, Ando M. Off-pump coronary artery bypass surgery in a renal transplant patient. *Jpn. J. Thorac. Cardiovasc. Surg.,* 2006;54:532-4.

[112] Shayan H, Rocha R, Wei L, et al. Midterm Outcomes of Off-Pump and On-Pump Coronary Artery Revascularization in Renal Transplant Recipients. *J. Card. Surg.,* 2011.

[113] Carrier M, Perrault LP, Jeanmart H, Martineau R, Cartier R, Page P. Randomized trial comparing off-pump to on-pump coronary artery bypass grafting in high-risk patients. *Heart Surg. Forum.,* 2003;6:E89-92.

[114] Celik JB, Gormus N, Topal A, Okesli S, Solak H. Effect of off-pump and on-pump coronary artery bypass grafting on renal function. *Renal. Fail,* 2005;27:183-8.

[115] Kobayashi J, Tashiro T, Ochi M, et al. Early outcome of a randomized comparison of off-pump and on-pump multiple arterial coronary revascularization. *Circulation,* 2005;112:I338-43.

[116] Sajja LR, Mannam G, Chakravarthi RM, et al. Coronary artery bypass grafting with or without cardiopulmonary bypass in patients with preoperative non-dialysis dependent renal insufficiency: a randomized study. *J. Thorac. Cardiovasc. Surg.,* 2007;133:378-88.

[117] Tang AT, Knott J, Nanson J, Hsu J, Haw MP, Ohri SK. A prospective randomized study to evaluate the renoprotective action of beating heart coronary surgery in low risk patients. *Eur. J. Cardiothorac. Surg.,* 2002;22:118-23.

In: Off-Pump Coronary Artery Bypass Grafting
Editors: S.G. Raja and M. Amrani
ISBN 978-1-62081-575-5

Chapter 7

CEREBRAL OUTCOMES AFTER OFF-PUMP CORONARY ARTERY BYPASS GRAFTING

Diederik van Dijk
Anesthesiologist and Intensivist, Department of Anesthesiology and Intensive Care, University Medical Center Utrecht, Utrecht, The Netherlands

ABSTRACT

Several studies have demonstrated potentially harmful side effects of cardiopulmonary bypass (CPB) on the brain. This includes macro-emboli caused by aortic manipulation and micro-emboli from cardiotomy suction. CPB also initiates a profound inflammatory response, which increases the permeability of the blood-brain barrier and is associated with temporary brain swelling. Hence, cerebral complications of coronary artery bypass grafting (CABG) have been largely attributed to the use of CPB. These complications are broadly categorized as stroke (type I neurologic outcomes) and postoperative cognitive decline (type II neurologic outcomes). Many randomized clinical trials comparing cerebral outcomes after off-pump and on-pump CABG have been performed. Early individual studies and an early meta-analysis indicated that off-pump CABG might decrease the risk of stroke. However, an up to date meta-analysis of 11 high quality clinical trials, including 4121 randomized patients, does not even show a trend towards a lower stroke rate after off-pump CABG (relative risk 1.05; 95% CI 0.56 – 1.96). The randomized studies evaluating cognitive decline after off-pump and on-pump CABG also failed to demonstrate a benefit of avoiding CPB. It seems that natural ageing contributes much more to long-term cognitive decline than undergoing off-pump or on-pump CABG. Failure of CPB avoidance to improve cerebral outcomes can be due to several reasons. This chapter provides an overview of cerebral outcomes following on- pump and off-pump CABG and offers explanations for the failure of off-pump CABG to improve cerebral outcomes.

INTRODUCTION

Cerebral complications of coronary artery bypass grafting (CABG) have been largely attributed to the use of cardiopulmonary bypass (CPB) [1-3]. This seems reasonable because several studies have demonstrated potentially harmful side effects of CPB on the brain. Cannulation and cross-clamping of the ascending aorta may induce atheromatous macro-emboli, which are held responsible for perioperative stroke [4]. The CPB itself and cardiotomy suction are sources of cerebral micro-emboli, which can be confirmed with transcranial Doppler [3]. Post-mortem examination of the brains of patients who had undergone on-pump cardiac surgery also reveals evidence of cerebral micro-emboli [5]. During CPB episodes of low blood pressure may occur, to a degree that is usually not considered acceptable in patients undergoing non-cardiac surgery. CPB also initiates a profound inflammatory response [1, 6-8] and increases the permeability of the blood-brain barrier. Brain swelling can be observed in patients who undergo magnetic resonance imaging immediately after on-pump CABG surgery [9]. Serum concentrations of S-100 protein, a biochemical marker of cerebral injury, are elevated after on-pump CABG [10]. Because of all these potentially negative effects of CPB on the brain, many regard the use of CPB as the culprit in cerebral complications following cardiac surgery.

TWO TYPES OF CEREBRAL COMPLICATIONS

Based on a study of CABG patients from 24 US institutions by Roach and associates, cerebral complications can be classified into two categories [1]. Type I outcomes are defined as focal neurological injury, or stupor, or coma at hospital discharge. Type II outcomes are defined as deterioration in intellectual function, disorientation, memory deficit, or seizures, without evidence of focal injury.

Type I outcomes largely reflect perioperative stroke, which occurs on average in around 2% of CABG patients [1,2] but in as much as 9% of patients older than 75 years [11]. When a formal pre- and postoperative neurological examination is performed, a higher incidence of new focal injury can be found, but often without affecting patients in functional terms [12].

Type II outcomes occur in around 3 percent of patients [1] and largely reflect postoperative cognitive decline (POCD) [2, 13, 14]. Again, a more thorough examination of patients reveals a higher incidence of cognitive injury. Whereas Roach et al [1] based type II outcomes on clinical data and hospital-discharge summaries evaluated by an expert panel, POCD is more often diagnosed with repeated administration of a battery of psychometric tests [2, 13, 15,16]. Compared to an expert panel, psychometric tests are believed to be much more sensitive for detecting subtle cognitive changes [15]. It is, therefore, not surprising that studies evaluating POCD with psychometric tests have consistently reported a higher incidence of POCD than the 3 percent type II outcomes found by Roach et al [1]. Depending on the timing of neuropsychological assessments and the definition of POCD, the reported incidence of POCD after CABG surgery varies between 10 and 70 percent [13, 16]. Only a small proportion of patients, however, experience relevant POCD and become sufficiently disabled to prevent return to employment [1].

As both type I and type II neurological outcomes are attributed to the use of CPB, it has been anticipated that off-pump coronary artery (OPCAB) grafting would reduce the incidence of both types of cerebral complications. Studies comparing cerebral outcomes after off-pump and on-pump CABG are summarized and interpreted in the next sections.

THE EFFECT OF OFF-PUMP CABG ON STROKE RATE

Several randomized clinical trials comparing off-pump and on-pump CABG have been performed. These studies were invariably underpowered to quantify a possible effect of off-pump CABG on the incidence of perioperative stroke. An early meta-analysis which also included randomized studies of poor methodological quality, indeed found a benefit of off-pump CABG on stroke rate [17]. This meta-analysis included 2895 patients enrolled in 26 randomized trials and reported a spectacular 49% reduction in stroke rate after off-pump CABG, compared to on-pump CABG (relative risk 0.51; 95% CI 0.27 – 0.95) [17]. However, two meta-analyses published in 2008 and 2009 also assessed the quality of the randomized trials [18,19]. Only in a minority of these randomized trials, the randomization procedure was adequate and the outcome assessment blinded [18]. The methodological quality of the randomized studies was inversely associated with the effect size of the intervention being studied. In five trials with adequate randomization and blinded outcome assessment, Møller et al. found a relative risk for stroke of 0.97 (95% CI 0.54 – 1.73) [18]. Figure 1 shows forest plot of an up to date meta-analysis of 11 high quality randomised studies. This includes the ROOBY trial published in 2009 [20]. In a pooled sample of 4121 patients randomised to off-pump CABG *versus* on-pump CABG, the incidence of stroke was 0.94% and 0.91%, respectively (relative risk 1.05; 95% CI 0.56 – 1.96).

	Off-pump		On-pump			Odds Ratio	
Study or Subgroup	Events	Total	Events	Total	Weight	M-H, Fixed, 95% CI	Year
Czerny	0	40	0	40		Not estimable	2001
Angelini-A	1	100	3	101	15.3%	0.33 [0.03, 3.23]	2002
Angelini-B	2	100	3	100	15.3%	0.66 [0.11, 4.04]	2002
Nathoe	1	142	2	139	10.4%	0.49 [0.04, 5.42]	2003
Muneretto	0	88	0	88		Not estimable	2003
Lee	0	30	1	30	7.7%	0.32 [0.01, 8.24]	2003
Widimsky	0	208	0	192		Not estimable	2004
Puskas	2	100	2	100	10.2%	1.00 [0.14, 7.24]	2004
Lingaas	0	60	0	60		Not estimable	2006
Karolak	0	150	0	150		Not estimable	2007
Shroyer	14	1104	8	1099	41.1%	1.75 [0.73, 4.19]	2009
Total (95% CI)		**2122**		**2099**	**100.0%**	**1.05 [0.56, 1.96]**	
Total events	20		19				
Heterogeneity: Chi² = 3.47, df = 5 (P = 0.63); I² = 0%							
Test for overall effect: Z = 0.15 (P = 0.88)							

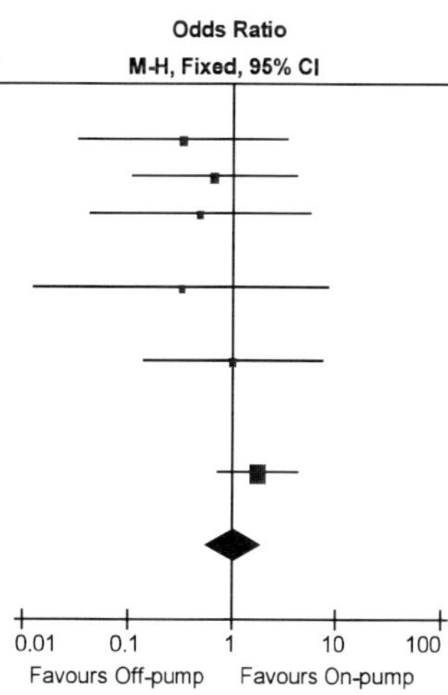

Figure 1. Forest plot of 11 high quality randomized clinical trials: Intervention effect of off-pump *versus* on-pump coronary artery bypass grafting on stroke. CI denotes confidence integral; M-H denotes Mantel-Haenszel.

Although this meta-analysis suggests that there is not even a trend towards a lower stroke rate after off-pump CABG, the confidence interval is wide and it is still possible that an adequately powered randomized study would show a benefit (or harm) of off-pump CABG on stroke rate. It would require a sample size of around 5,000 patients to demonstrate statistically significant reduction in the incidence of stroke from 2% after on-pump CABG to 1% off-pump CABG. It is obvious that such a large randomized trial would be difficult to perform. The largest trial conducted thus far included 2,203 patients [20].

A way to overcome the problem of low statistical power in randomized studies evaluating a rare event such as stroke, is to use information from observational studies, which may include much larger patient samples. These studies rely on statistical methods such as stratification, matching, and regression analyses to adjust for baseline differences in treatment groups. An interesting technique for adjustment is the propensity score method, which achieves a kind of pseudo randomization between off-pump and on-pump patients.

A meta-analysis of 22 studies with propensity score analysis, including a total sample of 55,290 patients, found an odds ratio of 0.49 (95% CI 0.41 – 0.58) for the effect of off-pump surgery on stroke rate [21].More statistically significant information, with much larger patient samples but lower level of evidence, can be obtained with retrospective studies based on existing databases.

An example of such a study is the analysis of the 2004 Nationwide Inpatient Sample (NIS), which was based on 63,047 discharge records of patients who underwent isolated CABG [22]. Of these patients, 14,389 underwent off-pump CABG; the rest had on-pump CABG. The incidence of stroke was 1.7% and 1.8%, respectively (relative risk 0.95; 95% CI 0.83 – 1.10) [22]. Another study of 30,426 patients registered in the California Coronary Artery Bypass Graft (CABG) Outcomes Reporting Program (CCORP) did find a benefit of OPCAB on stroke rate [23]. The observed incidence of stroke was 1.08% after off-pump CABG and 1.42% after on-pump CABG, despite a higher predicted risk in the off-pump patients (adjusted odds ratio: 0.76, 95% CI 0.59 - 0.98). However, intraoperative conversion of off-pump CABG to CPB was associated with the highest postoperative stroke rate [23].

In summary, the number of high quality clinical trials comparing stroke after off- vs. on-pump CABG is limited. A meta-analysis of 11 high quality randomised studies reveals no effect of off-pump CABG on stroke rate. Although more than 4000 patients have been included in these trials, the number of strokes was sparse, which increases the risk of random errors (‘play of chance’).

Some non-randomized studies with much larger patient samples report a benefit of off-pump CABG on stroke rate, but even after correction for confounding variables, these studies remain liable to many sorts of bias. There is no evidence that off-pump CABG reduces the incidence stroke.

The Effect of Off-Pump CABG on Postoperative Cognitive Decline

The assessment of possible neurocognitive injury after CABG is laborious and expensive. It requires the administration of a psychometric test battery, both before and after the operation [16]. Therefore, the sample size of studies evaluating the incidence of POCD is usually smaller than the sample size of studies evaluating the incidence of stroke. The first large randomized study comparing cognitive outcomes after off-pump *versus* on-pump

CABG study was the Octopus trial, which included 281 patients [24]. The patients underwent a battery of ten psychometric tests one day before and three and twelve months after operation. The test battery was administered by psychologists blinded for randomization and included tests for motor skills, verbal memory capacity, attention, visuospatial capacity and information processing. Cognitive decline was defined as a decrease in an individual's performance of at least 20% from baseline, in at least 20% of the tests. At three month follow-up, the incidence of cognitive decline was 21% after off-pump and 29% and on-pump surgery (relative risk 0.65; 95% CI 0.36 - 1.16) [24]. A post-hoc analysis of the 3-month cognitive outcome using a more reliable and conservative definition of POCD showed a difference in cognitive outcome favoring OPCAB. The incidence of POCD was 3.9% after off-pump and 11.7% after on-pump surgery (relative risk 0.34; 95% CI 0.12 – 0.90) [25]. However, at one and five year follow-up, there was no difference between the two groups, regardless of the definition applied [24, 26]. The Octopus Trial included young and relatively healthy patients. It was then hypothesized that the wrong patients were studied and that elderly patients would benefit much more from off-pump CABG because POCD is strongly age-dependent. Therefore, 120 elderly participants (mean age 76 years) of the randomised Best Bypass Surgery trial underwent psychometric testing before surgery and at 3-month follow-up. Irrespective of the definition of POCD that was applied, this study also failed to demonstrate a difference in the incidence of POCD [27]. The relatively large ROOBY trial also included a cognitive assessment that covered the domains of attention, memory, and visuospatial skills [20]. However, of the 2203 randomized patients, only 1156 completed the baseline test and the one-year follow-up test. There was no significant difference between the two treatment groups in one-year cognitive outcome [20].

Several other randomized trials have been performed, some of them with a sample size as small as 40 patients [28]. Because all trials conducted differ in the composition of the psychometric test battery, the timing of assessment, and definitions of POCD, a valid meta-analysis of the data from these trials is impossible. Remarkably, two attempts have been made though, and both have been published [29, 30]. There are also non-randomized studies comparing early and long-term cognitive outcome after off-pump and on-pump CABG [31,32]. Taking all the currently available evidence into account, it must be concluded that there is probably some benefit of off-pump CABG on cognitive outcome in the first few months after surgery. However, there seems to be no measurable effect of off-pump *versus* on-pump CABG on long-term cognitive outcome.

Why is the Effect of Off-Pump CABG on the Risk of Cerebral Complications So Disappointing?

The use of CPB is associated with micro-emboli, macro-emboli, episodes of hypotension and a profound inflammatory response [2-8]. Despite these disturbing side-effects of CPB, however, randomized studies fail to show a difference in the frequency of cerebral complications between patients undergoing surgery with and without CPB [24, 27]. Several possible explanations can be offered for failure of avoiding CPB to improve cerebral outcomes.

It has often been suggested that the randomized studies failing to demonstrate benefits of off-pump CABG have recruited the wrong patients. The favorable effects of off-pump technique may be more marked in older patients, with more extensive aortic disease and comorbidities [11, 33]. A randomized study in elderly patients evaluating POCD at 3 month follow-up failed to confirm this hypothesis [27] and also subgroup analyses of randomized studies reporting stroke could not confirm that elderly patients benefit more from off-pump CABG than young patients. A non-randomised study in octogenarians, though, found a spectacular decrease in stroke rate from 9 to 0 percent ($p < 0.0005$) by avoiding CPB [33]. In another non-randomised cohort of patients with diabetes who underwent off-pump CABG ($n = 540$) or on-pump CABG ($n = 475$), the incidence of stroke was 0.7% versus 2.3%, respectively ($p = 0.13$) [34].

Another explanation might be that the off-pump technique is a new source of cerebral complications. Exposure of the posterior cardiac wall frequently leads to transient episodes of elevated central venous pressure and concurrent decreased systemic blood pressure, resulting in a decreased cerebral perfusion pressure [35].

It is also possible that better cerebral outcomes can only be achieved with off-pump CABG, when manipulation of the aorta is completely avoided. In 2011, a meta-analysis has been published of six studies comparing a total of 4458 "anaortic" off-pump CABG patients with 4458 off-pump patients in whom an aortic side-clamp had been used for anastomosis of a coronary graft to the aorta [36]. The rate of stroke for "anaortic" off-pump CABG was 0.31% compared with 1.35% for off-pump procedures with aortic side-clamp ($p = 0.001$) [36]. However, all studies included in this meta-analysis were non-randomised and it is likely that the "anaortic" patients had a lower *a priory* stroke risk.

A fourth explanation is that cerebral micro-emboli from CPB do not cause permanent injury. With transcranial Doppler, it is difficult to distinguish gaseous micro-emboli from solid microemboli [2,3]. It is possible that the majority of the cerebral emboli detected with Doppler during on-pump CABG are gaseous micro-emboli, which may dissolve within seconds and could have minimal effects on brain function [3]. Likewise, cerebral edema after CPB may have a benign course. None of the patients with brain swelling immediately after CABG, had oedema during repeated magnetic resonance imaging six days later [9].

It is also conceivable that advances in CPB technology have resulted in improved cerebral outcomes. It is, therefore, possible that in contemporary practices the risk of cerebral complications is largely determined by factors other than CPB. This may include the inflammatory response to major surgery, certain anaesthetic drugs, the presence of generalized atherosclerotic disease, and advanced age [2]. Moller et al [14]. demonstrated a 10% incidence of cognitive decline after non-cardiac surgery, independent of regional or general anaesthesia, suggesting that surgical trauma could be a source of cognitive decline. For the development of long-term cognitive decline, even the causal role of CABG surgery in itself is now uncertain, regardless of the use of CPB. Selnes et al. [32] compared cognitive outcomes at 6 year follow-up between 152 CABG surgery patients and 92 non-surgical cardiac comparison patients. Compared to baseline performance, mild late cognitive decline was observed for both groups, but there were no differences between the surgical and non-surgical patients. The Octopus Study group [37] performed a largely similar study, and compared 281 CABG surgery patients to 112 healthy subjects without coronary artery disease. At five-year follow-up, a statistically significant difference in cognitive decline between the CABG surgery patients and the healthy subjects could not be demonstrated. Both studies suggest that natural ageing contributes much more to long-term POCD than undergoing CABG surgery [32, 37].

A final possible explanation for the finding that avoiding CPB does not result in less cerebral complications, is that the studies carried out so far lacked statistical power. The confidence intervals of individual randomized studies and even the meta-analyses are wide, because cerebral complications of cardiac surgery are rare events. Although many studies have reported high incidences of POCD, it has become clear that the psychometric tests used to detect POCD have limited precision and may overestimate the incidence of POCD [25,38]. The tests are administered to patients at baseline, usually the day before their surgery, and a second time after their surgery. When a patient's postoperative performance is lower than his preoperative performance by some degree (for example -1 SD or -20%), he is classified as having POCD. However, most psychometric tests were never designed to detect within-subject cognitive decline over time and it has become apparent that there is considerable natural variation in test performance when subjects undergo the same test twice [25,38]. It appears to be very difficult to discriminate true cognitive decline from natural variations in psychometric test performance. Studies in healthy subjects have shown that most classical definitions of POCD generate a high rate of false positive results and, thus, overestimate the incidence of POCD [25,38]. An alarming prevalence of POCD of more then 30% one year after coronary bypass surgery, decreases to 10% when applying a more reliable definition [25]. Thus, both stroke and true POCD are rare events and therefore thousands instead of hundreds of patients need to be randomized to prove or rule out an effect of off-pump CABG on cerebral outcomes.

CONCLUSION

The randomized studies carried out so far indicate no favorable effect of off-pump *versus* on-pump CABG on stroke rate or long-term cognitive outcome. Because many of these studies were statistically underpowered, it is possible that future randomized studies with very large patient samples, or recruiting specific subgroups of patients, may find a more favorable effect of OPCAB grafting.

REFERENCES

[1] Roach GW, Kanchuger M, Mangano CM, et al, for the Multicenter Study of Perioperative Ischemia Research Group and the Ischemia Research and Education Foundation Investigators. Adverse cerebral outcomes after coronary bypass surgery. *N. Engl. J. Med.*, 1996;335:1857-1863.

[2] Newman MF, Mathew JP, Grocott HP, et al. Central nervous system injury associated with cardiac surgery. *Lancet*, 2006;368:694-703.

[3] Martin KK, Wigginton JB, Babikian VL, et al. Intraoperative cerebral high-intensity transient signals and postoperative cognitive function: a systematic review. *Am. J. Surg.*, 2009;197:55-63.

[4] Hartman GS, Yao FS, Bruefach M 3rd, et al. Severity of aortic atheromatous disease diagnosed by transesophageal echocardiography predicts stroke and other outcomes

associated with coronary artery surgery: a prospective study. *Anesth. Analg.*, 1996;83:701-708.

[5] Moody DM, Brown WR, Challa VR, et al. Brain microemboli associated with cardiopulmonary bypass: a histologic and magnetic resonance imaging study. *Ann. Thorac. Surg.*, 1995;59:1304-1307.

[6] Moat NE, Shore DF, Evans TW. Organ dysfunction and cardiopulmonary bypass: the role of complement and complement regulatory proteins. *Eur. J. Cardiothorac. Surg.*, 1993;7:563-573.

[7] Asimakopoulos G, Smith PL, Ratnatunga CP, Taylor KM: Lung injury and acute respiratory distress syndrome after cardiopulmonary bypass. *Ann. Thorac. Surg.*, 1999;68:1107-1115.

[8] Zanardo G, Michielon P, Paccagnella A, et al. Acute renal failure in the patient undergoing cardiac operation. Prevalence, mortality rate, and main risk factors. *J. Thorac. Cardiovasc. Surg.*, 1994;107:1489-1495.

[9] Harris DN, Bailey SM, Smith PL, et al. Brain swelling in first hour after coronary artery bypass surgery. *Lancet,* 1993;342:586-587.

[10] Lloyd CT, Ascione R, Underwood MJ, et al. Serum S-100 protein release and neuropsychologic outcome during coronary revascularization on the beating heart: a prospective randomized study. *J. Thorac. Cardiovasc. Surg.*, 2000;119:148-154.

[11] Newman MF, Wolman R, Kanchuger M, et al. Multicenter preoperative stroke risk index for patients undergoing coronary artery bypass graft surgery. Multicenter Study of Perioperative Ischemia (McSPI) Research Group. *Circulation*, 1996;94:II74-II80.

[12] Baker RA, Andrew MJ, Knight JL. Evaluation of neurologic assessment and outcomes in cardiac surgical patients. *Semin Thorac Cardiovasc Surg.*, 2001;13:149-157.

[13] Van Dijk D, Keizer AMA, Diephuis JC, et al. Neurocognitive dysfunctions following coronary artery bypass surgery: a systematic review. *J. Thorac. Cardiovasc. Surg.*, 2000;120:632-639.

[14] Moller JT, Cluitmans P, Rasmussen LS, et al. Long-term postoperative cognitive dysfunction in the elderly ISPOCD1 study: ISPOCD investigators. International Study of Post-Operative Cognitive Dysfunction. *Lancet,* 1998;351:857-861.

[15] Murkin JM, Newman SP, Stump DA, Blumenthal JA. Statement of consensus on assessment of neurobehavioral outcomes after cardiac surgery. *Ann. Thorac. Surg.*, 1995;59:1289-1295.

[16] Sauër AM, Kalkman C, Van Dijk D. Postoperative cognitive decline. *J. Anesth.*, 2009;23:256-259.

[17] Sedrakyan A, Wu AW, Parashar A, Bass EB, Treasure T. Off-pump surgery is associated with reduced occurrence of stroke and other morbidity as compared with traditional coronary artery bypass grafting: a meta-analysis of systematically reviewed trials. *Stroke,* 2006;37:2759-2769.

[18] Møller CH, Penninga L, Wetterslev J, Steinbrüchel DA, Gluud C. Clinical outcomes in randomized trials of off- vs. on-pump coronary artery bypass surgery: systematic review with meta-analyses and trial sequential analyses. *Eur. Heart. J.*, 2008;29:2601-2616.

[19] Feng ZZ, Shi J, Zhao XW, Xu ZF. Meta-analysis of on-pump and off-pump coronary arterial revascularization. *Ann. Thorac. Surg.*, 2009;87:757-765.

[20] Shroyer AL, Grover FL, Hattler B, et al. On-pump versus off-pump coronary artery bypass surgery. *N. Engl. J. Med.*, 2009;361:1827-1837.
[21] Kuss O, von Salviati B, Börgermann J. Off-pump versus on-pump coronary artery bypass grafting: a systematic review and meta-analysis of propensity score analyses. *J. Thorac. Cardiovasc. Surg.*, 2010;140:829-835.
[22] Chu D, Bakaeen FG, Dao TK, Lemaire SA, Coselli JS, Huh J. On-pump versus off-pump coronary artery bypass grafting in a cohort of 63,000 patients. *Ann. Thorac. Surg.*, 2009;87:1820-1826.
[23] Li Z, Denton T, Yeo KK, Parker JP, White R, Young JN, Amsterdam EA. Off-pump bypass surgery and postoperative stroke: California coronary bypass outcomes reporting program. *Ann. Thorac. Surg.*, 2010;90:753-759.
[24] Van Dijk D, Jansen EWL, Hijman R, et al. Cognitive outcome after off-pump and on-pump coronary bypass surgery: results from a randomized study. *JAMA*, 2002;287:1405-1412.
[25] Keizer AM, Hijman R, Kalkman CJ, Kahn RS, van Dijk D. The incidence of cognitive decline after (not) undergoing coronary artery bypass grafting: the impact of a controlled definition. *Acta. Anaesthesiol. Scand.*, 2005;49:1232-1235.
[26] Van Dijk D, Spoor M, Hijman R, et al. Cognitive and cardiac outcomes 5 years after off-pump vs on-pump coronary artery bypass graft surgery. *JAMA*, 2007;297:701-708.
[27] Jensen BO, Hughes P, Rasmussen LS, Pedersen PU, Steinbrüchel DA. Cognitive outcomes in elderly high-risk patients after off-pump versus conventional coronary artery bypass grafting: a randomized trial. *Circulation*, 2006;113:2790-2795.
[28] Diegeler A, Hirsch R, Schneider F, et al. Neuromonitoring and neurocognitive outcome in off-pump versus conventional coronary bypass operation. *Ann. Thorac. Surg.*, 2000;69:1162-1166.
[29] Cheng DC, Bainbridge D, Martin JE, Novick RJ. Does off-pump coronary artery bypass reduce mortality, morbidity, and resource utilization when compared with conventional coronary artery bypass? a meta-analysis of randomized trials. *Anesthesiology*, 2005;102:188-203.
[30] Takagi H, Tanabashi T, Kawai N, Umemoto T. Cognitive decline after off-pump versus on-pump coronary artery bypass graft surgery: meta-analysis of randomized controlled trials. *J. Thorac. Cardiovasc. Surg.*, 2007;134:512-513.
[31] Liu YH, Wang DX, Li LH, et al. The effects of cardiopulmonary bypass on the number of cerebral microemboli and the incidence of cognitive dysfunction after coronary artery bypass graft surgery. *Anesth. Analg.*, 2009;109:1013-1022.
[32] Selnes OA, Grega MA, Bailey MM, et al. Cognition 6 Years after surgical or medical therapy for coronary artery disease. *Ann. Neurol.*, 2008;63:581-590.
[33] Ricci M, Karamanoukian HL, Abraham R, et al. Stroke in octogenarians undergoing coronary artery surgery with and without cardiopulmonary bypass. *Ann. Thorac. Surg.*, 2000;69:1471-1475.
[34] Emmert MY, Salzberg SP, Seifert B, et al. Is off-pump superior to conventional coronary artery bypass grafting in diabetic patients with multivessel disease? *Eur. J. Cardiothorac. Surg.*, 2011;40:233-239.
[35] Nierich AP, Diephuis J, Jansen EW, Borst C, Knape JT. Heart displacement during off-pump CABG: how well is it tolerated? *Ann. Thorac. Surg.*, 2000;70:466-472.

[36] Edelman JJ, Yan TD, Bannon PG, Wilson MK, Vallely MP. Coronary artery bypass grafting with and without manipulation of the ascending aorta--a meta-analysis. *Heart Lung. Circ.,* 2011;20:318-324.

[37] Van Dijk D, Moons KGM, Nathoe HM, et al. Cognitive outcomes five years after NOT undergoing coronary artery bypass graft surgery. *Ann. Thorac. Surg.,* 2008:85:60-64.

[38] Selnes OA, Pham L, Zeger S, McKhann GM. Defining cognitive change after CABG: decline versus normal variability. *Ann. Thorac. Surg.,* 2006;82:388-390.

In: Off-Pump Coronary Artery Bypass Grafting
Editors: S.G. Raja and M. Amrani
ISBN 978-1-62081-575-5

Chapter 8

Gastrointestinal Outcomes of Off-Pump Coronary Artery Bypass Surgery

Shahzad G. Raja
Cardiac Surgeon, Harefield Hospital, London, UK

Abstract

Gastrointestinal complications secondary to cardiac surgery on cardiopulmonary bypass are rare, but result in a significantly high mortality rate. Although the pathogenesis of gastrointestinal lesions is complex and multifactorial, the major factor implicated in cardiac surgery is reduced systemic blood flow, which leads to inappropriate oxygen delivery and energy deficit. Cardiopulmonary bypass is associated with a broad range of systemic complications, including nonpulsatile flow, hemolysis, activation of the inflammatory cascade, anticoagulation, hypothermia, and, finally, reduced end-organ perfusion. Furthermore, cardiopulmonary bypass can increase gastrointestinal permeability and, as a consequence, enhance the release of cytokines that will lead to mucosal damage and microcirculation problems. Off-pump coronary artery bypass surgery is believed to reduce end organ damage seen after conventional coronary artery bypass grafting leading to less morbidity. This chapter provides an overview of incidence, predictors, pathogenesis, pathology, and management of gastrointestinal complications after surgery on cardiopulmonary bypass and focuses on the impact of off-pump coronary artery bypass surgery on gastrointestinal complications.

Introduction

The etiology and risk factors contributing to gastrointestinal (GI) complications after coronary artery bypass grafting (CABG) have been defined extensively [1]. The combined stress of anesthesia, surgery, anticoagulation, hypothermia, and cardiopulmonary bypass (CPB) triggers a hormonal stress response and a massive defense reaction compounded by haemodilution and nonpulsatile flow, which as a whole can lead to organ damage [2].

Like all other organ systems, the GI system is exposed to vasoactive substances and microembolism during CPB, but usually few clinical manifestations occur. Most of the GI complications after CABG have been attributed to low cardiac output and visceral hypoperfusion resulting in mucosal ischemia and necrosis. Stress ulceration, mucosal atrophy, bacterial overgrowth from stress ulcer prophylaxis, and loss of barrier function with increased permeability may lead to bacterial translocation, sepsis, and multiorgan failure [3]. CPB causes reduction in mucosal blood flow and leads to mesenteric sequestration of neutrophils and stimulates systemic inflammatory response [4].

It has been demonstrated that significant intestinal mucosal ischaemia can occur during CPB despite the normal indices of global perfusion. Factors released during CPB such as vasopressin, catecholamines, thromboxane A2 and B2 lead to redistribution of blood flow away from the mucosa because of regional vasoconstriction, and may contribute to mucosal ischaemia leading to GI complications [5].

Off-pump coronary artery bypass (OPCAB) surgery has been argued to reduce the inflammatory response during CABG [6-8]. Based on this argument, it is believed that OPCAB surgery can reduce end organ damage seen after conventional CABG leading to less morbidity [9]. There are numerous studies in the literature comparing the outcomes between off-pump and on-pump coronary artery revascularization techniques [10]. However, there are few data comparing GI complications following these two different methods of myocardial revascularization. This chapter provides an overview of incidence, pathogenesis, predictors and clinical features of GI complications after surgery on cardiopulmonary bypass and attempts to evaluate the current best available evidence on the impact of off-pump coronary artery bypass on gastrointestinal complications.

Incidence of Gastrointestinal Complications after Cardiac Surgery

Over the past three decades multiple studies have addressed the issue of gastrointestinal (GI) complications following cardiac surgery [1,3-5,13-39]. These complications, although rare, are often severe and can be associated with a high mortality. GI complications result in prolonged hospital stays and an increased cost of hospitalization. In the literature, the reported incidence of GI complications after cardiac operations varies between 0.29% and 5.5% [11-13]. Mortality also varies between studies with a low of 11% and a high of 72% [1,14]. Most series suggest the incidence is between 1% and 2% with a mortality of 30% (Table 1).

Predictors and Pathogenesis of Gastrointestinal Complications after Cardiac Surgery

Careful analysis of the existing world medical literature on this issue revealed 10 studies that have been conducted using multivariate analysis to identify the independent determinants of GI complications in cardiac surgery [3,27-30,36-40] (Table 2).

Although the pathogenesis of GI complications after cardiac surgery is complex and multifactorial, the major factor implicated in cardiac surgery is reduced systemic blood flow, which leads to inappropriate oxygen delivery and energy deficit [36]. The GI organs are at particular risk for ischemic events for several reasons, and oxygen shunting and consequent distal hypoxia can occur at the tip of intestinal villi even under normal conditions [36,41]. The GI tract does not have the ability to autoregulate to compensate for reductions in blood pressure [36].

Table 1. Incidence of gastrointestinal complications after cardiac surgery

Author	Year	No. of patients	No. of GI complications	Incidence (%)	Deaths	Mortality (%) of GI complications
Andersson et al.[38]	2005	6119	50	0.8	13	26
Mangi et al.[39]	2005	8709	46	0.5	27	59
Yoshida et al.[24]	2005	549	17	3.1	0	0
McSweeney et al	2004	2417	148	6.1	26	18
D'Ancona et al.[36]	2003	11058	147	1.3	29	20
Byhahn et al.[25]	2000	1116	23	2.1	20	87
Zacharias et al.[27]	2000	4463	113	2.5	26	23
Fitzgerald et al.[22]	2000	14521	187	1.3	163	87
Perugini et al. [29]	1997	1477	31	2.1	6	19
Lazar et al.[21]	1995	2054	29	1.4	8	28
Spotnitz et al.[29]	1995	1831	39	2.1	14	36
Ott et al	1995	8448	55	0.7	38	69
Mercado et al.[20]	1994	4923	64	1.3	10	16
Christenson et al.[3]	1994	3174	73	2.3	12	16
Tsiotos et al.[33]	1994	19246	116	0.6	30	26
Huddy et al.[19]	1991	4473	39	0.9	22	56
Ohri et al.[30]	1991	4629	33	0.7	4	12
Rosemurgy et al.[13]	1988	7140	21	0.3	4	19
Krasna et al.[35]	1988	1279	33	2.6	11	33
Moneta et al.[34]	1985	2428	27	1.1	3	11
Hanks et al.[16]	1982	5080	43	0.9	25	58
Pinson et al.[15]	1983	5682	142	2.5	13	9

Furthermore, due to persistent vasoconstriction, splanchnic hypoperfusion may continue even after hemodynamic stability has been gained [36].

Preoperative, intraoperative, and postoperative variables may all influence abdominal perfusion [38]. Comorbidities, such as low left ventricular ejection fraction [3,27,28] and peripheral vascular disease [27], may all cause splanchnic hypoperfusion and have actually been identified as determinants of GI complications in patients undergoing cardiac surgery (Table 2). However, cardiopulmonary bypass is the main predictor of gastrointestinal complications after cardiac surgery [42].

CPB, routinely used in cardiac surgery, provokes a systemic inflammatory reaction, characterized by fever, leucocytosis, and tachycardia that, in 1% to 2% of all cases, leads to multiple organ dysfunction syndrome [43,44]. The inflammatory stimulus is primarily related to the bioincompatibility of the materials used in the circuit, which activates various humoral cascades and blood elements, and to the maldistribution of blood flow, which can lead to ischaemic damage in sensitive organs like the intestine [45]. Gut involvement and the possible translocation of bacteria into the bloodstream can amplify the inflammatory response [46].

Table 2. Predictors of gastrointestinal complications after cardiac surgery from studies undertaking multivariate analysis

Author	Year	Predictors		
		Preoperative	Intraoperative	Postoperative
Christenson et al.[3]	1994	NYHA classes III & IV, LVEF < 40%, age > 70 years, reoperation, and urgent operation		MI, low CO necessitating substantial inotropic support or IABP
Raja et al.[40]	2003		CPB & cardioplegic arrest	
Zacharias et al.[27]	2000	Age > 70 years, triple vessel disease, NYHA class IV, PVD, CHF, reoperation	CPB duration	Substantial inotropic support, need for transfusions, IABP, re-exploration
Perugini et al.[28]	1997		CPB duration	
Spotnitz et al.[29]	1995			IABP
Ohri et al.[30]	1991		CPB duration	
D'Ancona et al.[36]	2003	Preoperative chronic renal failure	Valve surgery	Prolonged mechanical ventilation, postoperative renal failure, sepsis, and sternal infection
McSweeney et al.[37]	4004	Decreased LVEF, hyperbilirubinemia, thrombocytopenia, prolonged PTT, and reoperation	Combined CABG and intracardiac or proximal aortic surgery, and intraoperative transfusion	Inotropic support
Andersson et al.[38]	2005	Age > 80 years, active smoker need for preoperative inotropic support, NYHA class III-IV,	CPB time > 150 min	Postoperative AF, postoperative CHF, reoperation for bleeding, and postoperative vascular complications
Mangi et al.[39]	2005	Peripheral vascular disease		IABP

NYHA, New York Heart Association; CPB, cardiopulmonary bypass; CO, cardiac output; MI, myocardial infarction; LVEF, left ventricular ejection fraction; IABP, intra-aortic balloon pump; PTT, partial thromboplastin time; CHF, congestive heart failure; CABG, coronary artery bypass grafting.

Translocation into the bloodstream of intestinal bacteria and their toxic byproducts according to the "gut motor hypothesis" [47] functions as an "undrained intestinal abscess" [48]. This triggers multiple organ dysfunction syndrome, which is the main cause of death among intensive care unit patients [48].

CPB causes an ischemic damage of the gastric mucosa reflected by a reduction of the gastric intramucosal pH (pHi) after CPB [46,50,51]. The prolonged and marked suffering of the intestinal mucosa is further substantiated by the increased ^{51}Cr-EDTA (chromium-labeled test) urinary excretion for the first 24 perioperative hours and postoperative increase of the partial pressure of carbon dioxide gradient between the gastric mucosa and arterial blood (Pg

– Pa) [46]. Postoperative increase of gastric Pg - Pa is even more significant because it is considered more reliable than pHi to assess gastrointestinal perfusion and oxygenation and is well correlated to mortality and complications after coronary artery bypass graft and valve replacement [52]. In conditions of increased permeability, ^{51}Cr-EDTA passes through defective tight junctions of epithelial cells lining the mucosa: urinary ^{51}Cr-EDTA levels are thus a marker of the permeability of the small intestine as well as of the colon [53]. These findings suggest "patchy" splanchnic perfusion, which primarily affects the stomach and the colon leading to bacterial translocation from the gut, which is a possible cause of bacteraemia and predisposes to infectious complications, among them multiple organ failure [54].

SPECIFIC GASTROINTESTINAL COMPLICATIONS AFTER CARDIAC SURGERY

Gastrointestinal Bleeding

GI bleeding is the single most common GI complication after cardiac surgery. The risk of bleeding complications after cardiac surgery is significant due to the level of anticoagulation often required for operations utilizing CPB. The overall mean incidence of GI bleeding (both upper and lower) among all GI complications occurring after cardiac surgery is reported to be around 35% [12]. The mortality associated with GI bleeding after cardiac surgery is around 19%.

Most episodes of upper GI bleeding (UGIB) are related to duodenal and gastric sources [12]. The occurrence of UGIB in one study was 0.9% with a mortality of 15% compared to a mortality of 2.3% among the nonbleeding control group [20]. The incidence in another study was 0.9% and the mortality rate of that group was 35% [55]. This demonstrates that, despite a low incidence, the mortality associated with UGIB is high, particularly if surgical intervention is necessary to control massive bleeding. Halm et al. identified several risk factors associated with UGIB including prolonged CPB time, prolonged aortic cross-clamp time as well as prolonged mechanical ventilation [55]. Blood transfusions and early endoscopic evaluation are recommended to identify the source of bleeding and to determine appropriate therapy. This may involve endoscopic clipping, injecting, or fulgurating the vessel. An operation may be necessary if the bleeding cannot be arrested [12].

The causes of lower GI bleeding (LGIB) are mostly secondary to diverticulosis, arteriovenous malformations (AVMs), and colitis [12]. Only 9% of all GI bleeding after cardiac surgery is due to LGIB. The associated mortality is 17.4% [12]. Bleeding diverticula and vascular malformations are the most common causes, with the incidence reported to be 40% and 30% respectively [56]. Bleeding from arteriovenous malformations and diverticula is often self-limiting. Other causes such as colitis (10% to 15%), neoplasia (5% to10%), and anorectal bleeding (10% to 5%) may also occur [56,57]. One must also keep in mind that 10% of presumed LGIB is caused by an upper GI source [57].

If the patient is hemodynamically stable, the first step in diagnosis may be a technetium-99 tagged red blood cell scan. If a source of bleeding is recognized, the patient can undergo arteriography with the goal of embolization. Colonoscopy can also be undertaken to evaluate lower GI bleeding. Though technically difficult in a patient without an adequate bowel preparation, the overall diagnostic yield is 69% to 80% and it can lead to a therapeutic intervention [58].

Patients who have massive GI bleeding (>1000 ml in the first 24 hours or 5 total units of blood transfused), or are hemodynamically unstable due to hypovolemia should be evaluated for operative intervention. If the location of the bleeding has been identified, either by endoscopy, arteriography, or perhaps by definitive bleeding scan, partial resection is appropriate. Diagnosis can also be made during laparotomy by intraoperative endoscopy, including enteroscopy to search for a small bowel cause if no colonic source is discovered [59]. If the source still has not been identified, then subtotal colectomy, possibly with fecal diversion, may be necessary. Increased mortality and morbidity is associated with patients who undergo subtotal colectomy when compared with those who receive partial colectomy [60]. Therefore, early identification and localization of the source of bleeding should be aggressively pursued once bleeding presents [61].

The use of potent antiplatelet agents such as clopidogrel has increased significantly in the past 10 years. Many publications have examined the overall risk of bleeding in patients taking clopidogrel perioperatively, but few have reported on the incidence of GI bleeding after cardiac surgery. In one prospective study of safety and efficacy, 135 consecutive patients undergoing off-pump CABG were given clopidogrel (75 mg/day) and aspirin (325 mg/day) within six hours after surgery. Among the reported complications during that study there was one patient (0.7%) who was taken off the regimen for GI bleeding [62].

Ischemic Bowel

Ischemic bowel represents about 14% of all GI complications following cardiac operations and occurs after 0.16% of all cardiac operations. The mortality associated with ischemic bowel after cardiac surgery is significant, with an average of about 50%, but it has been as high 100% in some series [12]. Many factors have been implicated in the development of ischemic bowel including advanced age, emergent operations, presence of peripheral vascular disease, and perioperative hypotension [63-65]. The presence of leukocytosis along with LGIB, hyperkalemia, and unexplained lactic acidosis are suggestive but not specific for ischemic bowel [66]. This obviously contributes to delayed diagnosis and increased morbidity. As with any other abdominal complication, the presence of sedatives and prolonged mechanical ventilation in many of these patients poses a diagnostic challenge.

Two types of intestinal ischemia may present in this population, each with a different management approach: Nonocclusive mesenteric ischemia is due to hypoperfusion and is more common. Occlusive mesenteric arterial disease results from emboli or thrombus formation and is usually associated with an acute onset leading to a rapid clinical deterioration [34,66].

In nonocclusive disease, the presentation is often delayed and slower in onset and is without evidence of vascular obstruction. It is seen frequently in patients who have hypoperfusion syndrome or are on inotropic pressor support. The pathogenesis of this process is poorly understood but likely involves low cardiac output and diffuse mesenteric vasoconstriction that leads to intestinal hypoxia and possible necrosis [67]. In the absence of peritonitis or unexplained acidosis as an indication for emergency laparotomy, mesenteric angiography remains the gold standard though CT angiogram has become a fast and noninvasive alternative. In nonocclusive mesenteric ischemia, the characteristic angiogram shows the "string of sausages" sign in the major branches of the superior mesenteric artery.

The initial treatment of nonocclusive mesenteric ischemia includes aggressive resuscitation with efforts towards improving myocardial performance, maximizing hemodynamics to enhance intestinal perfusion, and reducing vasospasm to minimize the direct ischemic insult on the bowel and reperfusion injury. Broad spectrum antibiotics should be initiated empirically [68]. If the diagnosis of nonocclusive ischemia is made and the patient does not improve despite optimized hemodynamics, intraarterial transcatheter papaverine infusion can be utilized.

Occlusive disease should be treated, if diagnosed early, with the use of thrombolytics, embolectomy, or mesenteric bypass. Endovascular techniques (i.e., angioplasty, stenting, and thrombolytics) in conjunction with laparotomy can be used in this critically ill patient population. The use of locally delivered thrombolytics has been advocated, but there are no formal recommendations for the use of these agents in post-CABG patients [69]. Retrograde open mesenteric stenting has been advocated by a number of groups for the treatment of occlusive mesenteric ischemia as an alternative to mesenteric bypass [64,70-72]. In the case of open operative intervention, embolectomy and/or revascularization should precede bowel resection. This is done to minimize the amount of bowel that needs to be resected. A second look laparotomy may be necessary. Though it is possible to attempt a laparoscopic approach in these patients [73], generally laparotomy is an expeditious approach with the option to palpate the mesenteric vessels and to use fluorescein and/or doppler signals to assess bowel perfusion.

Peptic Ulcer

The average incidence of perforated duodenal or gastric ulcer post cardiac surgery is about 6% of all GI complications associated with a mortality of 36% [12]. All patients have to be treated surgically and the type of operation varies. There are many potential surgical options to treat a bleeding peptic ulcer if necessary. In the case of a bleeding duodenal ulcer the general surgeon may opt to oversew the ulcer and perform a vagotomy with pyloroplasty or a vagotomy and antrectomy operation. If the patient is unstable, the definitive procedure may be deferred and the ulcer simply oversewn. In the case of a bleeding gastric ulcer, definitive operations include biopsy, oversew and vagotomy, and pyloroplasty or distal gastrectomy. Again, if the patient is unstable, the surgeon may opt to biopsy and oversew initially [74].

Peptic ulcer prophylaxis became routine following cardiac surgery after the publication of a retrospective study by Mead and Folk in 1969 [56]. This study demonstrated a decrease in UGIB from 22% to 1.9% after routine use of antacids. A recent prospective randomized trial of GI prophylaxis divided patients into three groups of 70 patients who were given teprenone (mucosal protective agent), ranitidine (H_2 blocker), or rabeprazole (proton pump inhibitor [PPI]) beginning postoperative day 1 [75]. All patients underwent gastric fiberoscopy between postoperative days 5 and 7. They reported a clinically overt incidence of UGIB of 3.8%, which included four patients from the mucosal protection group, four from the H_2 blocker group, and none from the PPI group. Two of the patients, one from the mucosal protection group and one from the H_2 blocker group, died from complications of

UGIB. Incidence of hemorrhagic gastritis and active ulceration was also significantly lower in the group treated with a PPI, as were reports of epigastric pain. This evidence along with literature from adult critical care suggests the use of a PPI for prophylaxis. In the event a patient develops a significant UGIB endoscopic evaluation is warranted. If perforation of a viscus occurs prompt surgical exploration is required. There are a number of surgical options for perforated peptic ulcer; if the patient is unstable the surgeon may opt for placing an omental patch and deferring a definitive operation. Definitive operations for duodenal ulcers include omental patch with highly selective vagotomy and omental patch with vagotomy and pyloroplasty. For perforated gastric ulcers definitive operations include wedge excision with vagotomy and pyloroplasty and distal gastrectomy. There has emerged a role for nonoperative management of perforated peptic ulcers in selected patients. In patients fit for an operation, nonoperative management may be employed if the diagnosis is in doubt or if there is evidence the perforation has sealed. In patients unfit for surgery, either due to age, comorbidities, or presence of hemodynamic instability, the surgeon may opt for a trial of nasogastric drainage, circulatory support, and intravenous antibiotics [76].

Pancreatitis

Pancreatitis represents approximately 11% of GI complications after cardiac surgery; this corresponds to 0.13% incidence after all cardiac operations [12]. The vast majority of these patients are managed nonoperatively with supportive measures, and the mortality rate is 20% [12]. The characteristic symptoms of back pain, mid-epigastric pain, nausea, and vomiting are unusual (or difficult to elicit) in the postcardiac surgery setting [77]. The presence of hyperamylasemia is quite common after cardiac operations, occurring in 30% to 40% of patients undergoing cardiac surgery. However, only 1% to 3% of these patients develop clinically significant pancreatitis [78].

Specific risk factors for pancreatic injury after CPB have been evaluated in several studies. These risk factors include the presence of renal insufficiency (both preoperative and postoperative), valve surgery, prolonged CPB time, prolonged aortic cross-clamp time hypotension, vasoactive drug requirements, and low cardiac output syndrome [79]. A study by Fernandez Del Castillo et al. found that pancreatic cell injury after CPB seems to be more common in patients who received more than 800 mg/m^2 of calcium chloride perioperatively [80].

Patients can be divided into three subgroups [12]. The first consists of patients with isolated hyperamylasemia with a normal lipase and the absence of physical findings that suggests pancreatitis. These patients require no specific therapy. The second subgroup has hyperamylasemia as well as elevated lipase with no significant findings on physical examination or on imaging studies, and fall into the category of subclinical pancreatitis. These patients should be monitored closely while receiving routine postoperative care. If there are any signs or symptoms suggestive of progression to clinically overt pancreatitis the patient should be made NPO (nothing per mouth), CT imaging completed, and intravenous hydration initiated. Finally, in patients who develop obvious clinical pancreatitis enteral feeding distal to the ligament of Treitz or total parenteral nutrition (if there is a contraindication to enteral feeding) should be initiated to supply all nutrients if a prolonged period of gut rest is anticipated. Currently there is thought to be no role for empiric antibiotic therapy in acute pancreatitis without infection or necrosis [81]. CT imaging should be performed to evaluate any clinical changes suggestive of pancreatic infection or necrosis. Collections presenting in patients with a worsening clinical picture should undergo percutaneous aspiration in order to identify any infectious processes that require early aggressive drainage.

Hyperbilirubinemia and Liver Failure

The incidence of post-CPB hyperbilirubinemia (usually defined as a bilirubin level greater than 2.5 to 3 mg/dL) ranges from 9% to 40% with a mean of 25%, though often is not catastrophic [82]. The mean incidence of liver failure in literature is reported to be 2.2% of GI complications and 0.026% of all cardiac operations, and the mean mortality of hyperbilirubinemia is 4% and of liver failure is 56% [12]. Liver failure is defined as the loss of synthetic and metabolic functions of the liver, and is characterized by decreased production of albumin and clotting factors and the development of hepatic encephalopathy.

In one prospective observational study, 25% of patients undergoing cardiac surgery with CPB developed postoperative hyperbilirubinemia and the mortality was 4.1%. Over half (56.2%) had a peak bilirubin on postoperative day 1, 33.5% on postoperative day 2, and 10.3% on postoperative day 7 [82]. Typically conjugated bilirubin is elevated more significantly than the unconjugated form [82,83]. The type of surgery is significant, as patients undergoing a valve replacement and combined valve–CABG are at highest risk as compared with CABG alone or repair of congenital defects. Other risk factors include elevated preoperative bilirubin, severe preoperative elevation of right atrial pressure, number of units of perioperative blood transfused, hypotension/hypoxia, prolonged CPB time, aortic cross clamp time, and use of IABP [82-84]. Medications can also lead to drug-induced cholestasis. Medications used postcardiac surgery that have been implicated in cholestatic jaundice include ampicillin (and other penicillin antibiotics), cimetidine, and erythromycin. Use of halothane anesthesia was once considered a cause of postoperative liver dysfunction, but was not significant in a study by Mastoraki et al. [83]. The suspected causes include preoperative heart failure contributing to liver congestion (causing decreased ability to metabolize bilirubin and decreased bile transport), hemolysis from bypass, field suction, mechanical prostheses, transfused blood, liver hypoxia, and possibly ischemia/reperfusion injury to the liver.Postoperative hyperbilirubinemia is associated with increased mortality, increased time on mechanical ventilation, and longer ICU stays. In some patients liver failure will develop secondary to multisystem organ failure of nonhepatic origin. In patients with primary liver dysfunction, there appears to be two clinical paths that lead to these worsened outcomes: patients in whom the bilirubin continues to rise through the first postoperative week, and the development of liver failure secondary to sepsis or multisystem organ failure [84]. The bilirubin should be followed in patients with a preoperative elevation and those with multiple risk factors.Management generally involves interventions to improve liver perfusion, removal of hepatotoxic medications, laboratory evaluation to search for an underlying hematologic disorder, and abdominal ultrasound to assess for biliary obstruction, portal venous thrombosis or fluid collection/abscess. Specific treatment is then directed to the underlying cause [85].

Impact of Off-Pump Coronary Artery Bypass Grafting on Gastrointestinal Complications

The development and application of OPCAB technology has largely been driven by the hope of decreasing the incidence and/or severity of the adverse outcomes associated with cardiopulmonary bypass by performing CABG surgery without CPB. Impetus for this technology over the last decade has been provided by a number of studies that have reported the safety and efficacy of OPCAB [86-91]. In fact, randomized controlled trials (RCTs) demonstrate that OPCAB surgery yields results at least comparable to on-pump surgery in the early and mid-term postoperative periods, and that OPCAB surgery has advantages in a number of areas [92-99].

Table 3. Incidence of gastrointestinal complications after on-pump and off-pump coronary artery bypass surgery

Author	Year	No of Patients		Study type	Incidence of GI Complications(%)		*p* value
		CPB	OPCAB	(Level of evidence)	CPB	OPCAB	
Croome et al.[100]	2009	2010	441	Retrospective (Level III)	1.49%	0.91%	0.34
Emmiler et al.[101]	2009	1967	658	Retrospective (Level III)	0.4%	0.2%	0,28
Berson et al.[102]	2004	360	1,080	Retrospective (Level III)	1%	1%	0.407
Karthik et al.[103]	2004	211	211	Retrospective (Level III)	2.5%	1%	0.18
Racz et al.[104]	2004	59,044	9,135	Retrospective (Level III)	0.9%	1.2%	0.003
Sanisoglu et al.[105]†	2004	600	546	Retrospective (Level III)	2.4%	2.4%	0.963
Mack et al.[106]	2004	10,118	7,283	Retrospective (Level III)	4.8%	3.6%	0,02
Muneretto et al.[107]	2003	88	88	RCT (Level II)	3.4%	0%	ns
Raja et al.[40]†	2003	150	150	RCT (Level II)	7.3%	0.6%	<0.0001
Puskas et al.[108]	2003	100	100	RCT (Level II)	3%	2%	0.682
Poirier et al.[109]	2003	4,657	6,748	Retrospective (Level III)	1.2%	1,1%	ns
Musleh et al.[110]	2003	1,210	1,117	Retrospective (Level III)	1.2%	1.6%	0.347
Zamvar et al.[111]	2002	247	120	Retrospective (Level III)	1.21%	1.66%	ns

† Studies specifically investigating the incidence of gastrointestinal complications after on-pump and off-pump coronary artery bypass surgery.

CPB, cardiopulmonary bypass; OPCAB, off-pump coronary artery bypass; RCT, randomized controlled trial; ns, not significant.

Interestingly, as shown in Table 3, there are a limited number of studies, which specifically compare the incidence of gastrointestinal complications after OPCAB and conventional CABG on CPB. A literature search identified a total of 13 studies [40,100-111] that compare the incidence of GI complications after OPCAB and conventional CABG on CPB (Table 3).

Out of these only one RCT [40] specifically compares the incidence of GI complications after OPCAB and conventional CABG. In this RCT the overall incidence of gastrointestinal complications in the selected population [150 CPB patients, 114 men, mean age 64 (45-75) years and 150 OPCAB patients, 113 men, mean age 64 (38-66) years with no previous abdominal surgery] was 4% (n=12), with 11 patients in the on-pump group and one patient in the off-pump group ($p<0.0001$); 9(6%) patients in the on-pump group and none in the off-pump group died. Patients who developed gastrointestinal complications had significantly prolonged periods of both CPB (192.4± 83.2 vs 112.1±49.6 minutes, $p<0.0001$) and aortic cross clamping (105.3±45.6 vs 68.2± 35.6 minutes, $p<0.0001$). Patients with low cardiac output, new onset AF, postoperative need for vasopressor support, postoperative blood loss, and those needing redo thoracotomy within the first postoperative day had an increased incidence of gastrointestinal complications. Results from the univariate analysis for the association of each risk factor with post-operative gastrointestinal complications revealed that the use of CPB with cardioplegic arrest, renal insufficiency, emergency surgery, left ventricular ejection fraction<50%, low cardiac output, need for inotropic support, new onset AF, postoperative blood loss, and redo thoracotomy<24hr were all predictors of gastrointestinal complications after myocardial revascularization. However, stepwise multivariate regression analysis indicated the use of CPB inclusive of cardioplegic arrest as the only independent predictor of postoperative gastrointestinal complications (Odds Ratio 7.4; Confidence Interval 3.4 to 17.9).

On the contrary, recent retrospective studies by Croome et al. [100], Sanisoglu et al. [105] and Musleh et al.[110], specifically comparing the impact of OPCAB and CPB on the incidence of GI complications, have failed to show any difference in terms of GI complications between on- and off-pump groups undergoing CABG surgery. They attribute this to a similar degree of intraoperative injury to the gastric mucosa during OPCAB, with a worsening trend for OPCAB patients in the early postoperative period [112]. Several studies have documented the presence of significant transient hemodynamic impairment during distal anastomoses in OPCAB [113]. Significant drops in cardiac output may occur despite relatively well-preserved systemic arterial pressures. Hemodynamic deterioration is worse during grafting of the less accessible coronary targets that require extensive cardiac manipulation for adequate exposure. Cardiac verticalization results in compression of the right heart chambers against the surrounding fibrous pericardium and pleura and mechanical dysfunction of the right ventricle [114]. Moreover, despite a preserved mean arterial pressure, elevation of the central venous pressure due to a combination of Trendelenburg posture and cardiac elevation results in significant drops in perfusion pressure [112]. It is speculated that perhaps it is the cumulative effect of these transient episodes of reduced cardiac output and reduced perfusion pressure in the course of distal anastomoses during OPCAB which results in a degree of ischaemic injury to the gastric mucosa at least comparable to CPB [112].

Lastly, although the total incidence of GI complication after on-pump and off-pump CABG appears to be about the same, closer inspection of the available data suggests that the type of GI complication is different. Patients done off-pump tend to have a lower incidence of mesenteric ischemia, but they tend to make up for that with higher incidence of GI bleeding, peptic ulcer disease, and diverticulitis [40,100,101,105,110].

Implications for Clinical Practice

The morbidity and mortality associated with the development of post cardiac surgery GI complications impose an imperative for the identification of preventive strategies as well emphasizing the need for early recognition of cases that do occur. The technique of OPCAB has successfully reduced the vascular complication rates in patients with stroke, renal failure, and peripheral vascular disease [103,108]. Theoretically, the avoidance of cardiopulmonary bypass-induced mesenteric hemodynamic lability as well as the avoidance of cannulation-related embolic events should also diminish the likelihood of bypass-related GI complications. Unfortunately, available evidence from RCTs and retrospective studies is conflicting in this regard and has failed to demonstrate the superiority of OPCAB in protecting against GI complications (Table 3). This may be in part due to the selection bias inherent in studies investigating outcome and off-pump operation and by the already low percentage of overall patients suffering GI complications [39]. Other strategies that may help prevent mesenteric ischemia include routine epiaortic ultrasonography to identify and avoid debris in the aorta; institution of a screening program for heparin-induced thrombocytopenia (HIT) and active prophylaxis against HIT with iloprost and dipyridamole; the use of internal mammary-based pedicled grafts; and proximal anastomotic devices to avoid clamping the aorta in such patients; and paying meticulous attention to hemodynamic management in the perioperative period [39].

Early recognition of impending GI complication(s) due to the insult of mesenteric ischemia is an important determinant of survival [115]. Awareness of the predictors of GI complications and presenting clinical complaints allows the physician to intervene prior to laboratory manifestation of end-organ damage.

As the overwhelming majority of cases of mesenteric ischemia occur during the initial hours to days following operation, fast-track extubation pathways and/or minimal sedation [116] theoretically may enable earlier recognition of a catastrophic GI event [39]. This opens a window for both more sophisticated diagnostic imaging such as computed tomographic angiography or magnetic resonance angiography and for intervention. Early laparotomy guided by the clinical scenario may therefore result in early intraoperative recognition of a correctable ischemic event: isolated superior mesenteric artery/large vessel occlusion or segmental colonic necrosis. Patients at high-risk of GI bleeding must receive prophylactic proton pump inhibitors. In settings in which early extubation may not be feasible, the use of invasive monitoring systems such as continuous gastric wall pH monitoring has been advocated, [117] but the efficacy and role of such strategies in routine postoperative care remain untested [39].

The prognosis associated with postoperative GI complication following heart operation remains grim. Mesenteric ischemia follows cardiac surgery in susceptible patients at a period of hours to days, whereas a more diverse group of intra-abdominal disease (diverticulitis, cholecystitis, pancreatitis, peptic ulcer) occurs days to weeks following operation. Routine surgical management is indicated in this latter group of patients, but perioperative preventive strategies are likely to be of greater benefit in the former. Laboratory markers of widespread ischemic insult, often used to make the diagnosis of mesenteric ischemia, unfortunately appear after the closure of a window for therapeutic intervention [39].

These values may help to provide a better framework for surgical decision-making and family counseling, but ultimately techniques to reduce the occurrence of and/or preemptively diagnosis postcardiotomy mesenteric ischemia will be necessary to decrease its associated mortality.

Conclusion

At present there is a paucity of RCTs to specifically compare the impact of OPCAB and CPB on the incidence of GI complications with the current best available evidence suggesting a comparable incidence of GI complications after on-pump and off-pump CABG. Awareness of the predictors of GI complications after cardiac surgery is important so that cardiac surgeons can alter their operative strategy or early postoperative management decisions based on identification of such variables. Finally, when confronted with a patient who has a postoperative course, which deviates from the expected and also has risk factors for GI complication(s), the treating physician must have a heightened index of suspicion so that early recognition of problem with prompt institution of life-saving treatment can be ensured.

References

[1] Ott MJ, Buchman TG, Baumgartner WA. Postoperative abdominal complications in cardiopulmonary bypass patients: a case-controlled study. *Ann. Thorac. Surg.*, 1995;59:1210-3.

[2] Laffeay JG, Boylan JF, Cheng DC. The systemic inflammatory response to cardiac surgery: implications for the anesthesiologist. *Anesthesiology,* 2002;97:215-52.

[3] Christenson JT, Schmuziger M, Maurice J, et al. Gastrointestinal complications after coronary artery bypass grafting. *J. Thorac. Cardiovasc. Surg.*, 1994;108:899-906.

[4] Tofukuji M, Stahl GL, Metais C, et al. Mesenteric dysfunction after cardiopulmonary bypass: role of complement C5a. *Ann. Thorac. Surg.*, 2000;69:799-807.

[5] Tao W, Zwischenberger JB, Nguyen TT, et al. Gut mucosal ischemia during normothermic cardiopulmonary bypass results from blood flow redistribution and increased oxygen demand. *J. Thorac. Cardiovasc. Surg.*, 1995;110:819-28.

[6] Okubo N, Hatori N, Ochi M, et al. Comparison of m-RNA expression for inflammatory mediators in leukocytes between on-pump and off-pump coronary artery bypass grafting. *Ann. Thorac. Cardiovasc. Surg.*, 2003;9:43-9.

[7] Ascione R, Lloyd CT, Underwood MJ, et al. Inflammatory response after coronary revascularization with or without cardiopulmonary bypass. *Ann. Thorac. Surg.*, 2000;69:1198-204.

[8] Matata BM, Sosnowski AW, Galinanes M. Off-pump bypass graft operation significantly reduces oxidative stress and inflammation. *Ann. Thorac. Surg.*, 2000;69:785-91.

[9] Ascione R, Al-Ruzzeh S, Amer K, et al. Subsystem organ function during coronary surgery. *Perfusion,* 2002;17:295-303.

[10] Reston JT, Tregear SJ, Turkelson CM. Meta-analysis of short-term and mid-term outcomes following off-pump coronary artery bypass grafting. *Ann. Thorac. Surg.,* 2003;76:1510-5.

[11] Yapici N, Ince C. Gastrointestinal complications and its predictors after cardiac surgery. Turk. J. Gastroenterol., 2010;21:3-6.

[12] Rodriguez R, Robich MP, Plate JF, Trooskin SZ, Sellke FW. Gastrointestinal complications following cardiac surgery: a comprehensive review. J. Card. Surg., 2010;25:188-97.

[13] Rosemurgy AS, McAllister E, Karl RC. The acute surgical abdomen after cardiac surgery involving extracorporeal circulation. Ann. Surg., 1988;207:323-6.

[14] Welling RE, Rath R, Albers JE, Glaser RS. Gastrointestinal complications after cardiac surgery. Arch. Surg., 1986;121:1178-80.

[15] Pinson CW, Alberty RE: General surgical complications after cardiopulmonary bypass surgery. *Am. J. Surg.,* 1983;146:133-137.

[16] Hanks JB, Curtis SE, Hanks BB, *et al.* Gastrointestinal complications after cardiopulmonary bypass. *Surgery,* 1982;92:394-400.

[17] Aranha GV, Pickleman J, Pifarre R, *et al.* The reasons for gastrointestinal consultation after cardiac surgery. *Am. Surg.,* 1984;50:301-304.

[18] Reath DB, Maull KI, Wolfgang TC: General surgical complications following cardiac surgery. *Am. Surg.,* 1983;49:11-14.

[19] Huddy SP, Joyce WP, Pepper JR. Gastrointestinal complications in 4473 patients who underwent cardiopulmonary bypass surgery. *Br. J. Surg.,* 1991;78:293-296.

[20] Mercado PD, Farid H, O'Connell TX, *et al.* Gastrointestinal complications associated with cardiopulmonary bypass procedures. *Am. Surg.,* 1994;60:789-792.

[21] Lazar HL, Hudson H, McCann J, *et al.* Gastrointestinal complications following cardiac surgery. *Cardiovasc. Surg.,* 1995;3:341-344.

[22] Fitzgerald T, Kim D, Karakozis S, *et al.* Visceral ischemia after cardiopulmonary bypass. *Am. Surg.,* 2000;66:623-626.

[23] Yilmaz AT, Arslan M, Demirkilc U, *et al.* Gastrointestinal complications after cardiac surgery. *Eur. J. Cardiothorac. Surg.,* 1996;10:763-767.

[24] Yoshida K, Matsumoto M, Sugita T, *et al.* Gastrointestinal complications in patients undergoing coronary artery bypass grafting. *Ann. Thorac. Cardiovasc. Surg.,* 2005;11:25-28.

[25] Byhahn C, Strouhal U, Martens S, *et al.* Incidence of gastrointestinal complications in cardiopulmonary bypass patients. *World J. Surg.,* 2001;25:1140-1144.

[26] Harjola PT, Siltanen P, Appelqvist P, et al. Abdominal complications after open heart surgery. *Ann. Chir. Gynaecol. Fenn.,* 1968;57:272-4.

[27] Zacharias A, Schwann TA, Parenteau GL, et al. Predictors of gastrointestinal complications in cardiac surgery. *Tex. Heart Inst. J.,* 2000;27:93-9.

[28] Perugini RA, Orr RK, Porter D, et al. Gastrointestinal complications following cardiac surgery. An analysis of 1477 cardiac surgery patients. *Arch. Surg.,* 1997;132:352-7.

[29] Spotnitz WD, Sanders RP, Hanks JB, et al. General surgical complications can be predicted after cardiopulmonary bypass. *Ann. Surg.,* 1995;221:489-96.

[30] Ohri SK, Desai JB, Gaer JA, et al. Intraabdominal complications after cardiopulmonary bypass. *Ann. Thorac. Surg.,* 1991;52:826-31.
[31] Simic O, Strathausen S, Hess W, et al. Incidence and prognosis of abdominal complications after cardiopulmonary bypass. *Cardiovasc. Surg.,* 1999;7:419-24.
[32] Leitman IM, Paull DE, Barie PS, et al. Intra-abdominal complications of cardiopulmonary bypass operations. *Surg. Gynecol. Obstet.,* 1987;165:251-4.
[33] Tsiotos GG, Mullany CJ, Zietlow S, et al. Abdominal complications following cardiac surgery. *Am. J. Surg.,* 1994;167:553-7.
[34] Moneta GL, Misbach GA, Ivey TD. Hypoperfusion as a possible factor in the development of gastrointestinal complications after cardiac surgery. *Am. J. Surg.,* 1985;149:648-50.
[35] Krasna MJ, Flancbaum L, Trooskin SZ, et al. Gastrointestinal complications after cardiac surgery. *Surgery,* 1988;104:773-80.
[36] D'Ancona G, Baillot R, Poirier B, et al. Determinants of gastrointestinal complications in cardiac surgery. *Tex. Heart. Inst. J.,* 2003;30:280-5.
[37] McSweeney ME, Garwood S, Levin J, et al; Investigators of the Ischemia Research and Education Foundation; Multicenter Study of Perioperative Ischemia Research Group. Adverse gastrointestinal complications after cardiopulmonary bypass: can outcome be predicted from preoperative risk factors? *Anesth. Analg.,* 2004;98:1610-7.
[38] Andersson B, Nilsson J, Brandt J, et al. Gastrointestinal complications after cardiac surgery. *Br. J. Surg.,* 2005;92:326-33.
[39] Mangi AA, Christison-Lagay ER, Torchiana DF, et al. Gastrointestinal complications in patients undergoing heart operation: an analysis of 8709 consecutive cardiac surgical patients. *Ann. Surg.,* 2005;241:895-901.
[40] Raja SG, Haider Z, Ahmad M. Predictors of gastrointestinal complications after conventional and beating heart coronary surgery. *Surgeon,* 2003;1:221-228.
[41] Mutlu GM, Mutlu EA, Factor P. GI complications in patients receiving mechanical ventilation. *Chest,* 2001;119:1222-41.
[42] Raja SG, Haider Z, Ahmad M. Cardiopulmonary bypass is the main predictor of gastrointestinal complications after cardiac surgery. *Tex. Heart Inst. J.,* 2004;31:108.
[43] Edmunds LH. Inflammatory response to cardiopulmonary bypass. *Ann. Thorac. Surg.,* 1998;66:12-16.
[44] Royston D. The inflammatory response and extracorporeal circulation. *J. Cardiothorac. Vasc. Anesth.*, 1997;113:341-354.
[45] Ohri SK. Systemic inflammatory response and the splanchnic bed in cardiopulmonary bypass. *Perfusion,* 1996;11:200-212.
[46] Rossi M, Sganga G, Mazzone M, et al. Cardiopulmonary bypass in man: role of the intestine in a self-limiting inflammatory response with demonstrable bacterial translocation. *Ann. Thorac. Surg*., 2004;77:612-8.
[47] Deitch EA. Multiple organ failure: pathophysiology and potential failure of therapy. *Ann. Surg.,* 1992;216:117-128.
[48] Nieuwenhuijzen GA, Goris RJ. The gut: the 'motor' of multiple organ dysfunction syndrome? *Curr. Opin. Clin. Nutr. Metab. Care,* 1999;2:399-404.
[49] Bone RC. Toward a theory regarding the pathogenesis of the systemic inflammatory response syndrome: what we do and do not know about cytokine regulation. *Crit. Care. Med.,* 1996;24:163-72.

[50] Andersen LW, Landow L, Baek L, et al. Association between gastric intramucosal pH and splanchnic endotoxin, antibody to endotoxin, and tumor necrosis factor-alpha concentrations in patients undergoing cardiopulmonary bypass. *Crit. Care. Med.*, 1993;21:210-217.

[51] Riddington DW, Venkatesh B, Boivin CM, et al. Intestinal permeability, gastric intramucosal pH, and systemic endotoxemia in patients undergoing cardiopulmonary bypass. *JAMA*, 1996;275:1007-1012.

[52] Bennett-Guerrero E, Panah MH, Bodian CA, et al. Automated detection of gastric luminal partial pressure of carbon dioxide during cardiovascular surgery using the Tonocap. *Anesthesiology*, 2000;92:38-45.

[53] Jenkins AP, Nukajam WS, Menzies IS, et al. Simultaneous administration of lactulose and 51Cr-ethylenediaminetetraacetic acid. A test to distinguish colonic from small-intestinal permeability change. *Scand. J. Gastroenterol.*, 1992;27:769-73.

[54] Feltis BA, Wells CL. Does microbial translocation play a role in critical illness?. *Curr. Opin. Crit. Care.*, 2000;6:117-122.

[55] Halm U, Halm F, Thein D, *et al. Helicobacter pylori* infection: A risk factor for upper gastrointestinal bleeding after cardiac surgery? *Crit. Care. Med.*, 2000;28:110-113.

[56] Mead J, Folk F. Gastrointestinal bleeding after cardiac surgery. *N. Engl. J. Med.*, 1969;281:799.

[57] Eisen GM, Dominitz JA, Faigel DO, *et al.* An annotated algorithm for the evaluation of choledocholithiasis. *Gastrointest. Endosc.*, 2001;53:864-866.

[58] Jensen DM, Machicado GA: Diagnosis and treatment of severe hematochezia. The role of urgent colonoscopy after purge. *Gastroenterology*, 1988;95:1569-1574.

[59] Jakobs R, Hartmann D, Benz C, *et al.* Diagnosis of obscure gastrointestinal bleeding by intra-operative enteroscopy in 81 consecutive patients. *World J. Gastroenterol.*, 2006;12:313-316.

[60] Hoedema RE, Luchtefeld MA. The management of lower gastrointestinal hemorrhage. *Dis. Colon. Rectum.*, 2005;48:2010-2024.

[61] Green BT, Rockey DC. Acute gastrointestinal bleeding. *Semin. Gastrointest. Dis.*, 2003;14:44-65.

[62] Shennib H, Endo M, Benhameid O: A feasibility study of the safety and efficacy of a combined clopidogrel and aspirin regimen following off-pump coronary artery bypass grafting. *Heart Surg. Forum*, 2003;6:288-291.

[63] Sakorafas GH, Tsiotos GG: Intra-abdominal complications after cardiac surgery. *Eur. J. Surg.*, 1999;165:820-827.

[64] Abboud B, Daher R, Boujaoude J. Acute mesenteric ischemia after cardio-pulmonary bypass surgery. *World. J. Gastroenterol.*, 2008;14:5361-5370.

[65] Ghosh S, Roberts N, Firmin RK, *et al.* Risk factors for intestinal ischaemia in cardiac surgical patients. *Eur. J. Cardiothorac. Surg.*, 2002;21:411-416.

[66] Allen KB, Salam AA, Lumsden AB: Acute mesenteric ischemia after cardiopulmonary bypass. *J. Vasc. Surg.*, 1992;16:391-395.

[67] Khan TA, Bianchi C, Ruel M, *et al.* Differential effects on the mesenteric microcirculatory response to vasopressin and phenylephrine after cardiopulmonary bypass. *J. Thorac. Cardiovasc. Surg.*, 2007;133:682-688.

[68] Berland T, Oldenburg WA. Acute mesenteric ischemia. *Curr. Gastroenterol. Rep.*, 2008;10:341-346.

[69] Abboud B, Daher R, Sleilaty G, *et al.* Is prompt exploratory laparotomy the best attitude for mesenteric ischemia after cardiac surgery? *Interact Cardiovasc. Thorac. Surg.*, 2008;7:1079-1083.
[70] Demirpolat G, Oran I, Tamsel S, *et al.* Acute mesenteric ischemia: Endovascular therapy. *Abdom. Imaging*, 2007;32:299-303.
[71] Moyes LH, McCarter DH, Vass DG, *et al.* Intraoperative retrograde mesenteric angioplasty for acute occlusive mesenteric ischaemia: A case series. *Eur. J. Vasc. Endovasc. Surg.*, 2008;36:203-206.
[72] Wyers MC, Powell RJ, Nolan BW, *et al.* Retrograde mesenteric stenting during laparotomy for acute occlusive mesenteric ischemia. *J. Vasc. Surg.*, 2007;45:269-275.
[73] Burpee SE, Kurian M, Murakame Y, *et al.* The metabolic and immune response to laparoscopic versus open liver resection. *Surg. Endosc.*, 2002;16:899-904.
[74] Reuben BC, Neumayer LA: Variations reported in surgical practice for bleeding duodenal ulcers. *Am. J. Surg.*, 2006;192:e42-e45.
[75] Hata M, Shiono M, Sekino H, *et al.* Prospective randomized trial for optimal prophylactic treatment of the upper gastrointestinal complications after open heart surgery. *Circ. J.*, 2005;69:331-334.
[76] Jamieson GG. Current status of indications for surgery in peptic ulcer disease. *World J. Surg.*, 2000;24:256-258.
[77] Herline AJ, Pinson CW, Wright JK, *et al.* Acute pancreatitis after cardiac transplantation and other cardiac procedures: Case-control analysis in 24,631 patients. *Am. Surg.*, 1999;65:819-825.
[78] Rattner DW, Gu ZY, Vlahakes GJ, *et al.* Hyperamylasemia after cardiac surgery. Incidence, significance, and management. *Ann. Surg.*, 1989;209:279-283.
[79] Lefor AT, Vuocolo P, Parker FB Jr, *et al.* Pancreatic complications following cardiopulmonary bypass. Factors influencing mortality. *Arch. Surg.*, 1992;127:1225-1230.
[80] Fernandez-del Castillo C, Harringer W, Warshaw AL, *et al.* Risk factors for pancreatic cellular injury after cardiopulmonary bypass. *N. Engl. J. Med.*, 1991;325:382-387.
[81] Frossard JL, Steer ML, Pastor CM: Acute pancreatitis. *Lancet*, 2008;371:143-152.
[82] An Y, Xiao YB, Zhong QJ. Hyperbilirubinemia after extracorporeal circulation surgery: A recent and prospective study. *World. J. Gastroenterol.*, 2006;12:6722-6726.
[83] Mastoraki A, Karatzis E, Mastoraki S, *et al.* Postoperative jaundice after cardiac surgery. *Hepatobiliary Pancreat. Dis. Int.*, 2007;6:383-387.
[84] Chu CM, Chang CH, Liaw YF, *et al.* Jaundice after open heart surgery: A prospective study. *Thorax*, 1984;39:52-56.
[85] Faust TW, Reddy KR: Postoperative jaundice. *Clin. Liver. Dis.*, 2004;8:151-166.
[86] Al-Ruzzeh S, Ambler G, Asimakopoulos G, et al. Off-Pump Coronary Artery Bypass (OPCAB) surgery reduces risk-stratified morbidity and mortality: a United Kingdom Multi-Center Comparative Analysis of Early Clinical Outcome. *Circulation*, 2003;108 Suppl 1:II1-8.
[87] Mack MJ, Duhaylongsod FG. Through the open door! Where has the ride taken us? *J. Thorac. Cardiovasc. Surg.*, 2002;124:655-9.
[88] Magee MJ, Jablonski KA, Stamou SC, et al. Elimination of cardiopulmonary bypass improves early survival for multivessel coronary artery bypass patients. *Ann. Thorac. Surg.*, 2002;73:1196-1202.

[89] Patel NC, Grayson AD, Jackson M, et al. The effect off-pump coronary artery bypass surgery on in-hospital mortality and morbidity. *Eur. J. Cardiothorac. Surg.,* 2002;22:255-60.

[90] Plomondon ME, Cleveland JC Jr, Ludwig ST, et al. Off-pump coronary artery bypass is associated with improved risk-adjusted outcomes. *Ann. Thorac. Surg.,* 2001;72:114-119.

[91] Cleveland JC Jr, Shroyer AL, Chen AY, et al. Off-pump coronary artery bypass grafting decreases risk-adjusted mortality and morbidity. *Ann. Thorac. Surg.,* 2001;72: 1282-1288.

[92] Puskas JD, Williams WH, Mahoney EM, et al. Off-pump vs conventional coronary artery bypass grafting: early and 1-year graft patency, cost, and quality-of-life outcomes: a randomized trial. *JAMA,* 2004;291:1841-9.

[93] Straka Z, Widimsky P, Jirasek K, et al. Off-pump versus on-pump coronary surgery: final results from a prospective randomized study PRAGUE-4. *Ann. Thorac. Surg.,* 2004;77:789-93.

[94] Legare JF, Buth KJ, King S, et al. Coronary bypass surgery performed off pump does not result in lower in-hospital morbidity than coronary artery bypass grafting on pump. *Circulation,* 2004;109:887-892.

[95] Gerola LR, Buffolo E, Jasbik W, et al. Off-pump versus on-pump myocardial revascularization in low-risk patients with one or two vessel disease: perioperative results in a multicenter randomized controlled trial. *Ann. Thorac. Surg.,* 2004;77:569-573.

[96] Puskas JD, Williams WH, Duke PG, et al. Off-pump coronary artery bypass grafting provides complete revascularization with reduced myocardial injury, transfusion requirements, and length of stay: a prospective randomized comparison of two hundred unselected patients undergoing off-pump versus conventional coronary artery bypass grafting. *J. Thorac. Cardiovasc. Surg.,* 2003;125:797-808.

[97] Nathoe HM, van Dijk D, Jansen EW, et al. A comparison of on-pump and off-pump coronary bypass surgery in low-risk patients. *N. Engl. J. Med.,* 2003;348:394-402.

[98] Angelini GD, Taylor FC, Reeves BC, et al. Early and midterm outcome after off-pump and on-pump surgery in Beating Heart Against Cardioplegic Arrest Studies (BHACAS 1 and 2): a pooled analysis of two randomised controlled trials. *Lancet,* 2002; 359:1194-1199.

[99] van Dijk D, Nierich AP, Jansen EW, et al. Early outcome after off-pump versus on-pump coronary bypass surgery: results from a randomized study. *Circulation,* 2001;104:1761-1766.

[100] Croome KP, Kiaii B, Fox S, et al. Comparison of gastrointestinal complications in on-pump versus off-pump coronary artery bypass grafting. Can. J. Surg., 2009;52:125-8.

[101] Emmiler M, Yaveri A, Koçoğullari CU, et al. Gastrointestinal ischemia related mortality in patients undergoing off- or on-pump coronary artery bypass grafting. Heart Surg. Forum., 2009;12:E79-84.

[102] Berson AJ, Smith JM, Woods SE, et al. Off-pump versus on-pump coronary artery bypass surgery: does the pump influence outcome? *J. Am. Coll Surg.,* 2004;199:102-8.

[103] Karthik S, Musleh G, Grayson AD, et al. Coronary surgery in patients with peripheral vascular disease: effect of avoiding cardiopulmonary bypass. *Ann. Thorac. Surg.,* 2004;77:1245-9.

[104] Racz MJ, Hannan EL, Isom OW, et al. A comparison of short- and long-term outcomes after off-pump and on-pump coronary artery bypass graft surgery with sternotomy. *J. Am. Coll Cardiol.*, 2004;43:557-64.
[105] Sanisoglu I, Guden M, Bayramoglu Z, et al. Does off-pump CABG reduce gastrointestinal complications? *Ann. Thorac. Surg.*, 2004;77:619-25.
[106] Mack MJ, Pfister A, Bachand D, et al. Comparison of coronary bypass surgery with and without cardiopulmonary bypass in patients with multivessel disease. *J. Thorac. Cardiovasc. Surg.*, 2004;127:167-73.
[107] Muneretto C, Bisleri G, Negri A, et al. Off-pump coronary artery bypass surgery technique for total arterial myocardial revascularization: a prospective randomized study. *Ann. Thorac. Surg.*, 2003;76:778-82.
[108] Puskas JD, Williams WH, Duke PG, et al. Off-pump coronary artery bypass grafting provides complete revascularization with reduced myocardial injury, transfusion requirements, and length of stay: A prospective randomized comparison of two hundred unselected patients undergoing off-pump versus conventional coronary artery bypass grafting. *J. Thorac. Cardiovasc. Surg.*, 2003;125:797-808.
[109] Poirier B, Baillot R, Bauset R, et al. Abdominal complications associated with cardiac surgery. Review of a contemporary surgical experience and of a series done without extracorporeal circulation. *Can. J. Surg.*, 2003;46:176-82.
[110] Musleh GS, Patel NC, Grayson AD, et al. Off-pump coronary artery bypass surgery does not reduce gastrointestinal complications. *Eur. J. Cardiothorac. Surg.*, 2003;23:170-4.
[111] Zamvar VY, Khan NU, Madhavan A, et al. Clinical outcomes in coronary artery bypass graft surgery: comparison of off-pump and on-pump techniques. *Heart Surg. Forum*, 2002;5:109-13.
[112] Velissaris T, Tang A, Murray M, et al. A prospective randomized study to evaluate splanchnic hypoxia during beating-heart and conventional coronary revascularization. *Eur. J. Cardiothorac. Surg.*, 2003;23:917-24.
[113] Watters MPR, Ascione R, Ryder IG, et al. Haemodynamic changes during beating heart coronary surgery with the Bristol Technique. *Eur. J. Cardiothorac. Surg.*, 2001;19:34-40.
[114] Grundeman PF, Borst C, Verlaan CW, et al. Exposure of circumflex branches in the tilted, beating porcine heart: echocardiographic evidence of right ventricular deformation and the effect of right or left heart bypass. *J. Thorac.Cardiovasc. Surg.*, 1999;118:316-323.
[115] Clavien PA, Muller C, Harder F. Treatment of mesenteric infarction. *Br. J. Surg.*, 1987;74:500-3.
[116] Flynn M, Reddy S, Shepherd W, et al. Fast-tracking revisited: routine cardiac surgical patients need minimal intensive care. *Eur. J. Cardiothorac. Surg.*, 2004;25:116-22.
[117] Fiddian-Green RG, Baker S. Predictive value of the stomach wall pH for complications after cardiac operations: comparison with other monitoring. *Crit. Care Med.*, 1987;15:153-6.

In: Off-Pump Coronary Artery Bypass Grafting
Editors: S.G. Raja and M. Amrani
ISBN 978-1-62081-575-5

Chapter 9

OUTCOMES OF OFF-PUMP CORONARY ARTERY BYPASS GRAFTING IN HIGH RISK PATIENTS

Domenico Calcaterra,[1] Tomas A. Salerno[2] and Marco Ricci[2]
[1]Department of Cardiothoracic Surgery,
University of Iowa Carver College of Medicine, Iowa City, IA, US
[2]Division of Cardiothoracic Surgery, University of Miami
Miller School of Medicine/Jackson Memorial Hospital, Miami, FL, US

ABSTRACT

Previous reports have demonstrated that advanced age, chronic lung disease, diabetes, renal dysfunction, atheromatous aorta and severe left ventricular dysfunction are important independent predictors of operative mortality and morbidity after coronary artery bypass grafting (CABG). In addition, cardiopulmonary bypass (CPB) is associated with diffuse systemic inflammatory responses during and after cardiac surgery and may contribute to the morbidity associated with CABG. Off-pump coronary artery bypass (OPCAB) grafting has emerged as an alternative technique allowing coronary revascularization without the risk associated with CPB. The debate on whether off-pump coronary artery bypass grafting (CABG) is superior to "on-pump" CABG in patients requiring coronary interventions remains on-going. In low risk patients, the benefits of off-pump CABG remain unclear. However, there seems to be a benefit in high risk patients. This chapter discusses the potential benefits of off-pump CABG in high risk patients.

INTRODUCTION

Since its introduction in the 1960s, coronary artery bypass surgery using cardiopulmonary bypass and cardioplegic arrest (on-pump) has represented the standard method for treatment of symptomatic multi-vessel coronary artery disease. Off-pump coronary artery revascularization became popular in the 1980s and 1990s with the goal of preventing the complications related to the use of cardiopulmonary bypass. However, the use of this technique was limited initially by the technical difficulty of the operation, until recent years when the introduction of new devices (stabilizers, mister blower, intra-coronary shunts) and the refinement of anesthesia and surgical techniques, has allowed complete revascularization of the heart. For these reasons, off-pump coronary artery surgery has gained renewed interest and many centers around the world elected to use it as the preferential method for coronary artery revascularization in the modern era.

Despite that, the controversy between advocates of one or the other technique has not yet been settled. Several randomized studies comparing outcomes between on-pump and off-pump techniques have shown contradictory results and definitely not a clear advantage of one technique over the other in the treatment of low risk patients. Off-pump surgery seems to be associated with reduced need for blood transfusions, shorter ventilation time, diminished release of myocardial enzymes and probably overall reduction of hospital costs but at expense, according to some, of completeness of revascularization and 1-year graft patency. This has generally led to general equivalency of outcomes in low risk patients. Part of this problem is likely related to the fact that conventional revascularization on-pump has resulted in very satisfactory outcomes with very low morbidity and mortality, a benchmark difficult to match or surpass. High risk patients, however, seem to have improved outcomes, according to most reports, with the off-pump technique.

What follows is a discussion of the aspects related to the potential benefit of off-pump CABG in high-risk patients with coronary artery disease.

ADVANTAGES OF OFF-PUMP CABG

The activation of a systemic inflammatory response and the formation of gaseous, lipoprotein, and particulate emboli associated with cardiopulmonary bypass are responsible for the organ dysfunction affecting the heart, brain, lungs and kidneys. Impairment of the coagulation system affects postoperative bleeding and blood product transfusion requirement with further risk of lung and kidney injury [1]. Also, clamping of the aorta and cardioplegic arrest can be detrimental in patients at higher operative risk and with depressed ventricular function. Therefore, it is intuitive that avoiding the use of CPB and particularly cardioplegic arrest and the resulting myocardial ischemic injury may be beneficial, especially in patients with limited myocardial reserve and pre-existing organ ventricular dysfunction. However, the question remains as to whether off-pump coronary artery revascularization is able to provide the same quality of bypass grafting and outcome as achieved with conventional on-pump techniques. Conventional CABG has been demonstrated to be effective in the treatment of symptomatic multivessel coronary artery disease but it still carries significant risks, in terms of mortality (2-5%), cerebrovascular accidents (2-4%), blood transfusion requirement (30-90%), atrial fibrillation (30%), and neurocognitive dysfunction (50-75%) [2].

One of the largest randomized trials published in 2009 and including 2203 low risk patients showed no benefit of off-pump CABG with regards to death, myocardial infarction and stroke [3]. The rate of graft patency (82.6% versus 87.8%, $P<0.01$) and completeness of revascularization (2.9+/-0.9 and 3.0+/-1.0, $P=0.002$) were lower in the off-pump group. However, the findings from this study could have been impacted by the fact that as many as

759 patients did not undergo follow-up angiograms. Also, it remains unclear whether the operating surgeons were experienced enough with off-pump CABG procedures.

Table 1. Mortality and morbidity in low-risk patients

Clinical Outcomes

Outcome	n (N)	OPCAB %	CCAB %	OR [95%CI]	NNT [95%CI]	Heterogeneity p-value	Heterogeneity I^2	P for Overall Effect
Death, 30d	3082 (29)	1.2	1.0	1.02 [0.58-1.80]	–	1.0	0	0.9
Death, 1-2y	1135 (6)	2.3	2.6	0.88 [0.41-1.88]	–	0.9	0	0.8
Atrial Fibrillation, 30d	2425 (17)	17.6	26.8	0.58 [0.44-0.77]	11 [8-17]	0.07	36	<0.0001
Transfused Patients, 30d	2412 (17)	28.4	42.5	0.43 [0.29-0.65]	7 [6-10]	<0.0001	46	<0.0001
Respiratory Infections, 30d	896 (7)	4.6	9.9	0.41 [0.23-0.74]	19 [12-52]	0.3	21	<0.0001
Inotropes, in hospital	1655 (16)	15.1	23.6	0.48 [0.32-0.73]	12 [8-21]	0.04	43	<0.0001
Cognitive Dysfunction, 2-6mos	393 (3)	20.3	31.8	0.56 [0.35-0.89]	10 [6 to 11]	0.19	39	0.01

Resource Utilization

Outcome	N	WMD [95%CI]	Heterogeneity p-value	Heterogeneity I2	P for Overall Effect
Hospital LOS, d	1384 (17)	–1.0 days [–1.5 to –0.5]	<0.0001	66	<0.0001
ICU LOS, d	1266 (15)	–0.3 days [–0.6 to –0.1]	<0.0001	78	0.003
Ventilation Time, h	1425 (20)	–3.4 hrs [–5.1 to–1.7]	<0.0001	97	<0.0001

NNT = number needed to treat; WMD = weighted mean difference

NNT = number needed to treat; Redo/Urgent = Repeat, urgent, or emergent coronary bypass surgery; WMD = weighted mean difference

(Modified from "Off-pump versus Conventional artery bypass grafting: a meta-analysis and consensus statement from the 2004 ISMIC consensus conference" Innovations 2005:1: 3-27. with permission)

There have been more than 30 randomized clinical trials and several meta-analyses[4,5], including more than 3000 patients, comparing off-pump CABG versus the conventional procedure. In randomized trials of low risk patients, there was no difference in 30-day mortality (Table1) [6-8], but two meta-analyses of mixed-risk groups that also included non-randomized data found reduced risk of mortality at 30 days with off-pump versus on pump procedures. Reston and co-authors showed a 36% reduction in early mortality in a large cohort of patients from 43 class A and B studies combined[5]. Similarly, Wijeysundera and co-authors found a 21% early mortality reduction from the analysis of 14 class B studies [9]. However, this difference disappeared when combined analysis of class A and B studies were done. No difference in 1 to 3 years mortality was found in six randomized controlled studies including 1135 patients. A meta-analysis of these trials confirmed these results (OR 0.88, 95% CI 0.41-1.88; p= 0.8) [10].

Two recent meta-analyses of randomized controlled trials in low risk patients demonstrated similar outcome for both operations in terms of mortality, myocardial infarction and need for repeat revascularization at 1 and 2 years and lesser incidence of perioperative complications (stroke 50%, atrial fibrillation 30%, wound infection 48%, acute renal dysfunction 70%) [11,12].

Many randomized trials also showed a significant reduction in blood product transfusion requirements, inotropic support, intubation time, respiratory infections, and hospital stay following off-pump CABG compared to on-pump CABG [13 14]. A meta-analysis of randomized trials in mixed-risk population showed reduced incidence of blood transfusion requirement (OR 0.43, 95% CI 0.29-0.65, $p < 0.0001$ in 2412 patients), inotrope requirements (OR 0.48, 95% CI 0.32-0.73, $p < 0001$ in 1655 patients), respiratory infection (OR 0.41, 95%

CI 0.23-0.74, 0.0001 in 896 patients), and atrial fibrillation (OR 0.58, 95% CI 0.44-0.77, p = 0001 in 2425 patients)[6]. Randomized trials have shown no difference in terms of stroke, myocardial infarction, acute renal failure, intra-aortic balloon pump requirement, incidence of superficial and deep sternal wound infection, recurrence of angina, or need for re-intervention [6].

Other retrospective studies and two meta-analyses of those studies showed a 40 and 45% reduced incidence of stroke in off-pump versus on-pump CABG[5-9]. Also, a reduction in incidence of myocardial infarction (OR 0.58, 95% CI 0.44-0.76, p < 0.00009 in 24,322 patients), atrial fibrillation (OR 0.69, 95% CI 0.58-0.81, p < 0.00001, in 22,092 patients), renal failure (OR 0.62, 95% CI 0.58-0.78, p =0.00003 in 20,845 patients), re-operation for bleeding (OR 0.54, 95% CI 0.44-0.67, p < 0.0001, in 33,000 patients), wound infection (OR 0.155, 95% CI 0.37-0.83, p = 0.004, in 16,039 patients), and need for re-intervention (OR 3.63, CI 1.91-6.78, p = 0.0001, in 2823 patients) [6].

Another controversial aspect is the prevention of neurocognitive impairment that has been speculated to be one of the major advantages of off-pump procedures. The use of cardiopulmonary bypass has been advocated to be cause of post-operative neurocognitive impairment ("pump head") because of brain hypoperfusion during pump run, formation of macro- and micro-emboli originating from the CPB circuit, systemic inflammatory response syndrome causing cerebral edema and damage to the blood-brain barrier [1]. The term "pump head" has been used to describe a deterioration of intellectual function and memory loss after CPB and is reported to have incidence between 20 and 60 %. Randomized trials looking at cognitive outcomes at 1 month and 2 to 6 month periods gave opposite conclusions [3,15,16]and a meta-analysis of 4 randomized trials looking at neurocognitive outcome at 1 year showed no difference in off-pump versus conventional CABG .In summary, the literature seems unable to give a clear answer on the superiority of one or the other technique in the treatment of coronary artery disease in low risk patients. It appears that surgeon preference and level of comfort with using one or the other technique is the major determinant of off-pump techniques utilization. Off-pump procedures may be technically more difficult and outcomes are partly affected by surgeon's level of experience. Accordingly, there is a longer and steeper learning curve. Grafting of circumflex artery branches, especially if calcified and of small caliber can represent a real challenge. Therefore, low risk patients have probably comparable outcomes in terms of perioperative and 1 to 3-year mortality irrespective of what technique is used. In this setting, the possible advantages of "off-pump" surgery may be outweighed by the risk of incomplete revascularization and lower long term graft patency compared to "on-pump" surgery, which are probably proportionally related to degree of experience of the surgeon with the "off-pump" technique.High risk patients are considered by advocates of off-pump surgery the perfect target population for this technique.

The assumption is that the risks related to the use of cardiopulmonary bypass and cardioplegic arrest are amplified in patients with depressed ventricular function, poor organ reserve and advanced age. The definition of high risk patients in the literature is broad and includes different patient subgroups. Euroscore > 5, left ventricular (LV) dysfunction, atheromatous aorta, increased age (above 70), left main disease, diabetes, renal dysfunction, chronic obstructive pulmonary disease (COPD), hepatic disease, bleeding disorders and patients who refuse blood products define the high risk population. In the off-pump versus conventional coronary artery bypass grafting Consensus Statement[3], mortality of 2.8 vs

4.7% after off-pump versus conventional bypass surgery was identified (OR 0.58, 95% CI 0.49-0.68; $p < 0.0001$) (Table 2).

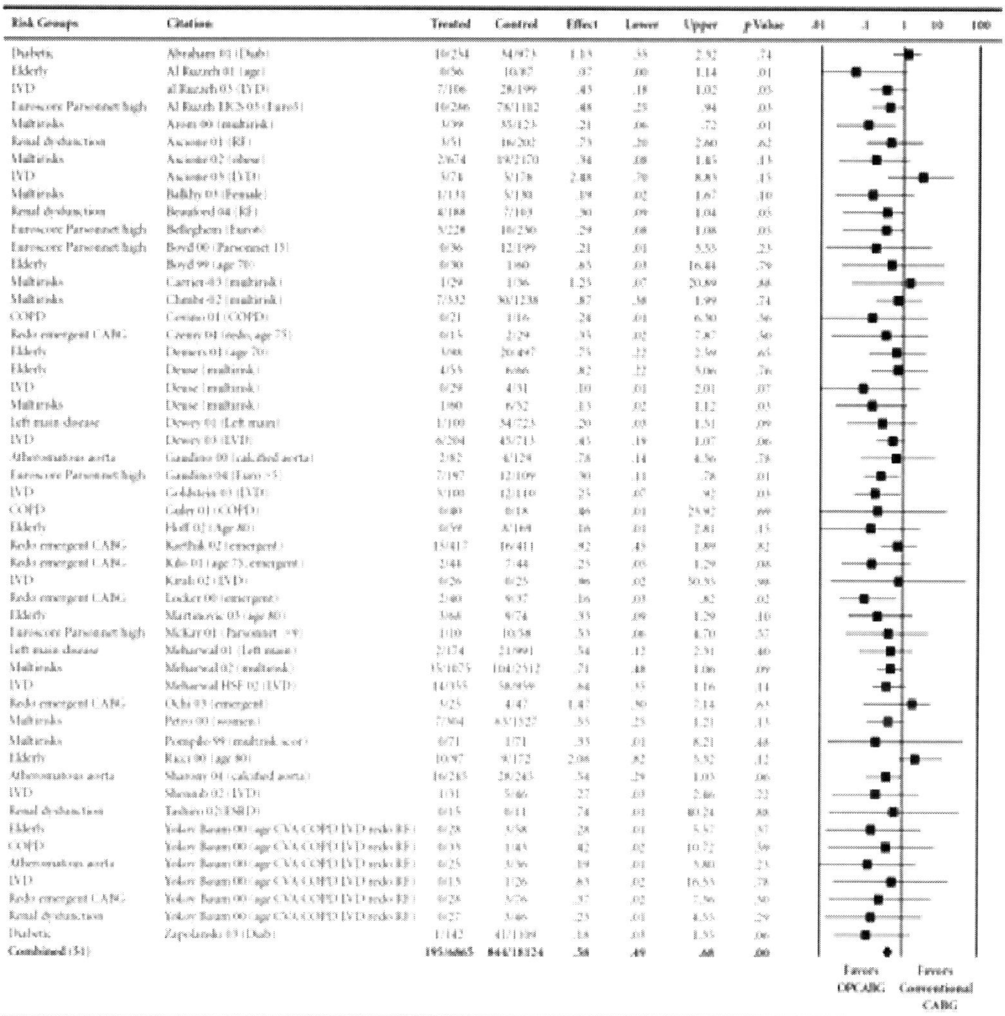

Figure 1. Meta-analysis of clinical outcomes for off-pump vs on-pump CABG in high-risk patients (30day death, stroke, myocardial infarction, atheromatous aorta, atrial fibrillation, transfusions, renal dysfunction, inotropes, IABP, reoperation for bleeding, COPD, diabetes, left main disease. (Modified from "Off-pump versus Conventional artery bypass grafting: a meta-analysis and consensus statement from the 2004 ISMIC consensus conference." Innovations 2005:1: 3-27. with permission).

In addition, pooled analysis showed that mortality was reduced for patients with Euroscore > 5, LV dysfunction, atheromatous aorta (Table 2). In contrast, no effect on early mortality was seen for off-pump CABG versus conventional bypass surgery for patients with increased age, left main disease, diabetes, renal dysfunction and COPD (Figure 1). In the same article, looking at postoperative morbidity, the pooled analysis of all high risk groups combined showed that off-pump CABG significantly reduced overall risk for stroke, myocardial infarction, atrial fibrillation, transfusions, renal dysfunction, inotrope requirement, intra-aortic balloon pump (IABP), and operation for bleeding compared to on-pump surgery (Figure 1). No significant difference was identified for incidence of wound infection (deep or superficial) and pulmonary complications. The consensus is based on the review of 42 non-randomized and 3 randomized trials [17-18].

Table 2. Thirty-day mortality in high-risk patients

						Heterogeneity		
Risk Groups	n (N)	OPCAB %	CCAB %	OR [95%CI]	NNT	p-value [95%CI]	I^2	P for Overall Effect
All Hi-Risk Pts	**24,989 (51)**	**2.8**	**4.7**	**0.58 [0.49-0.68]**	**53**	**0.4**	**3**	**<0.0001**
LVD	**3,223 (9)**	**3.8**	**6.9**	**0.55 [0.38-0.80]**	**32**	**0.3**	**14**	**0.001**
Elderly	1,672 (8)	4.1	5.6	0.79[0.46-1.36]	-	0.2	35	0.4
Left Main	1,988 (2)	1.1	3.2	0.34[0.12-1.25]	-	0.4	0	0.1
Diabetics	2,478 (2)	2.8	3.6	0.92[0.47-1.81]	-	0.07	68	0.8
Renal Dysfunction	643 (4)	2.4	7.2	0.45[0.19-1.03]	-	1.0	0	0.06
Euroscor5+	**2,456 (5)**	**2.6**	**7.1**	**0.39 [0.24-0.63]**	**22**	**0.8**	**0**	**<0.0001**
Multirisks	**10,374 (9)**	**2.6**	**3.8**	**0.60 [0.45-0.81]**	**83**	**0.2**	**27**	**<0.0001**
Aorta, atheromatous	**762 (3)**	**5.1**	**8.5**	**0.54 [0.30-0.98]**	**-**	**0.7**	**0**	**0.04**
Redo/Urgent	1,213 (6)	3.9	6.4	0.65[0.37-1.12]	-	0.3	35	0.1
COPD	171 (3)	0	2.6	0.35[0.05-2.55]	-	0.9	0	0.3

*Meta-analysis of 45 trials including 26,349 highrisk patients (3 randomized and 42 nonrandomized trials)

COPD = chronic obstructive pulmonary disease; Euroscore5+ = High Euroscore/Parsonnet; LOS = Length of stay; LVD = left ventricular dysfunction; NNT = number needed to treat; Redo/Urgent = Repeat, urgent, or emergent coronary bypass surgery; WMD = weighted mean differenceTable 3b: 30-day Stroke in High-Risk Patients [Level B/A]*

(Modified from "Off-pump versus Conventional artery bypass grafting: a meta-analysis and consensus statement from the 2004 ISMIC consensus conference. " Innovations 2005:1: 3-27. with permission)

One of these trials [17], comparing off-pump versus on-pump in high risk patients, showed significant better outcome for composite end-points including death, neurological injury, renal failure, respiratory failure, and operative myocardial infarction in favor of off-pump surgery (p = 0.02). The study included 65 patients prospectively randomized who met multiple criteria for being high-risk, such us, age greater than 65, hypertension, diabetes, elevated serum creatinine, left ventricular ejection fraction below 45%, chronic pulmonary disease, unstable angina, congestive heart failure, redo surgery, anemia and carotid artery disease.

EUROSCORE GREATER THAN 5

The literature currently available seems to suggest, although for the most part based on retrospective analyses, the advantage of off-pump versus on-pump coronary artery bypass in the treatment of patients with multiple risk factors. These results of these studies seem to offer more consistent data in support of off-pump coronary artery surgery compared to studies recruiting low risk patients where results are often contradictory and biased by the surgical group preference and experience. These data on high risk populations seem to identify specific patients subgroups that may benefit from off-pump surgery: patients with Euroscore > 5, left ventricular dysfunction, elderly, patients with atheromatous aorta, acute myocardial infarction (MI), chronic lung disease, liver disease, renal dysfunction, diabetes and patients who refuse blood product transfusions. The results at 3 years of the Best Bypass Surgery Trial were recently published [19]. This single center prospective randomized trial study looked at primary outcome in terms of a composite of major adverse cardiac events (MACCE), including all-cause mortality, acute MI, cardiac arrest with successful resuscitation, low cardiac output syndrome/cardiogenic shock, stroke, and coronary re-intervention. Three-hundred forty-one patients with three vessel disease and EuroScore > 5 were randomly assigned to undergo off-pump or on-pump CABG. The procedures were performed by three surgeons experienced with both techniques in a surgical center where 20-25 % of all coronary artery revascularization procedures are performed off-pump. There were no statistically significant differences in the primary outcome of MACCE between the two groups. A non-significant reduction in 30-day mortality was observed in the off-pump group: 3.4 versus 6.7 % (RR 0.5; 95 % CI o.19-1.34; p=0.21). However, the tendency towards the superiority of off-pump CABG disappeared during the extended follow-up, where off-pump CABG turned out to have significantly increased mortality compared to the on-pump group (24 versus 15%; 95 % CI 1.02-2.73; p = 0.04). Myocardial infarction was detected in 13 off-pump patients compared to 23 on pump patients (7 versus 14 %; 95 % CI 0.27-1.04; p = 0.06). Of these, nine patients in the off-pump group compared to 13 patients on the on-pump group had a myocardial infarction within the first postoperative 48 hours.

ELDERLY PATIENTS

In 2 non-randomized retrospective studies, Hoff [20] and Hirose [21] looked at a specific subgroup of older adult patients, respectively older than 75 and 80. Patient outcome in terms of postoperative mortality and incidence of complications were compared between patients undergoing off-pump revascularization versus patients undergoing traditional surgery. Incidence of stroke, prolonged respiratory failure, bleeding, transfusions, and ICU and hospital length of stay were all higher in the standard CABG group. Re-operation for bleeding, MI, renal failure, wound infection, and operative mortality were not significantly different. Ricci and Salerno [22], analyzed retrospectively a group of 269 octogenarians undergoing coronary artery revascularization with off-pump or on-pump technique. Patients in the off-pump group had a statistically significant lower incidence of stroke (0 versus 9.3%; p = 0.04) and overall postoperative complications (85.6 versus 75%; p = 0.04) compared to the on-pump group. Nevertheless, patients in the off-pump group experienced a trend for higher 30-day mortality which was not statistically significant and could have been influenced by the significantly higher proportion of redo operations in the off-pump cohort (16.5 versus 4.7%; p = 0.002). In a recent publication, LaPar and co-authors [23] looked retrospectively at a large cohort of patients (80 and older) undergoing coronary artery revascularization. A total of 1993 patients were stratified in two groups: conventional coronary artery bypass (1589) and off-pump bypass (404). Compared to off-pump CABG, conventional bypass surgery required more blood transfusions (2 +/- 1.7 versus 1.6+/- 1.9; p = 0.05), and had higher incidence of atrial fibrillation (28.4 versus 21.5 %; p = 0.003), prolonged ventilation (14.7 versus 11.4 %; p = 0.05), and major postoperative complications (20.1 versus 15.6 %; p = 0.04). Postoperative stroke (2.6 versus 1.7 %; p = 0.21), renal failure (8.1 versus 6.2 %; p = 0.12), and postoperative length of stay were similar. However, despite more complications in patients having conventional bypass, mortality and hospital costs were similar between the two groups.

Left Ventricular Dysfunction

Three recent studies [24-26] have reviewed in a retrospective non-randomized fashion the outcomes of patients with coronary artery disease and ejection fraction (EF) < 35% undergoing surgical revascularization with off-pump or on-pump technique. In 2 of the 3 studies, standard CABG patients had significantly more grafts performed compared to the off-pump group. There were no significant differences in MI, renal failure, bleeding, wound infections, or stroke. Thirty-day mortality rates tended to be higher in the standard CABG patient group (14.1 versus 6.6%; p = 0.05). In one study, mid-term survival at 1, 2 and 3 years was slightly higher (92 versus 85%, 90 versus 82% and 87 versus 73 %) in the standard CABG group. However, these differences were not statistically significant. Sharoni and co-authors [26], reviewed retrospectively a group of 353 patients with EF < 35% undergoing coronary artery bypass. A group of 144 off-pump patients was compared to 209 patients operated with standard on-pump method. Patients in the off-pump group were more likely to be women, to have congestive heart failure, chronic obstructive pulmonary disease, hypertension and diabetes. The groups did not differ significantly in length of stay, major postoperative complications rates, or mortality. On the other hand, comparison of the impact of the procedure on the surgical method over time showed an increase in the use of off-pump CABG (13 versus 67%), without impact on morbidity or mortality. The conclusion of the study was that off-pump CABG is feasible and applicable for patients with depressed ventricular function and that this high risk group can potentially benefit from the off-pump approach.

Atheromatous Aorta

Off-pump surgery does not prevent manipulation of the aorta because it requires application of side-biting clamp to the ascending aorta for completion of proximal anastomoses but prevents the need for aortic cannulation. This has been advocated by some as a possible advantage of off- pump techniques in reducing the risk of cerebrovascular accidents. Many reports in the literature, although retrospective, seem to show the advantage of off-pump procedures in reducing the risk of stroke compared to conventional coronary surgery. Djaiani [27] and colleagues, published a result of a small study where a group of patients (n = 13) with aortic atheroma > 2 mm undergoing on-pump revascularization was compared to a risk-adjusted prospective cohort of patients (n = 13) undergoing off-pump surgery.

Transesophageal echocardiography and epiaortic scanning were performed to assess the proximal thoracic aorta in the two groups. Patients were evaluated for new ischemic brain lesions utilizing DW-MRI three to seven days after surgery. The average maximum thickness of the atheroma was comparable in the two groups (5.0 +/- 2.0 mm versus 4.8 +/- 1.9 mm). The prevalence of new ischemic brain lesions on DW-MRI was 0% in the off-pump versus 61% in the on-pump group (p = 0.001). Despite the small sample the study provides valuable data that can support the lower incidence of stroke in off-pump surgery. In two different retrospective non-randomized studies Sharony and colleagues [26,28] addressed the question of whether coronary artery revascularization in patients with severely atheromatous aorta should be performed off-pump. Mortality and stroke were higher in the standard CABG group.

Chronic Lung Disease

In a recent publication Kerendi [29] and co-authors tried to determine whether off-pump lowers the incidence of pulmonary complications among patients with chronic lung disease when compared with on-pump surgery. Of 7,060 patients undergoing coronary artery revascularization, 4,693 underwent off-pump CABG and 2,367 underwent traditional CABG. In the off-pump group 720 patients (15.3%) had chronic lung disease compared to 264 patients (11.2%) in the on-pump group. Off-pump surgery was performed in 73.2% of patients with chronic lung disease compared to 66.5% in those without ($p < 0.0001$). Chronic lung disease was associated with a greater incidence of prolonged ventilation, reintubation, pneumonia, ICU length of stay. After propensity score adjustment, off-pump surgery was associated with a significantly reduced incidence of prolonged ventilation, pneumonia, ICU stay and mortality.

Liver Disease

Cardiopulmonary bypass activates production and release of multiple vasoactive substances and cytotoxic mediators that affect the coagulation system, immune response, vascular resistance, vascular permeability, fluid balance and overall function of multiple organs. Therefore, off-pump revascularization may be advantageous in avoiding complications related to the use of cardiopulmonary bypass in patients with liver disease. The literature provides paucity of data regarding the outcome of patients with cirrhosis undergoing cardiac surgery. The general consensus [30-31] is that Child-Turcotte-Pugh class A carries a mortality of 10 to 25%, whereas Class B has mortality between 40 and 80 % and class C has a mortality of approximately 100 %. In the small series published, the reported experience with off-pump coronary artery revascularization is limited although significant. Hayashida [32]and Filsoufi [33]report respectively, 3 (all Child B) and 5 cases (mixed A and B class) performed off-pump. Mortality was 0%. These data may suggest that the avoidance of cardiopulmonary bypass may be beneficial in these patients, who present with significant preoperative organ dysfunction and hematologic disturbances [33]. In our experience of 6 consecutive patients with cirrhosis (4 Child A, and 3 Child B), all undergoing off-pump coronary artery revascularization, no mortality was recorded.

Renal Dysfunction

Postoperative acute renal failure is a serious complication of coronary artery revascularization and is associated with remarkable increase of morbidity and mortality [34,35]. Based on the patient population studied and the definition of renal failure used, the incidence of acute renal failure is reported to be from 1 to 30% and the associated reported risk of death ranges from 7 to 38% [36]. In a small controlled randomized trial including 22 low-risk patients undergoing coronary revascularization

(10 off pump vs 12 on-pump), Loef and associates [37] showed that "off-pump" procedures induced significantly fewer changes in microalbuminuria ($p < 0.01$), free sodium clearance ($p < 0.05$), free water clearance ($p < 0.01$), N-acetyl glucosaminidase activity ($p < 0.01$), and free hemoglobin ($p < 0.01$) compared to on-pump. These findings seem to suggest that off-pump CABG can potentially offer better renal protection than conventional coronary surgery performed using cardiopulmonary bypass and cardioplegic arrest. These findings were contradicted, however, by the results of another small randomized controlled trial by Tang and co-authors [38], who enrolled 40 low-risk patients with normal renal function undergoing coronary artery bypass surgery. This study showed that, although no changes in serum markers of renal dysfunction occurred, a similar degree of renal tubules and glomerular injury was present after both conventional and off-pump coronary revascularization. Accordingly, the larger retrospective analysis published [39] and looking at whether off-pump coronary artery bypass surgery prevented renal dysfunction in patients at high risk for renal failure (preoperative creatinine clearance < 60 ml/min), failed to show an advantage in favor of off-pump surgery. The conclusion of the study is that preoperative renal function should not be a deciding factor when determining whether or not a patient undergoes off-pump coronary artery surgery. These findings seem to suggest that off-pump surgery offers no added protection to low-risk individuals against perioperative renal dysfunction even in patient with pre-existing renal function impairment. However, findings may differ in high risk patients [40 41], with normal or compromised preoperative renal function, in whom the avoidance of cardiopulmonary bypass, by eliminating activation of the systemic inflammatory response and the multi-organ dysfunction possibly associated with it, might prevent renal hypoperfusion and damage with progressive impairment of renal function.

DIABETES

Diabetes mellitus is a well-established predictor for adverse outcome after both surgical and percutaneous revascularization [42]. Affected patients often present with advanced and more diffuse disease, often in association with renal dysfunction and peripheral vascular disease, compared to nondiabetic patients. In a recently published non-randomized retrospective study Emmert and colleagues [43] looked at 1015 diabetic patients who underwent myocardial revascularization. Patients underwent either off-pump coronary artery bypass (n = 540, 53%) or conventional coronary artery bypass grafting (n = 475; 47%). Data collection was performed prospectively and data analysis was done by propensity score-adjusted regression analysis. Off-pump patients had a significantly lower mortality rate (1.1 % versus 3.8 %; OR = 0.28; CI 95 % 0.11-0.72; $p = 0.008$) and suffered from significantly less major adverse cardiac events (MACCE: death, myocardial infarction, recurrent angina, stroke) (8.3% versus 17.9%; OR 0.41; CI 95% 0.28-0.61; $p < 0.001$) and major noncardiac adverse events (MNCAE: respiratory failure, prolonged ventilation, reoperation for bleeding) (99.4 % versus 18.5 %; OR 0.46; CI 95 % 0.31-0.66; $p < 0.001$). In particular, "off-pump" patients showed significant benefit with regard to stroke (0.7 versus 2.3 %; $p = 0.043$), reoperation for bleeding (3.9 versus 6.7 %; $p = 0.044$), need for IABP placement (0.2 versus

2.5 %; $p = 0.011$), frequency of prolonged ventilation (7.3 versus 14.3 %; $p = 0.01$). Also, the frequency of myocardial infarction (91.3 versus 3.2 %; $p = 0.12$), graft occlusion (1.4 versus 2.1 %; $p = 0.52$), and renal failure (4.1 versus 6.3 %; $p = 0.63$) was lower in the off-pump group, but failed to achieve statistical significance. The study concluded that off-pump coronary artery bypass offers a lower mortality and superior postoperative outcomes in diabetic patients with multivessel disease.

PATIENTS REFUSING TRANSFUSION OF BLOOD AND BLOOD PRODUCTS

It is estimated that at least 50% of cardiac surgery patients require blood product transfusions in the course of their hospitalization [44]. The use of cardiopulmonary bypass causes hemodilution, depletion of coagulation factors and platelet dysfunction[1,45]. Moreover, cardiac surgery for its own nature exposes to high risk of bleeding and 3 to 5% of patients require surgical exploration because of postoperative hemorrhage [46]. Increased blood loss, reoperation for bleeding, and requirement of blood product transfusions is a consistent finding in prospective randomized trials, matched cohort studies and retrospective analysis of patients undergoing on-pump versus off-pump coronary artery revascularization [47,48]. Therefore, it appears that off-pump surgery offers an advantage compared to on-pump surgery in the treatment of patients who do not accept blood and blood-product transfusions. In our experience of 8 Jehovah's witnesses patients who underwent off-pump coronary bypass surgery between November 2008 and May 2011, there were no mortality and no re-exploration for bleeding (unpublished data, Calcaterra D).

CONCLUSION

At present, in the long-standing controversy between on-pump and off-pump coronary artery revascularization, a strong body of evidence is lacking in support of the superiority of one technique over the other, at least in low risk patients. In the low risk patient population, no difference in 30-day and 1 to 3-year mortality were identified in prospective randomized trials (Level A)[6]. It has been suggested that a difference in mortality, if present, may be difficult to determine as it would require a large cohort of patients to reach statistical significance [10]. For instance, a 30-day mortality difference of 0.2 % between the two groups, as seen in pooled analysis of randomized trials [6], requires a pool of 85,000 patients to be significant [6,8]. Nevertheless, in a mixed-risk population, off-pump is associated with reduced risk of perioperative atrial fibrillation, blood transfusions, inotropic requirement, and respiratory infections (Level A) [6]. Also, level B evidence exists for potential reduction in additional perioperative morbidity, including stroke, myocardial infarction, renal failure, reoperation for bleeding, wound infection, and re-intervention [6]. The number of grafts performed and completeness of revascularization is slightly reduced with "off-pump" procedures (evidence level A and B) [6], but this does not translate in increased need for revascularization or re-intervention. In contrast, the results of the ROOBY trial showed that completeness of revascularization and 1-year graft patency was better for the on-pump group but level of the experience of the surgeons with off-pump technique and the fact that 759 of the 2127 patient alive at one year did not undergo follow-up angiogram provide major confounding factors to question the study results [3]. Another question that remains to be answered is whether the slightly lower number of grafts per patients generally reported in the literature has clinical significance. Based on the above, regarding the efficacy of off-pump versus on-pump coronary artery bypass surgery in low risk patients, off-pump is as effective and safe as on-pump surgery with a benefit seen in terms of decreased incidence of postoperative complications, blood transfusions, and inotropic requirement.

In high-risk patients undergoing coronary artery bypass surgery, observational studies seem to suggest a significant benefit of off-pump surgery as compared to on-pump CABG. The recently published Best Bypass Surgery Trial aimed to evaluate 30-day outcomes in 341 high-risk patients randomly assigned to undergo either on-pump or off-pump surgery. No significant differences in their composite primary outcome were seen. Within a 30-day follow up a statistically non-significant reduction in mortality was seen in the off-pump group (3.4 versus 6.7%; $p = 0.21$). The tendency towards superiority of off-pump disappeared during extensive follow-up (3.7 years) and the off-pump group turned out to have increased mortality (24 versus 14 %, $p = 0.04$). This trial, however, did not truly recruit high-risk patients and was performed in a center with no extensive experience with off-pump procedures (only 25% of all coronary artery bypass surgery operations were performed off-pump). Nevertheless, as discussed in this chapter, although based on the analysis of nonrandomized retrospective studies, the literature seems to support the advantage of off-pump coronary artery surgery in subgroups of high-risk patients, such as patients with EuroSCORE > 5, left ventricular dysfunction, elderly, patients with atheromatous aorta, acute MI, chronic lung disease, liver disease, renal dysfunction, diabetes, and patients not willing to accept blood product transfusions.

Multi-center, randomized controlled trials are needed to further support the observed advantage of off-pump surgery in the treatment of high risk patients. Currently, there are two multi-center prospective randomized trials underway aiming at evaluating the efficacy of off-pump surgery in high risk patients [49]. The CRISP trial is an international multi-center trial randomly assigning more than 5000 high risk patients to off-pump or on-pump coronary revascularization. The study design is “expertise-based”, where patients are randomly assigned to previously specified surgeons within the institution who favor and practice primarily either off-pump or on-pump surgery. The German Off-Pump Coronary Artery Bypass in Elderly (GOPCABE), is a multi-center trial randomly allocating 2000 patients older than 75 to undergo either off-pump or on-pump procedure.

In conclusion, from an unbiased revision of the literature, it can be stated that there is a substantial wealth of evidence demonstrating that off-pump surgery is a safe alternative to conventional coronary artery revascularization, with similar outcome for low risk patients. The greatest benefit of off-pump surgery is most likely to be seen in high risk patients and results from the ongoing prospective trials are eagerly awaited.

Off-pump surgery is technically demanding and should be performed in high-volume off-pump centers to obtain adequate proficiency and optimal outcomes. In our opinion, the procedure needs to be founded on the principles of (1) aiming at complete coronary revascularization with meticulous anastomotic technique, (2) maintaining adequate intraoperative hemodynamics through the use of an expert anesthesia technique, (3) using intra-coronary shunts during completion of distal anastomosis, and (4) obtaining graft patency assessment with intraoperative ultrasound flow measurement.

In the analysis of the controversy between on-pump and off-pump surgery in the literature, it appears obvious that the interpretation of study results seem always to be influenced by the authors' surgical preference and belief in one or the other technique. Similarly, we may be in the difficult position of not seeing our own personal bias towards off-pump coronary artery surgery based on the fact that our groups predominantly use the technique of off-pump surgery for coronary artery revascularization. Nevertheless, we believe that off-pump surgery, despite being technically challenging difficulty and with a steeper learning curve, offers major advantages compared to on-pump surgery in the treatment of coronary artery disease, particularly in the high risk patient population.

REFERENCES

[1] Murphy GJ, Angelini GD. Side Effects of Cardiopulmonary Bypass. *J. Card. Surg.,* 2004;19:481-488.

[2] SOS. Coronary artery bypass surgery versus percutaneous coronary intervention with stent implantation in patients with multivessel coronary artery disease (the Stent or Surgery trial): a randomised controlled trial. *Lancet,* 2002;360:965-970.

[3] Shroyer AL, Grover FL, Hattler B, et al. On-pump versus off-pump coronary-artery bypass surgery. *N. Engl. J. Med.,* 2009;361:1827-1837.

[4] Cheng DC, Bainbridge D, Martin JE, Novick RJ. Does off-pump coronary artery bypass reduce mortality, morbidity, and resource utilization when compared with conventional coronary artery bypass? A meta-analysis of randomized trials. *Anesthesiology,* 2005;102:188-203.

[5] Reston JT, Tregear SJ, Turkelson CM. Meta-analysis of short-term and mid-term outcomes following off-pump coronary artery bypass grafting. *Ann. Thorac. Surg.,* 2003;76:1510-1515.

[6] Puskas J, Cheng D, Knight J, et al. Off-pump versus conventional coronary artery bypass grafting: a meta-analysis and consensus statement from the 2004 ISMICS consensus conference. Innovations: *Technology and Techniques in Cardiothoracic and Vascular Surgery,* 2005;1:3.

[7] Puskas JD, Williams WH, Duke PG, et al. Off-pump coronary artery bypass grafting provides complete revascularization with reduced myocardial injury, transfusion requirements, and length of stay: A prospective randomized comparison of two hundred unselected patients undergoing off-pump versus conventional coronary artery bypass grafting. *J. Thorac. Cardiovasc. Surg.,* 2003;125:797-808.

[8] Puskas JD, Williams WH, O'Donnell R, et al. Off-pump and on-pump coronary artery bypass grafting are associated with similar graft patency, myocardial ischemia, and freedom from reintervention: long-term follow-up of a randomized trial. *Ann. Thorac. Surg.,* 2011;91:1836-1842.

[9] Wijeysundera DN, Beattie WS, Djaiani G, et al. Off-Pump Coronary Artery Surgery for Reducing Mortality and Morbidity: Meta-Analysis of Randomized and Observational Studies. *J. Am. Coll. Cardiol.,* 2005;46:872-882.

[10] Cheng DC, Bainbridge D, Martin JE, Novick RJ. Does off-pump coronary artery bypass reduce mortality, morbidity, and resource utilization when compared with conventional coronary artery bypass? A meta-analysis of randomized trials. *Anesthesiology,* 2005;102:188-203.

[11] Feng Z-Z, Shi J, Zhao X-W, Xu Z-F. Meta-analysis of on-pump and off-pump coronary arterial revascularization. *Ann. Thorac. Surg.,* 2009;87:757-765.

[12] Møller CH, Penninga L, Wetterslev J, Steinbrüchel DA, Gluud C. Clinical outcomes in randomized trials of off- vs. on-pump coronary artery bypass surgery: systematic review with meta-analyses and trial sequential analyses. *Eur.. Heart,* . 2008;29:2601-2616.

[13] van Dijk D, Nierich AP, Jansen EWL, et al. Early outcome after off-pump versus on-pump coronary bypass surgery. *Circulation,* 2001;104:1761 -1766.

[14] Hernandez F, Cohn WE, Baribeau YR, et al. Northern New England Cardiovascular Disease Study Group. In-hospital outcomes of off-pump versus on-pump coronary artery bypass procedures: a multicenter experience. *Ann. Thorac. Surg.,* 2001;72:1528-1533.

[15] Lee JD, Lee SJ, Tsushima WT, et al. Benefits of off-pump bypass on neurologic and clinical morbidity: a prospective randomized trial. *Ann. Thorac. Surg.,* 2003;76:18-26.

[16] Jensen BO, Hughes P, Rasmussen LS, Pedersen PU, Steinbrüchel DA. Cognitive outcomes in elderly high-risk patients after off-pump versus conventional coronary artery bypass grafting: a randomized trial. *Circulation,* 2006;113:2790-2795.

[17] Vicol C, Oberhoffer M, Nollert G, et al. First clinical experience with the HEARTSTRING, a device for proximal anastomoses in coronary surgery. *Ann. Thorac. Surg.,* 2005;79:1732-1737.

[18] Subramanian VA, Patel NU, Patel NC, Loulmet DF. Robotic assisted multivessel minimally invasive direct coronary artery bypass with port-access stabilization and cardiac positioning: paving the way for outpatient coronary surgery? *Ann. Thorac. Surg.,* 2005;79:1590-1596.

[19] Møller CH, Perko MJ, Lund JT, et al. No major differences in 30-day outcomes in high-risk patients randomized to off-pump versus on-pump coronary bypass surgery: the best bypass surgery trial. *Circulation,* 2010;121:498-504.

[20] Hoff SJ, Ball SK, Coltharp WH, et al. Coronary artery bypass in patients 80 years and over: is off-pump the operation of choice? *Ann. Thorac. Surg.,* 2002;74:S1340-1343.

[21] Hirose H, Amano A, Takahashi A. Off-pump coronary artery bypass grafting for elderly patients. *Ann. Thorac. Surg.,* 2001;72:2013-2019.

[22] Ricci M, Karamanoukian HL, Abraham R, et al. Stroke in octogenarians undergoing coronary artery surgery with and without cardiopulmonary bypass. *Ann. Thorac. Surg.,* 2000;69:1471-1475.

[23] LaPar DJ, Bhamidipati CM, Reece TB, et al. Is off-pump coronary artery bypass grafting superior to conventional bypass in octogenarians? *J. Thorac. Cardiovasc. Surg.,* 2011;141:81-90.

[24] Al-Ruzzeh S, Athanasiou T, George S, et al. Is the use of cardiopulmonary bypass for multivessel coronary artery bypass surgery an independent predictor of operative mortality in patients with ischemic left ventricular dysfunction? *Ann. Thorac. Surg.,* 2003;76:444-451.

[25] Sellke FW, DiMaio JM, Caplan LR, et al. Comparing on-pump and off-pump coronary artery bypass grafting. *Circulation,* 2005;111:2858–2864.

[26] Sharoni E, Song HK, Peterson RJ, Guyton RA, Puskas JD. Off pump coronary artery bypass surgery for significant left ventricular dysfunction: safety, feasibility, and trends in methodology over time--an early experience. *Heart,* 2006;92:499-502.

[27] Djaiani G, Fedorko L, Cusimano RJ, et al. Off-pump coronary bypass surgery: risk of ischemic brain lesions in patients with atheromatous thoracic aorta. *Can. J. Anaesth.,* 2006;53:795-801.

[28] Sharony R, Grossi EA, Saunders PC, et al. Propensity case-matched analysis of off-pump coronary artery bypass grafting in patients with atheromatous aortic disease. *J. Thorac. Cardiovasc. Surg.,* 2004;127:406-413.

[29] Kerendi F, Halkos ME, Puskas JD, et al. Impact of off-pump coronary artery bypass graft surgery on postoperative pulmonary complications in patients with chronic lung disease. *Ann. Thorac. Surg.,* 2011;91:8-15.

[30] Marui A, Kimura T, Tanaka S, et al. Coronary revascularization in patients with liver cirrhosis. *Ann. Thorac. Surg.,* 2011;91:1393-1399.

[31] Shaheen AAM, Kaplan GG, Hubbard JN, Myers RP. Morbidity and mortality following coronary artery bypass graft surgery in patients with cirrhosis: a population-based study. *Liver. Int.,* 2009;29:1141-1151.

[32] Hayashida N, Aoyagi S. Cardiac operations in cirrhotic patients. *Ann. Thorac. Cardiovasc. Surg.,* 2004;10:140-147.

[33] Filsoufi F, Salzberg SP, Rahmanian PB, et al. Early and late outcome of cardiac surgery in patients with liver cirrhosis. *Liver. Transpl.,* 2007;13:990-995.

[34] Chertow GM, Lazarus JM, Christiansen CL, et al. Preoperative renal risk stratification. *Circulation,* 1997;95:878-884.

[35] Conlon PJ, Stafford-Smith M, White WD, et al. Acute renal failure following cardiac surgery. Nephrology Dialysis *Transplantation,* 1999;14:1158 -1162.

[36] Stallwood MI, Grayson AD, Mills K, Scawn ND. Acute renal failure in coronary artery bypass surgery: independent effect of cardiopulmonary bypass. *Ann. Thorac. Surg.,* 2004;77:968-972.

[37] Loef BG, Epema AH, Navis G, et al. Off-pump coronary revascularization attenuates transient renal damage compared with on-pump coronary revascularization. *Chest,* 2002;121:1190-1194.

[38] Tang ATM, Knott J, Nanson J, et al. A prospective randomized study to evaluate the renoprotective action of beating heart coronary surgery in low risk patients. *Eur. J. Cardiothorac. Surg.,* 2002;22:118-123.

[39] Chukwuemeka A, Weisel A, Maganti M, et al. Renal dysfunction in high-risk patients after on-pump and off-pump coronary artery bypass surgery: a propensity score analysis. *Ann. Thorac. Surg.,* 2005;80:2148-2153.

[40] Raja SG, Amrani M. Evidence for efficacy of off-pump coronary artery bypass surgery: Facts and fads. J Thorac Cardiovasc Surg 2011;142:723.

[41] Raja SG. Pump or no pump for coronary artery bypass. *Tex. Heart Inst. J.,* 2005;32:489-501.

[42] Cohen Y, Raz I, Merin G, Mozes B. Comparison of factors associated with 30-day mortality after coronary artery bypass grafting in patients with versus without diabetes

mellitus. Israeli Coronary Artery Bypass (ISCAB) Study Consortium. *Am. J. Cardiol.*, 1998;81:7-11.

[43] Emmert MY, Salzberg SP, Seifert B, et al. Is off-pump superior to conventional coronary artery bypass grafting in diabetic patients with multivessel disease? *Eur. J. Cardiothorac. Surg.*, 2011;40:233-239.

[44] Ferraris VA, Ferraris SP, Saha SP, et al. Perioperative Blood Transfusion and Blood Conservation in Cardiac Surgery: The Society of Thoracic Surgeons and The Society of Cardiovascular Anesthesiologists Clinical Practice Guideline. *Ann. Thorac. Surg.*, 2007;83(5, Supplement):S27-S86.

[45] Moraca RJ, Wanamaker KM, Bailey SH, et al. Strategies and outcomes of cardiac surgery in Jehovah's Witnesses. *J. Card. Surg.*, 2011;26:135-143.

[46] Ereth MH, Nuttall GA, Oliver Jr WC, et al. Temperature and duration of cardiopulmonary bypass influence transfusion requirements. *J. Clin. Anesth.*, 1998;10:588-592.

[47] Ascione R, Williams S, Lloyd CT, et al. Reduced postoperative blood loss and transfusion requirement after beating-heart coronary operations: A prospective randomized study. *J. Thorac. Cardiovasc. Surg.*, 2001;121:689-696.

[48] Yokoyama T, Baumgartner FJ, Gheissari A, et al. Off-pump versus on-pump coronary bypass in high-risk subgroups. *Ann. Thorac. Surg*., 2000;70:1546-1550.

[49] Patel NN, Angelini GD. Off-pump coronary artery bypass grafting: for the many or the few? *J. Thorac. Cardiovasc. Surg*., 2010;140:951-953.e1.

In: Off-Pump Coronary Artery Bypass Grafting
Editors: S.G. Raja and M. Amrani
ISBN 978-1-62081-575-5

Chapter 10

OUTCOMES OF OFF-PUMP CORONARY ARTERY BYPASS GRAFTING IN ELDERLY

Shahzad G. Raja[1] and Mohamed Amrani[2]
[1]Cardiac Surgeon, Harefield Hospital, London, UK
[2]Senior Cardiac & Transplant Surgeon, Harefield Hospital, Honorary Senior Lecturer, Imperial College, London, UK

ABSTRACT

Worldwide the elderly population is growing at a very fast pace, and with it its burden of cardiovascular diseases. The incidence and severity of coronary artery disease increase with age. Compared with younger patients, the elderly have more severe disease, frequent comorbidities, and a higher perioperative mortality and morbidity. Current percutaneous and surgical myocardial revascularization therapies are quite efficient in improving life expectancy and relieving symptoms in this high risk subgroup of patients. Over the last decade, operative mortality has decreased significantly among the elderly patients undergoing coronary artery bypass grafting, even though prevalence of preoperative risk factors has constantly increased, shifting the emphasis from mortality to morbidity. Evidence from randomized controlled trials as well as observational studies suggests that off-pump coronary artery bypass surgery has the potential to attenuate occurrence of common and morbid complications after coronary artery bypass grafting in high risk patients. For elderly patients off-pump coronary artery bypass surgery can offer benefits in terms of operative mortality and reduction of common postoperative complications contributing to improve quality of life of these fragile patients. This chapter provides an overview of the age-related cardiovascular changes, epidemiology of coronary artery disease in the elderly and focuses on outcomes of surgical myocardial revascularization with special emphasis on the impact of off-pump coronary artery bypass surgery in elderly.

INTRODUCTION

The elderly population in the Western world is growing exponentially. The age group defined as "elderly" in the literature has gradually increased from ≥65 years to ≥80 years. The greatest increase in numbers undergoing heart surgery has occurred in the oldest group of persons, those aged ≥85 years [1]. Among the 25 000 coronary artery bypass grafting (CABG) operations performed every year in the United Kingdom, almost a quarter of the patients are aged >70 years, and 8% are >75 years [2]. This ageing surgical population, not unexpectedly, has a relatively greater prevalence of cerebrovascular disease, left ventricular dysfunction, diabetes mellitus, chronic obstructive pulmonary disease, renal impairment and peripheral arterial disease [3-5]. Therefore, such elderly people with multiple comorbidities tend to have a high rate of complications after CABG.3 Indeed, old age alone (ie, >75 years) is an independent risk factor for poor outcomes after CABG [4].

AGE-RELATED CARDIOVASCULAR CHANGES

In all, 80% of patients >80 years have identifiable cardiovascular disease [6]. Age-related changes occur in small and large vessels and in the heart itself, reducing physiological reserves. Most patients show no signs of impaired hemodynamic performance at baseline, but stresses of anesthesia will often uncover their limited cardiac reserve [6].

Heart

Aging is associated with numerous molecular, ionic, biophysical and biochemical changes in the heart [5,7,8]. These changes affect protein function, mitochondrial oxidative phosphorylation, calcium kinetics, excitation-contraction coupling, myofilament activation, contractile response, matrix composition and regeneration, cell growth and size, and apoptosis [5].

Age-related changes in cardiac morphology are mostly the result of alterations of intracellular molecular and biochemical pathways. In turn, many of the changes in cardiac function with advancing age develop in response to underlying alterations in morphology. Ultimately, cardiac ageing results in decreased mechanical and contractile efficiency, prolongation of the relaxation phase, stiffening of myocardial cells, mural connective tissue and valves, decreased number of myocytes, increased myocyte size, increased rate of myocyte apoptosis and blunted β-adrenoceptor-mediated contractile and inotropic response [9-11].

Vasculature

Aging affects various aspects of vascular morphology and function. The large arteries dilate, their walls thicken, the wall matrix changes, elastolytic and collagenolytic activity increases and smooth muscle tone increases. As a result, vascular stiffness increases with advancing age [8,12,13]. Increased vascular stiffness leads to elevated systolic arterial pressure and pulse-wave velocity, and to early reflected pulse pressure waves and late peak systolic pressure, thereby augmenting aortic impedance and cardiac mechanical load [8]. In this way, arterial stiffening triggers a variety of cardiac adjustments. Some of these adjustments are additional and are similar to the age-related intrinsic changes in cardiac morphology and may, therefore, be expected to worsen cardiac performance [13].

Coronary Circulation

Aging is associated with structural and functional changes in the coronary vasculature, which could affect myocardial perfusion with advancing age. The gradual age-related decline in coronary flow reserve may be a result of elevated baseline cardiac work and myocardial blood flow [14] or abnormal vasodilator capacity. Such a reduced dilator reserve may be the result of impaired endothelium-dependent dilation of large epicardial and resistance coronary vessels [15], decreased basal and stimulated release of nitric oxide by the coronary endothelium [16], or increased coronary vasoconstrictor effect of endothelin-1 (ET-1) [17]. Endothelin plasma concentrations increase with increasing age [18].

Age and Ischemic Heart Disease

Aging affects cardiovascular risk factors, incidence and clinical manifestation of cardiac disease, treatment strategies and prognosis [13]. Cardiovascular disease is superimposed on age-associated changes in cardiac and vascular characteristics. The final pathophysiological mechanism and clinical presentation result from an interaction between age-related changes in cardiovascular physiology and cardiovascular disease.

Chronic Ischemic Heart Disease

The diagnosis of ischemic heart disease may be more difficult in the elderly. Reduced physical activity with age limits the occurrence of demand angina. Possibly related to the age-related changes in myocardial compliance and diastolic relaxation, dyspnea, rather than pain, may dominate the clinical picture of myocardial ischemia and infarction. The predictive value of a negative exercise stress test is low in a population with a high prevalence of ischemic heart disease.

As many elderly people are unable to exercise to 85–90% of their predicted maximum heart rate, a pharmacological stress test with thallium scan or echocardiogram is often of greater diagnostic accuracy [13].

Although the goal and choice of anti-ischemic treatment are generally similar in young and old patients, the elderly must be expected to be more sensitive to the hypotensive effects of certain anti-ischemic drugs because of blunted baroreceptor reflex activity and sympathetic responsiveness, and increased myocardial and vascular stiffness. As a result of the same age-related decrease in sympathetic responsiveness, myocardial ischemia is less likely to be provoked by adrenergic-mediated increases in myocardial oxygen demand and the benefit derived from treatment with β-adrenoceptor blockers may be reduced.

Acute Myocardial Infarction

In the elderly, in-hospital and subsequent mortality, reinfarction and complications are all increased [19]. Likewise, perioperative myocardial infarction carries a considerably higher mortality in the elderly [13,20]. In addition, age is an independent predictor of adverse outcome following various therapeutic interventions, such as percutaneous transluminal angioplasty, coronary stenting and thrombolysis [13,21].

Increased mortality and morbidity in the elderly after myocardial infarction and therapeutic cardiovascular interventions have many causes. They include greater impairment of baseline left ventricular function, more advanced multivessel disease, higher rate of major complications [21], greater risk of cardiac rupture despite comparable infarct size (probably on the basis of age-related morphological changes), higher rate of vascular complications [21], increased incidence of non-cardiac complications (e.g. stroke and hemorrhage), greater likelihood of interventions being performed under emergency conditions [21], lower procedural success [21], more contraindications to thrombolytic therapy, longer times between onset of symptoms and presentation for evaluation and treatment, blunted catecholamine response, impaired renal and respiratory reserve, and coexisting diseases [13, 21,22].

Demographics of Ischemic Heart Disease in the Elderly

Expanded life span among the elderly population in both North America and western European countries has increased the prevalence of coronary artery disease. The population of the 85 years and older increases 10 times faster than the average population. Average life expectancy at 80 years exceeds 8 years and is still around 6 years at 89 years [23]. According to the US statistics, up to 25% of octogenarians are significantly affected by cardiovascular disease [23].

Over the next 20 years, the absolute number of American citizens reaching at least 85 years is expected to double passing from 9.3 millions to 19.5 millions, which will make the demand for cardiovascular medical care literally explode [24].

Age is the most powerful predictor of cardiovascular adverse events after acute coronary artery syndrome [25].

For each aging decade, in-hospital death rises by 70%. Although citizens of at least 75 years old represent only 6% of the US population, they are responsible for 60% of the in-hospital deaths related to myocardial infarction (MI). According to the World Health Organization (WHO), prevalence of cardiovascular disease will increase by 120% in men and by 137% in women during the next two decades mainly due to the aging of the current population [23]. Although the average age of the first MI is 65.8 years in men and 70 years in women, candidates from both sexes are expected to survive this event by more than 15 years

[25]. In spite of this astonishing demographic outbreak and the surge for medical care it will create, the elderly population still does not receive all the proper attention they deserve [26,27].

CORONARY REVASCULARIZATION IN THE ELDERLY

Selection of the most appropriate treatment pathway for elderly patients with ischemic heart disease requires careful evaluation of the risks and benefits of three forms of treatment: medical therapy, percutaneous coronary intervention (PCI) and CABG surgery, on an individual basis. Two recent studies have examined outcomes in the elderly when assigned to revascularization versus optimal medical therapy [28,29]. Trial of invasive versus medical therapy in elderly patients with chronic symptomatic coronary artery disease (TIME), a prospective randomized trial involving 305 patients with angina, found that, at 6 months revascularization, percutaneous or surgical, was associated with an improved quality of light (QOL) and fewer major cardiac events (19 vs 49%) than optimized medical treatment [28]. The authors concluded that elderly patients with symptoms not controlled by medication benefit from angiography with a view to revascularization. The Alberta Provincial PRoject for Outcome Assessment in Coronary Heart disease (APPROACH) observational study analyzed the absolute risk reduction in late mortality following CABG or PCI compared with medical therapy, based on a cardiac catheterization database of more than 6000 elderly patients with ischemic heart disease [29]. Intervention improved outcome in all groups compared with pharmacological therapy and persisted after accounting for potential selection biases; paradoxically, the greatest benefit was found in the oldest patients (>80 years of age), with survival improvements of 17.0% for CABG and 11.3% for PCI, respectively.

Recently, to appreciate how modern therapeutics could benefit the elderly with acute coronary syndrome, the CRUSADE (Can Rapid Risk Stratification of Unstable Angina Patients Suppress Adverse Outcomes with Early Implementation of the ACC/AHA Outcomes Guidelines) investigators revised the results of the study, including age/stratification designed to compare contemporary in-hospital treatment patterns and outcomes of elderly patients with non-ST-segment elevation acute coronary syndrome ACS with their younger counterparts [30]. Patients were clustered into four age groups: below 65, 65–74, 75–84, and above 85 years old. In-hospital death increased with age from 1.9% below 65 years to 11.5% above 85 years, even after adjustment for risk factors (odds ratio 3.00). Occurrence of other in-hospital events correlated with age, cardiac heart failure, stroke, recurrent MI, and transfusion need being the most common. Even though close to 60% of the 85 years and older had an in-hospital coronary angiogram, less than 20% had PCI performed compared with 50% in those below 65 years of age. On average, CABG was performed in 10% of the patients until the age of 80 years abruptly dwindling down after. Age correlated with a lesser use of aspirin, beta-blockers, heparin, clopidogrel, and platelet glycoprotein IIb/IIIa inhibitors, even though the use of these five guidelines-recommended therapies was associated with lower in-hospital mortality. This remained true even after correcting for other risk factors regardless of patient age. Authors concluded that future work was required to clarify treatment and prevention of ACS in the elderly.

OUTCOMES OF PCI IN THE ELDERLY

The results of both PCI and CABG are improving [31,32], although the exponential rise of PCI over the last decade has made it the principal method of coronary revascularization. In the elderly, PCI is beneficial, but the rate of complications increases disproportionately [32,33] and coronary anatomy is often less amenable. [34] A study of PCI in 8828 octogenarians during 1998–2000 found angiographic success in 93% with stents placed in 75% of patients [35]. Post-procedural mean length of stay was 3.3 days with an in-hospital mortality of 3.77%, decreasing to 1.35% in patients without recent MI ($p < 0.0001$).

Over the past decade, device technology of drug-eluting stents has evolved with a concomitant improvement in outcomes of PCI in the elderly. A recently published report from the randomized multicentre SPIRIT III trial comparing the outcomes in elderly and younger patients treated with everolimus-eluting stent (EES) versus paclitaxel-eluting stent (PES) has shown that implantation of both EES and PES appears to be safe in elderly patients [36]. However, currently published experience of the use of drug-eluting stents in the elderly is limited. Furthermore, the long-term outcomes of current PCI technology and the clinical relevance of incomplete revascularization following PCI in the elderly are yet to be determined.

OUTCOMES OF CONVENTIONAL CORONARY ARTERY BYPASS GRAFTING IN THE ELDERLY

Although old age is seen as a significant risk factor for conventional cardiac surgery, recent publications have reported favorable outcome in elderly patients. CABG in octogenarians relieves angina effectively [2,37]. The overall mortality after CABG in elderly patients has steadily declined over the years with improvements in surgical techniques. The crude survival rates after CABG in individuals aged >75 years in the UK has increased from 92.4% (n= 821) in 1998 to 94.1% (n= 1804) in 2001 [2]. Modern literature acknowledges an operative mortality between 2.7 and 6.4% for isolated CABG and a 5-year life expectancy of 65% [38-40]. A large study found a 34% reduction in risk-adjusted operative mortality in elderly people (1982–96), apart from confirming a time-related increase in the prevalence of older patients and an increase in the preoperative risk profile of these patients. But, when compared with patients of a younger age group, those aged >75 years continue to have poorer short-term outcomes [1]. In an analysis of 6057 patients who underwent isolated CABG between 1996 and 2002, the 30-day mortality rate and the incidence of postoperative complications was found to largely escalate with age [41]. In-hospital outcomes and cost were examined among 2272 elderly people (≥75 years) and 9745 younger patients (<75 years) who underwent CABG between 1997 and 2001 in another study [42]. After controlling for clinical differences, age ≥75 years was found to be associated with a longer length of hospital stay, higher mortality rates and higher in-hospital cost [42]. Recent data from prospective and randomized trials have even reported more favorable outcome with conventional CABG surgery over PCI, especially for diabetes and patients above 65 years of age [40,43]. Over time, prevalence of postoperative complications and use of hospital resource have significantly declined in this population [39]. Maganti et al. [39] have reported a regression in operative mortality among octogenarians from 7.1 to 3.2% along with a decreased incidence of postoperative complications such as stroke, low cardiac output, and use of intra-aortic balloon pump. Concomitantly, they documented an increased prevalence of risk factors such as diabetes, dyslipidemia, hypertension, and left main disease in this population.As CABG effectively relieves angina and may prolong survival, improved quality of life could be expected after surgery. Equally important to determining the overall quality of life is the need to determine the effect that CABG has on physical and mental health. Data available to help clinicians identify those elderly patients who are likely to have an improvement in quality of life after CABG are limited. Although hospitalisation may be longer for elderly patients, physiological, psychological and social recovery patterns through the first 6 weeks postoperatively have been reported to be similar to those of a younger age group [44]. In a study which used self-reported health questionnaires in 1744 patients aged >65 years undergoing CABG, significant improvements were noted in quality of life after a 6-month follow-up [45]. This benefit was present across all age groups and was found to be particularly magnified in patients who had a poorer preoperative health status. Hedeshian *et al*. [37] found that patients aged >70 years presented for CABG at a lower functional level than younger patients, but the marked improvement in functional capacity that occurred after surgery was comparable among all age groups. More recently, survivors among octogenarians who underwent isolated CABG were found to have an excellent quality of life for up to 5 years after surgery [45]. Hence, excellent long-term survival after CABG in elderly people may indeed be accompanied by an equally satisfactory quality of life in the majority.

Rationale for Use of Off-Pump Coronary Artery Bypass Grafting in Elderly

Off-pump coronary artery bypass (OPCAB) grafting, in recent years, has emerged as an effective surgical technique, and may be of particular benefit in high-risk populations including the elderly. Conventional CABG using cardiopulmonary bypass (CPB) and cardioplegic arrest has, for many years, represented the "gold standard" in coronary revascularisation.

However, over the past decade OPCAB has gained increasing popularity. Resurgence of interest in OPCAB is associated with the expectation that avoiding deleterious effects of the CPB pump leads to better outcomes and possibly decreased costs and resource utilization [46]. OPCAB is clearly associated with blunting of systemic inflammatory response syndrome (SIRS) [47]. SIRS results from a cascade of events generated by the contact of plasma proteases and blood cells with the gaseous interface and bioincompatible surfaces of the CPB machine.

High-risk patients including the elderly are particularly susceptible to damage by these inflammatory mediators [48,49]. There is overwhelming evidence from randomized controlled trials, propensity score analyses and observational studies that OPCAB is associated with reductions in the risks for stroke, atrial fibrillation, wound infection, and acute kidney injury. OPCAB also reduces transfusion and inotrope requirements, ventilation time, intensive care unit and hospital stays, and in-hospital and 1-year direct costs [50-56]. Since atrial fibrillation, decline of neurocognitive functions, delirium, stroke, increased length of stay, and renal failure are common complications more frequently encountered in this population [57,58], it makes sense to offer OPCAB surgery to the elderly patients.

OUTCOMES OF OFF-PUMP CORONARY ARTERY BYPASS GRAFTING IN THE ELDERLY

Advanced age is an independent risk factor for mortality after CABG surgery [57]. Avoiding CPB can hamper complications and mortality related to revascularization surgery [59-62].

Table 1. Studies comparing outcomes of on-pump and off-pump coronary artery bypass grafting in elderly

Author, reference (year)	No. of Patients OPCAB/CPB	Type of study	Level of evidence	Definition of elderly (years)	Exclusion criteria*
Saleh[66] (2011)	156/187	Retrospective†	2b	>80	3, 5
LaPar[67] (2011)	404/1589	Retrospective	2b	>80	3, 5
Tugtekin[71] (2007)	107/237	Retrospective	2b	>80	3
Meco[72] (2007)	78/41	Retrospective†	2b	>75	3
D'Alfonso[81] (2004)	73/41	Retrospective	2b	>80	ND
Deuse[87] (2003)	53/66	Retrospective	2b	>75	ND
Meharwal[88] (2002)	186/389	Retrospective	2b	>70	3, 4
Demaria[89] (2002)	62/63	Retrospective	2b	>80	ND
Hoff[90] (2002)	59/69	Retrospective	2b	>80	1, 2
Ascione[91] (2002)	219/771	Retrospective	2b	>70	ND
Hirose[93] (2001)	104/74	Retrospective	2b	>75	ND
Al-Ruzzeh[94] (2001)	56/87	Retrospective	2b	>75	2-4
Ricci[95] (2000)	97/172	Retrospective	2b	>80	Nil
Koutlas[96] (2000)	53/220	Retrospective	2b	>75	3, 5
Boyd[97] (1999)	30/70	Retrospective	2b	>70	ND

*Exclusion criteria: 1, emergency operation; 2, minimally invasive direct coronary artery bypass grafting; 3, coronary grafting in combination with other cardiac surgical procedures; 4, <2 grafts; 5, repeat surgery; 6, catastrophic stage: unstable hemodynamic status or severe ischemia that could not be stabilized with inotropes or intra-aortic balloon pump.

ND = not defined.

† Propensity matched analysis.

Elderly patients are particularly sensitive to the side effects of the CPB and require increased resource utilization compared with younger patients [63-65]. The current literature comparing on and off-pump technique in elderly is quite modest and reflects the difficulty to enroll these very fragile patients in prospective randomized studies. Nevertheless, many nonrandomized studies and subgroup analyses of randomized trials, have demonstrated potential benefit of avoiding CPB in the elderly population [66-97] (Table 1).

Mortality

Age is an independent predictor of postoperative morbidity and mortality among elderly patients undergoing CABG [64,98]. In such patients minimizing the invasiveness of the surgical procedure by avoiding the use of CPB is an attractive option to improve outcomes.

Table 2. Outcomes of on-pump and off-pump coronary artery bypass grafting in elderly

Author, reference (year)	No. of Patients OPCAB/CPB	Mortality(%) OPCAB/CPB	Stroke(%) OPCAB/CPB	AF(%) OPCAB/CPB	RF(%) OPCAB/CPB	LOS(days) OPCAB/CPB
Saleh[66] (2011)	156/187	4.7/6.5	1.9/5.4	28.2/43.9	13.5/15.5	10/9
LaPar[67] (2011)	404/1589	5.9/5.1	1.7/2.6	21.5/28.4	6.2/8.1	12.3/12.2
Tugtekin[71] (2007)	107/237	3.7/5.1	0/1.3	23.3/23.3	2.8/2.1	NR
Meco[72] (2007)	78/41	1.3/12.2*	0/4.9	21.8/26.8	0/12.2	10.5/23.3*
D'Alfonso[81] (2004)	73/41	6.8/14.6*	1.4/2.4	4.1/14.7	2.4/2.6	NR
Deuse[87] (2003)	53/66	7.5/9.1	0/0	NR	NR	9.6/9.7
Meharwal[88](2002)	186/389	2.2/4.6	0/0.5	10.2/18.5	1.1/2.1	5/8*
Demaria[89] (2002)	62/63	4.8/15.9*	0/6.3*	54.8/61.5	19.8/14.5	9/9.6
Hoff[90] (2002)	59/69	0/4.7	0/7.1*	23.3/30.8	0/1.8	6.3/11.5*
Ascione[91 (2002)	219/771	1.4/2.1	0.46/1	12.3/14	0.9/1.9	8.7/8.7
Hirose[93] (2001)	104/74	1.9/0	1/8.1*	NR	1.9/1.4	13.8/20
Al-Ruzzeh[94] (2001)	56/87	0/11*	0/5*	29/41	0/7*	9.7/10.7
Ricci[95] (2001)	97/172	5.2/10.3	0/9.3*	NR	4.1/4.1	9.1/10.8
Koutlas[96] (2000)	53/220	0/7.6*	2.2/2.3	26/26	0/3.5	4.4/8.4*
Boyd[97] (1999)	30/70	0/1.7	0/6.7	10/28.3*	NR	6.3/7.7*

AF = atrial fibrillation; NA = not reported; RF = renal failure.
* $p < 0.05$.

Panesar et al. [65] in an extensive review of the 1999-2005 literature targeting older patients, operated either on or off-pump, have come up with an exhaustive meta-analysis of the topic. They selected 1533 patients in the OPCAB group and 3388 in conventional group. Primary endpoint was operative mortality and stroke, and secondary endpoints were prevalence of atrial fibrillation, renal failure, and length of hospital stay. They categorized the patients into three distinct groups: above 70 years, above 75 years, and above 80 years old. At large, operative mortality was diminished in the OPCAB group ($p = 0.01$) and more specifically in the oldest group ($p = 0.007$).

Majority of the publications since 2005, analyzing impact of OPCAB and CPB on mortality in elderly, report similar in-hospital mortality rates for conventional CABG and OPCAB with the overall early mortality for this high-risk group ranging from 4.6% to 5.9% [66,67,69-71] (Table 2). However, some recent nonrandomized studies such as the propensity score analysis by Meco et al. [72] have shown that mortality is higher in the patient group operated with CPB as compared to patients operated without CPB (12.2% vs 1.3%, $p = 0.01$). Furthermore, their logistic regression analysis has shown that avoiding CPB is an independent protective factor for mortality and morbidity in the elderly.

Stroke

Coronary artery bypass surgery is associated with adverse neurological complications, of which stroke is the most debilitating. Despite the improvement in surgical techniques and cardioplegic agents, along with the introduction of membrane oxygenators and in-line filtration, there is a persistent stroke rate associated with CABG ranging from 1% to 5% [99,100]. It is estimated that 3000 to 15,000 patients each year suffer a stroke in the perioperative period after CABG [99,100]. Age is identified as an independent predictor of stroke [101,102]. The increasing risk with older age has been related to the higher prevalence of diseased aorta which may lead to perioperative atheroembolism from aortic arch plaque [103]. Indeed, the identification of an atherosclerotic ascending aorta has been reported as the single, most significant marker for an adverse cerebral outcome after CABG [103], reflecting the role of aortic atheroembolism as the main cause of ischemic stroke [104].

Over the last decade, prevalence of stroke after CABG surgery has significantly decreased in octogenarians, and recent reports quote a risk of 2% [39] (Table 2). Prevalence still remained twice as high as what is currently seen in younger patients [105]. Prevention definitely remains the key issue in the management of this complication [23]. Athanasiou et al. [62] in their meta-analysis of all observational studies, published in MEDLINE between 1999 and 2002, showed that the OPCAB technique was associated with significantly lower incidence of stroke in elderly patients compared with the CPB technique (1% vs 3%), with an odds ratio of 0.38% to 95% (confidence interval [CI], 0.22 to 0.65). Similar results have been reported by Panesar et al. [65]. Their meta-analysis showed a significant reduction in OPCAB patients above 70 years old compared with conventional CABG surgery. The strongest benefit was observed in the octogenarians. Even though history of previous stroke was more frequent in OPCAB surgery octogenarians patients (15.4 versus 8.9%), occurrence of new postoperative stroke was significantly higher with conventional surgery ($p = 0.002$). Less invasive nature of OPCAB with minimal manipulation of atheromatous aorta could account for the reduction of postoperative stroke in the elderly.

Cognitive Impairment

Cognitive deficits have been documented in a majority of patients after cardiac surgery [106]. Off-pump surgery has been shown to better preserve neurocognitive impairment than conventional CABG surgery [59,107-109]. The pathophysiology of these neurocognitive deficits appears to be multifactorial [110]. Prospective randomized trials specifically designed to explore the potential benefit of OPCAB surgery on postoperative neurocognitive functions have confirmed the benefit of OPCAB surgery in the first 3 months after surgery [59,70,74,107-109,111,112].

Interestingly, Jensen et al. [74] failed to show a difference in the incidence of cognitive dysfunction 3 months after either OPCAB or conventional CABG in a substudy of the randomized Best Bypass Surgery trial. In this study a total of 120 elderly patients (mean age 76 ± 4.5 years) underwent psychometric testing before surgery and at a mean of 103 ± 15 days postoperatively with a neuropsychological test battery that included 7 parameters from 4 tests. Cognitive dysfunction was defined as the occurrence of at least 2 of the 7 possible deficits. Secondary analysis was performed on the basis of the definition of a 20% decline in cognitive scores compared with baseline, and with z score analysis. Cognitive dysfunction was identified in 4 of the 54 patients (7.4%, 95% CI 2.1% to 17.9%) in the OPCAB group and 5 of the 51 patients (9.8%, 95% CI 3.3% to 21.4%) in the conventional CABG group. At 1 year follow-up the findings remained the same [70].

The reasons for the limited differences in cognitive outcome between the treatment groups observed in the study Jensen et al. [74] may be explained in several ways. When one examines the literature, the crucial step of finding a significant neurocognitive deficit is in determining the definition itself. The definition of a significant deficit varies, and the lower the threshold of "deficit" is determined to be, the more patients there will be who have a deficit. This level is arbitrary from research group to research group and varies from a deterioration of 1 SD in 1 or more tests, a deterioration of 20% or 25% in at least 1 or 2 tests, to the use of a standardized *z* score or composite *z* score [113]. The definition of cognitive dysfunction in the study by Jensen et al. [74] was more restrictive than the "20% criterion" and the definition with the *z* score. In the analyses of the test results from Jensen's study,74 the evaluation of cognitive function was based on differences between preoperative and postoperative performance. Therefore, the association between early and late cognitive outcome could be explained by regression toward the mean [114], because generally, the use of scores favors patients with poor preoperative performance because of the "protective" effect of low baseline performance [113].

Another explanation involves the short-term follow-up in Jensen's study [74], because it has been suggested that improved cognitive outcome with an OPCAB procedure may only become clear in the long term. van Dijk et al. [111] found an increasing incidence of cognitive decline from 3 to 12 months, and Newman et al. found cognitive decline in 24% of patients 6 months after conventional CABG, which increased to 42% after 5 years.

A final explanation might be that the OPCAB technique is a new source of cognitive dysfunction caused by decreased cerebral perfusion pressure during episodes of elevated central venous pressure and corresponding decreased arterial blood pressure, in connection with dislocation of the heart during surgical exposure of the posterior cardiac wall [116]. The influence of systemic mean arterial pressure during CPB and neurological outcome has been the subject of considerable debate. Commonly, a mean arterial pressure of 50 to 60 mm Hg when the patient is undergoing CPB is regarded as safe to avoid neurological complications [74].

Postoperative Atrial Fibrillation

Atrial fibrillation (AF) is the most common complication after cardiac surgery, with little change over the past 2 decades [117]. Postoperative AF increases hospital morbidity and mortality and has significant adverse effects on patient recovery. The lengthening of hospital stay and the consequent burden caused by the occurrence of postoperative AF has led to an extensive scrutiny of predisposing factor and preventive strategies [118,119].

Aging increases the prevalence of AF by 44% in every 10 years [23]. At least three recent meta-analyses have questioned the influence of OPCAB surgery on postoperative AF. The first one included all observational studies comparing on and off-pump revascularization on patients above 70 years of age and demonstrated a reduced incidence of postoperative AF in favor of OPCAB patients [105]. The second one included all randomized and propensity score-matched nonrandomized studies published between 2001 and 2003 comparing both techniques regardless of age [120]. Their results suggested that OPCAB surgery could reduce the incidence of postoperative AF in the general population (age <70 years), but the optimal 'protective effect' was not as strong as recorded in the older population. The meta-analysis on benefit of OPCAB in elderly by Panesar et al. [65] although targeting mostly in-hospital mortality and stroke, showed a benefit in favor of OPCAB for all groups above 70 years old confirming the findings of the other studies.

Postoperative Renal Dysfunction

Renal dysfunction is a serious complication after coronary artery bypass surgery with cardiopulmonary bypass. Cardiopulmonary bypass-related non-pulsatile flow, hypothermia, haemolysis, systemic inflammatory reactions and emboli are mentioned as possible causes for this postoperative renal dysfunction [54]. In addition advanced age is an important predictor of postoperative renal dysfunction after CABG [121]. A recent propensity-based study conducted on 2041 patients confirmed these findings [122]. However, a meta-analysis of 6 randomized controlled trials and 16 observational studies, comprising 27,806 patients, failed to show strong benefit in the elderly population regarding OPCAB and renal failure [123]. Currently, the evidence on this issue is limited (Table 2) and further studies are required to clarify this topic.

Resource Utilization

Advanced age is associated with diminished physiologic reserve and increased comorbid illnesses, including diabetes, chronic obstructive pulmonary disease, cerebrovascular disease, and peripheral vascular disease. These comorbidities lead to increased postoperative complications and resource utilization in this population. In an era of fiscal constraint and fixed resources, management of the elderly CABG patient poses significant medical and ethical challenges for both healthcare providers and healthcare administrators. Boyd et al. [97] have examined the cost of OPCAB and conventional CABG surgery in the geriatric population. They hypothesized that postoperative morbidity was responsible for longer intensive care unit (ICU) and hospital stays. They grouped together patients who had an ICU stay longer than 24 hours and/or a hospital stay longer than 8 days, and defined these individuals as adverse economic outcomes. The prevalence of adverse economic outcomes was four times higher in the CABG population (OPCAB 10% vs CABG 40%, $p < 0.005$). Furthermore, the reduction in hospital resources in the OPCAB patients resulted in an average savings of CAN $1,082 per patient in this group. These savings were based solely on decreases in hospital stay and ICU stay, and did not include additional savings yielded from decreased operating room equipment costs or blood product usage. Again the evidence on this topic is scant at present.

Quality of Life

The success of cardiac surgery is not solely judged by its effects on mortality but also by its neuropsychological and emotional consequences, and by its influence on health-related quality of life (HRQoL) [124]. Changes in cognitive function have been associated with reduced HRQoL 1 year [124] and 5 years after cardiac surgery in terms of lower general health and a less productive working status [125]. A randomized study, using a post-test only design, compared medical treatment to invasive treatment in 113 patients with inducible ischemic heart disease. At an average follow-up of 36 months, more invasively treated patients had concentration difficulties but better HRQoL scores in the physical variables. [126] CABG appears to have a beneficial effect on psychological function and HRQoL for the majority of patients [127].

Jensen et al. [73] have conducted to date the first and only randomized study to evaluate the effect of off-pump versus on-pump CABG on changes in various aspects of HRQoL in elderly moderate to high-risk patients during the first 3 months after the operation. After randomization and before heart surgery, 120 consecutive patients were asked to fill in the Medical Outcomes Study Short Form 36 (SF-36) and Major Depression Inventory diagnostic scale for self-report of HRQoL. Three months after surgery, the same questionnaires were mailed to the patients. The response rate was 96.5%. At baseline, the groups were comparable except for a difference in educational level. Both groups improved in all eight SF-36 domains from baseline to 3 months. No statistical differences were seen between the groups except for changes in mean difference of role limitation due to emotional problems, which was significantly ($p = .04$) improved in favor of the on-pump group. Depression scores remained unchanged within and between the two surgical groups. Both on-pump and off-pump patients improved in health-related quality of life scores after CABG surgery. No clinically relevant difference between the groups could be demonstrated. However, despite being a randomized study, generalizations of these findings is limited by the fact that it is a single centre experience and there is need for further studies to verify whether or not there is an improvement in HRQoL among OPCAB elderly patients compared to patients undergoing on-pump CABG.

Conclusion

The elderly are the fastest growing segment of the CABG patient population. These patients often have concomitant diseases, such as renal insufficiency, chronic obstructive pulmonary disease, peripheral vascular disease, prostatic enlargement complicated by urinary retention, and degenerative cerebral disease. The overall reduction in the operative mortality and morbidity after CABG due to recent technological advances in surgical and anesthetic techniques and improvements in postoperative care has made CABG a valid option of treatment for this group of patients. The decision for surgery is complex in this group of patients and one must take into account several elements, such as the lack of synchronism between physiological age and chronological age, the quality of life, and the risk– benefit ratio. Furthermore, the risk of death from a cardiac operation in elderly patients can be reduced to that of younger patients with consistent and careful application of modern techniques and clinical practices. OPCAB, due to its less invasive nature compared to conventional CABG, appears an attractive option to reduce procedure specific mortality and morbidity in the elderly. However, current observational studies with small numbers, examining the impact of avoiding CPB on early mortality and morbidity in the elderly, have yielded variable results. It is expected that adequately powered future studies, with randomized design, will provide more concrete evidence to verify the safety and efficacy of OPCAB in the elderly

References

[1] Ivanov J, Weisel RD, David TE, et al. Fifteen-year trends in risk severity and operative mortality in elderly patients undergoing coronary artery bypass graft surgery. *Circulation,* 1998; 97:673-680.

[2] Natarajan A, Samadian S, Clark S. Coronary artery bypass surgery in elderly people. *Postgrad. Med. J.,* 2007;83:154-8.

[3] Moshkovitz Y, Paz Y, Shabtai E, et al. Predictors of early and overall outcome in coronary artery bypass without cardiopulmonary bypass. *Eur. J. Cardiothorac. Surg.,* 1997;12:31-39.

[4] Loop FD, Lytle BW, Cosgrove DM, et al. Coronary artery bypass graft surgery in the elderly. Indications and outcome. *Cleve. Clin. J. Med.,* 1988;55:23-34.

[5] Lakatta EG. Changes in cardiovascular function with aging. *Eur. Heart J.,* 1990;11(Suppl C):22-29.

[6] Loran DB, Zwischenberger JB. Thoracic surgery in the elderly. *J. Am. Coll. Surg.,* 2004;199:773-784.

[7] Folkow B, Svanborg A. Physiology of cardiovascular aging. *Physiol. Rev.,* 1993;73:725-64.

[8] Lakatta EG. Cardiovascular aging research: the next horizons. *J. Am. Geriatr. Soc.,* 1999;47:613-25.

[9] Gajraj RJ, Doi M, Mantzaridis H, Kenny GNC. Comparison of bispectral EEG analysis and auditory evoked potentials for monitoring depth of anaesthesia during propofol anaesthesia. *Br. J. Anaesth.,* 1999;82:672-8.

[10] Lakatta EG. Cardiovascular regulatory mechanisms in advanced age. *Physiol. Rev.*, 1993;73: 413-67.

[11] Olivetti G, Melissari M, Capasso JM, Anversa P. Cardiomyopathy of the aging human heart. Myocyte loss and reactive cellular hypertrophy. *Circ. Res.*, 1991;68:1560-68.

[12] *Lakatta E. Aging effects on the vasculature in health: risk factors for cardiovascular disease. Am. J. Geriatr. Cardiol.*, 1994; 3:11-17.

[13] Priebe HJ. The aged cardiovascular risk patient. *Br. J. Anaesth.*, 2000;85:763-78.

[14] Czernin J, Müller P, Chan S, et al. Influence of age and hemodynamics on myocardial blood flow and flow reserve. *Circulation,* 1993;88:62-9.

[15] Egashira K, Inou T, Hirooka Y, et al. Effects of age on endothelium-dependent vasodilation of resistance coronary artery by acetylcholine in humans. *Circulation,* 1993;88:77-81.

[16] Amrani M, Goodwin AT, Gray CC, Yacoub MH. Ageing is associated with reduced basal and stimulated release of nitric oxide by the coronary endothelium. *Acta. Physiol. Scand.*, 1996;157:79-84.

[17] Goodwin AT, Amrani M, Marchbank AJ, Gray CC, Jayakumar J, Yacoub MH. Coronary vasoconstriction to endothelin-1 increases with age before and after ischaemia and reperfusion. *Cardiovasc. Res.*, 1999;41:554-62.

[18] Miyauchi T, Yanagisawa M, Iida K, et al. Age- and sex-related variation of plasma endothelin-1 concentration in normal and hypertensive subjects. *Am. Heart. J.*, 1992; 123:1092-3.

[19] Barakat K, Wilkinson P, Deaner A, Fluck D, Ranjadayalan K, Timmis A. How should age affect management of acute myocardial infarction? A prospective cohort study. *Lancet,* 1999;353:955-9.

[20] Detsky AS, Abrams, HB, McLaughlin JR, et al. Predicting cardiac complications in patients undergoing non-cardiac surgery. *J. Gen. Intern.*, Med 1986;1:211-19.

[21] Alfonso F, Azcona L, Perez-Vizcayno MJ, et al. Initial results and long-term clinical and angiographic implications of coronary stenting in elderly patients. *Am. J. Cardiol.*, 1999;83:1483-7.

[22] Paul SD, O'Gara PT, Mahjoub ZA. Geriatric patients with acute myocardial infarction: cardiac risk factor profiles, presentations, thrombolysis, coronary interventions and prognosis. *Am. Heart J.*, 1996;131:710-15.

[23] Cartier R. Off-pump coronary artery revascularization in octogenarians: is it better? *Curr. Opin. Cardiol.*, 2009;24:544-52.

[24] Centers for Disease Control and Prevention. Trends in aging: United States and worldwide. *Morb. Mortal. Wkly. Rep.*, 2003;52:101-104,106.

[25] Granger CB, Goldberg RJ, Dabbous O, et al. Global Registry of Acute Coronary Events Investigators. Predictors of hospital mortality in the Global Registry of Acute Coronary Events. *Arch. Intern. Med.*, 2003;163:2345-2353.

[26] Avezum A, Makdisse M, Spencer F, et al. GRACE Investigators. Impact of age on management and outcome of acute coronary syndrome: observations from the Global Registry of Acute Coronary Events (GRACE). *Am. Heart J.*, 2005; 140:67-73.

[27] Lee PY, Alexander KP, Hammill BG, et al. Representation of elderly persons and women in published randomized trials of acute coronary syndromes. *JAMA*, 2001; 286:708-713.

[28] TIME Investigators. Trial of invasive versus medical therapy in elderly patients with chronic symptomatic coronary-artery disease (TIME): a randomised trial. *Lancet,* 2001;358:951-7.

[29] Graham MM, Ghali WA, Faris PD, et al. Alberta Provincial Project for Outcomes Assessment in Coronary Heart Disease (APPROACH) Investigators. Survival after coronary revascularization in elderly. *Circulation*, 2002; 105:2378-2384.

[30] Alexander KP, Roe MT, Chen AY, et al. Evolution in cardiovascular care for elderly patients with non-ST-segment elevation acute coronary syndromes: results from the CRUSADE National Quality Improvement Initiative. *J. Am. Coll. Cardiol.,* 2005; 46:1479-1487.

[31] Peterson ED, Alexander KP, Malenka DJ, et al; American Heart Association Chronic CAD Working Group. American Heart Association Chronic CAD working group. Multicenter experience in revascularization of very elderly patients. *Am. Heart. J.,* 2004;148:486-92.

[32] Batchelor WB, Anstrom KJ, Muhlbaier LH, et al. Contemporary outcome trends in the elderly undergoing percutaneous coronary interventions: results in 7,472 octogenarians. National Cardiovascular Network Collaboration. *J. Am. Coll. Cardiol.,* 2000;36:723-30.

[33] De Gregorio J, Kobayashi Y, Albiero R, et al. Coronary artery stenting in the elderly: short-term outcome and long-term angiographic and clinical follow-up. *J. Am. Coll. Cardiol.,* 1998:32;577-583.

[34] Kowalchuk CJ, Siu SC, Lewis SM. Coronary artery disease in the octogenarian: angiographic spectrum and suitability for revascularization. *Am. J. Cardiol.,* 1990:66;1319-1323.

[35] Klein LW, Block P, Brindis RG, et al; ACC-NCDR registry. Percutaneous coronary interventions in octogenarians in the American College of Cardiology-National Cardiovascular Data Registry. Development of a nomogram predictive of in-hospital mortality. *J. Am. Coll. Cardiol.,* 2002:40;394-402.

[36] Hermiller JB, Nikolsky E, Lansky AJ, et al. Clinical and angiographic outcomes of elderly patients treated with everolimus-eluting versus paclitaxel-eluting stents: three-year results from the SPIRIT III randomised trial. *EuroIntervention,* 2011;7:307-13.

[37] Hedeshian M H, Namour N, Dziadik E, et al. Does increasing age have a negative impact on six-month functional outcome after coronary artery bypass? *Surgery,* 2002:132;239-244.

[38] Zingone B, Gatti G, Rauber E, et al. Early and late outcomes of cardiac surgery in octogenerians. *Ann. Thorac. Surg.,* 2009;87:71-78.

[39] Maganti M, Rao V, Brister S, Ivanov J. Decreasing mortality for coronary artery bypass surgery in octogenarians. *Can. J. Cardiol.,* 2009;25:e32–e35.

[40] Hlatky MA, Boothroyd DB, Bravata DM, et al. Coronary artery bypass surgery compared with percutaneous coronary interventions for multivessel disease: a collaborative analysis of individual patient data from ten randomised trials. *Lancet,* 2009;373:1190-1197.

[41] Mortasawi A, Arnrich B, Walter J, et al. Impact of age on the results of coronary artery bypass grafting. *Asian Cardiovasc. Thorac. Ann.,* 2004:12:324-329.

[42] Wilson M F, Baig M K, Ashraf H. Quality of life in octagenarians after coronary artery bypass grafting. *Am. J. Cardiol.,* 2005;95:761-764.

[43] Dacey LJ, Likosky DS, Ryan TJ Jr, et al. Northern New England Cardiovascular Disease Study Group. Long-term survival after surgery versus percutaneous intervention in octogenarians with multivessel coronary disease. *Ann. Thorac. Surg.,* 2007;84:1904-1911.

[44] Artinian N T, Duggan C, Miller P. Age differences in patient recovery patterns following coronary artery bypass surgery. *Am. J. Crit. Care.,* 1993;2:453-461.

[45] Rumsfeld J S, Magid D J, O'Brien M, et al. Changes in health-related quality of life following coronary artery bypass graft surgery. *Ann. Thorac. Surg.,* 2001;72:2026-2032.

[46] Raja SG, Dreyfus GD. Impact of off-pump coronary artery bypass surgery on post-operative pulmonary dysfunction: current best available evidence. *Ann. Card. Anaesth.,* 2006;9:17-24.

[47] Raja SG, Berg GA. Impact of off-pump coronary artery bypass surgery on systemic inflammation: current best available evidence. *J. Card. Surg.,* 2007;22:445-55.

[48] Marti L, Cervera C, Filella X, Marin JL, Almela M, Moreno A. Cytokine-release patterns in elderly patients with systemic inflammatory response syndrome. *Gerontology,* 2007;53:239-44.

[49] Deng M C, Dasch B, Erren M, et al. Impact of left ventricular dysfunction on cytokines, hemodynamics, and outcome in bypass grafting. *Ann. Thorac. Surg.,* 1996;62:184-190.

[50] Raja SG, Berg GA. Outcomes of off-pump coronary artery bypass surgery: current best available evidence. *Indian Heart J.,* 2007;59:15-27.

[51] Sedrakyan A, Wu AW, Parashar A, Bass EB, Treasure T. Off-pump surgery is associated with reduced occurrence of stroke and other morbidity as compared with traditional coronary artery bypass grafting: a meta-analysis of systematically reviewed trials. *Stroke,* 2006;37:2759-69.

[52] Parolari A, Alamanni F, Cannata A, et al. Off-pump versus on-pump coronary artery bypass: meta-analysis of currently available randomized trials. *Ann. Thorac. Surg.,* 2003;76:37-40.

[53] Reston JT, Tregear SJ, Turkelson CM. Meta-analysis of short-term and mid-term outcomes following off-pump coronary artery bypass grafting. *Ann. Thorac. Surg.,* 2003;76:1510-5.

[54] Raja SG, Dreyfus GD. Impact of off-pump coronary artery bypass surgery on postoperative renal dysfunction: current best available evidence. *Nephrology,* (Carlton) 2006;11:269-73.

[55] Raja SG, Dreyfus GD. Impact of off-pump coronary artery bypass surgery on postoperative bleeding: current best available evidence. *J. Card. Surg.,* 2006;21:35-41.

[56] Raja SG, Dreyfus GD. Current status of off-pump coronary artery bypass surgery. *Asian Cardiovasc Thorac. Ann.,* 2008;16:164-78.

[57] Mangano CM, Diamondstone LS, Ramsay JG, et al. Renal dysfunction after myocardial revascularization: risk factors, adverse outcomes, and hospital resource utilization. *Ann. Intern. Med.,* 1998;128:194-203.

[58] Amar D, Zhang H, Leung DH, et al. Older age is the strongest predictor of postoperative atrial fibrillation. *Anesthesiology,* 2002;96:352-356.

[59] Al-Ruzzeh S, George S, Bustami M, et al. Effect of off-pump coronary artery bypass surgery on clinical, angiographic, neurocognitive, and quality of life outcomes: randomised controlled trial. *Br. Med. J.,* 2006;332:1365.

[60] Stamou SC, Dangas G, Dullum MK, et al. Beating heart surgery in octogenarians: perioperative outcome and comparison with younger age groups. *Ann. Thorac. Surg.,* 2000;69:1140-1145.

[61] Guru V, Glasgow KW, Fremes SE, et al. The real-world outcomes of off-pump coronary artery bypass surgery in a public healthcare system. *Can. J. Cardiol.,* 2007;23:281-286.

[62] Athanasiou T, Al-Ruzzeh S, Kumar P, et al. Off-pump myocardial revascularization is associated with less incidence of stroke in elderly patients. *Ann. Thorac. Surg.,* 2004;77:745-753.

[63] Guerra M, Carlos Mota J. Adult cardiac surgery: impact on age group differences in preoperative risk factors and early mortality. *Rev. Port. Cir. Cardiotorac. Vasc.,* 2008;15:189-195.

[64] Scott BH, Seifert FC, Grimson R, Glass PS. Octogenarians undergoing coronary artery bypass graft surgery: resource utilization, postoperative mortality, and morbidity. *J. Cardiothorac. Vasc. Anesth.,* 2005;19:583-588.

[65] Panesar SS, Athanasiou T, Nair S, et al. Early outcomes in the elderly: a meta-analysis of 4921 patients undergoing coronary artery bypass grafting – comparison between off-pump and on-pump techniques. *Heart,* 2006;92:1808-1816.

[66] Saleh HZ, Shaw M, Fabri BM, Chalmers JA. Does avoidance of cardiopulmonary bypass confer any benefits in octogenarians undergoing coronary surgery? *Interact Cardiovasc. Thorac. Surg.,* 2011;12:435-9.

[67] LaPar DJ, Bhamidipati CM, Reece TB, Cleveland JC, Kron IL, Ailawadi G. Is off-pump coronary artery bypass grafting superior to conventional bypass in octogenarians? *J. Thorac. Cardiovasc. Surg.,* 2011;141:81-90.

[68] Serrão M, Graça F, Rodrigues R, Abecasis M, Bruges L, Calquinha J, Neves J, Bebocho MJ, Ferreira M, Queiroz e Melo J. Coronary artery bypass grafting in octogenarians: long-term results. *Rev. Port. Cardiol.,* 2010;29:989-98.

[69] Pinto E Silva AM, Campagnucci VP, Pereira WL, Rosa RF, Franken RA, Gandra SM, Rivetti LA. Off-pump myocardial revascularization in the elderly: analysis of morbidity and mortality. *Rev. Bras. Cir. Cardiovasc.,* 2008;23:40-5.

[70] Jensen BØ, Rasmussen LS, Steinbrüchel DA. Cognitive outcomes in elderly high-risk patients 1 year after off-pump versus on-pump coronary artery bypass grafting. A randomized trial. *Eur. J. Cardiothorac. Surg.,* 2008;34:1016-21.

[71] Tugtekin S, Kappert U, Alexiou K, Wilbring M, Nagpal AD, Matschke K. Coronary artery bypass grafting in octogenarians--outcome with and without extracorporeal circulation. *Thorac. Cardiovasc. Surg.,* 2007;55:407-11.

[72] Meco M, Biraghi T, Panisi P, Casselman F, Cosseta D, Cirri S. Aortocoronary bypass grafting in high-risk patients over 75 years. Propensity score analysis of on versus off-pump, early and midterm results. *J. Cardiovasc. Surg.,* (Torino) 2007;48:339-47.

[73] Jensen BØ, Hughes P, Rasmussen LS, Pedersen PU, Steinbrüchel DA. Health-related quality of life following off-pump versus on-pump coronary artery bypass grafting in elderly moderate to high-risk patients: a randomized trial. *Eur. J. Cardiothorac. Surg.,* 2006;30:294-9.

[74] Jensen BO, Hughes P, Rasmussen LS, Pedersen PU, Steinbrüchel DA. Cognitive outcomes in elderly high-risk patients after off-pump versus conventional coronary artery bypass grafting: a randomized trial. *Circulation,* 2006;113:2790-5.

[75] Kitamura H, Okabayashi H, Hanyu M, Nakano J, Nomoto T, Sakaguchi H, Jono H, Matsuo T. Early and late results and problems of coronary artery bypass grafting in patients over 80-year-old. *Kyobu Geka,* 2005;58:1034-7.

[76] Tomita S, Watanabe G. Performing off-pump coronary artery bypass grafting in elderly patients safely. *Kyobu Geka,* 2005;58(8 Suppl):641-6.

[77] Sugimoto T, Yamamoto K, Tanaka S, Saito N, Kikuchi C, Kasuya S, Oguma F. Off-pump versus conventional coronary artery bypass grafting in octogenarians. *Kyobu Geka,* 2005;58:96-103.

[78] Nakamura Y, Nakano K, Nakatani H, Gomi A, Sato A, Sugimoto K. Hospital and mid-term outcomes in elderly patients under-going off-pump coronary artery bypass grafting--comparison with younger patients--. *Circ. J.,* 2004;68:1184-8.

[79] Xue S, Xie B, Liu S, Xiao MD. Off-pump coronary artery bypass grafting in patients over the age of seventy. *Zhonghua Wai Ke Za Zhi,* 2004;42:661-3.

[80] Tanaka H, Narisawa T, Masuda M, Kishi D, Suzuki T. Coronary artery bypass in patients 80 years and older: comparison with a younger age group. *Ann. Thorac. Cardiovasc. Surg.,* 2004;10:85-9.

[81] D'Alfonso A, Mariani M A, Amerini A, et al. Off-pump coronary surgery improves in-hospital and early outcomes in octogenarians. *Ital. Heart. J.,* 2004;5:197–204.

[82] Carrier M, Perrault LP, Jeanmart H, Martineau R, Cartier R, Pagé P. Randomized trial comparing off-pump to on-pump coronary artery bypass grafting in high-risk patients. *Heart Surg. Forum.,* 2003;6:E89-92.

[83] Matsumoto Y, Endo M, Kasashima F, Abe Y, Kosugi I, Sasaki H. Off-pump coronary artery bypass grafting for octogenarians with acute coronary syndrome. *Kyobu Geka,* 2003;56(8 Suppl):682-7.

[84] Beauford RB, Goldstein DJ, Sardari FF, et al. Multivessel off-pump revascularization in octogenarians: early and midterm outcomes. *Ann. Thorac. Surg.,* 2003;76:12-7.

[85] Lin CY, Hong GJ, Lee KC, et al. Off-pump technique in coronary artery bypass grafting in elderly patients. *Aust. NZJ Surg.,* 2003;73:473-476.

[86] Shimokawa T, Minato N, Yamada N, et al Off-pump coronary artery bypass grafting in octogenarians. *Jpn. J. Thorac. Cardiovasc. Surg.,* 2003;51:86-90.

[87] Deuse T, Detter C, Samuel V, et al. Early and midterm results after coronary artery bypass grafting with and without cardiopulmonary bypass: which patient population benefits the most? *Heart Surg. Forum.,* 2003;6:77-83.

[88] Meharwal Z S, Trehan N. Off-pump coronary artery surgery in the elderly. *Asian Cardiovasc. Thorac. Ann.,* 2002;10:206-210.

[89] Demaria RG, Carrier M, Fortier S, et al. Reduced mortality and strokes with off-pump coronary artery bypass grafting surgery in octogenarians. *Circulation,* 2002;106(12 Suppl 1):I5–10.

[90] Hoff SJ, Ball SK, Coltharp WH, et al. Coronary artery bypass in patients 80 years and over: is off-pump the operation of choice? *Ann. Thorac. Surg.*, 2002;74:S1340-S1343.

[91] Ascione R, Rees K, Santo K, et al. Coronary artery bypass grafting in patients over 70 years old: the influence of age and surgical technique on early and mid-term clinical outcomes. *Eur. J. Cardiothorac. Surg.,* 2002;22:124-128.

[92] Ricci M, Karamanoukian HL, Dancona G, et al. On-pump and off-pump coronary artery bypass grafting in the elderly: predictors of adverse outcome. *J. Card. Surg.,* 2001;16:458-466.

[93] Hirose H, Amano A, Takahashi A. Off-pump coronary artery bypass grafting for elderly patients. *Ann. Thorac. Surg.,* 2001;72:2013-2019.

[94] Al-Ruzzeh S, George S, Yacoub M, et al. The clinical outcome of off-pump coronary artery bypass surgery in the elderly patients. *Eur. J. Cardiothorac. Surg.,* 2001;20:1152-1156.

[95] Ricci M, Karamanoukian HL, Abraham R, et al. Stroke in octogenarians undergoing coronary artery surgery with and without cardiopulmonary bypass. *Ann. Thorac. Surg.,* 2000;69:1471-5.

[96] Koutlas TC, Elbeery JR, Williams JM, et al. Myocardial revascularization in the elderly using beating heart coronary artery bypass surgery. *Ann. Thorac. Surg.,* 2000;69:1042-1047.

[97] Boyd WD, Desai ND, Del Rizzo DF, et al. Off-pump surgery decreases postoperative complications and resource utilization in the elderly. *Ann. Thorac. Surg.,* 1999;68:1490-1493.

[98] Johnson WM, Smith M, Woods SE, Hendy MP. Hiratzka LF. Cardiac surgery in octogenarians: does age alone influence outcomes? *Arch. Surg.,* 2005;140:1089-1093.

[99] Furlan AJ, Sila CA, Chimowitz MI, Jones SC. Neurologic complications related to cardiac surgery. *Neurol. Clin.,* 1992;10:145-166.

[100] Stamou SC, Dangas G, Dullum MK, et al. Beating heart surgery in octogenarians: perioperative outcome and comparison with younger age groups. *Ann. Thorac. Surg.,* 2000;69:1140-1145.

[101] Puskas JD, Winston D, Wright CE, et al. Stroke after coronary artery operations: incidence, correlates, outcome, and cost. *Ann. Thorac. Surg.,* 2000;69:1053-1056.

[102] McKhann G, Goldsborough M, Borowicz L, et al. Predictors of stroke risk in coronary artery bypass patients. *Ann. Thorac. Surg.,* 1997;63:516-521.

[103] Ascione R, Reeves BC, Chamberlain MH, et al. Predictors of stroke in the modern era of coronary artery bypass grafting: a case control study. *Ann. Thorac. Surg.,* 2002;74:474-480.

[104] Hammon JW, Stump DA, Kon ND, et al. Risk factors and solutions for the development of neurobehavioral changes after coronary artery bypass grafting. *Ann. Thorac. Surg.,* 1997;63:1613-1618.

[105] Athanasiou T, Aziz O, Mangoush O, et al. Do off-pump techniques reduce the incidence of postoperative atrial fibrillation in elderly patients undergoing coronary artery bypass grafting? *Ann. Thorac. Surg.,* 2004;77:1567-1574.

[106] Fearn SJ, Pole R, Wesnes K, et al. Cerebral injury during cardiopulmonary bypass: emboli impair memory. *J. Thorac. Cardiovasc. Surg.,* 2001;121:1150-1160.

[107] Diegeler A, Hirsch R, Schneider F, et al. Neuromonitoring and neurocognitive outcome in off-pump versus conventional coronary bypass operation. *Ann. Thorac. Surg.,* 2000;69:1162-1166.

[108] Zamvar V, Williams D, Hall J, et al. Assessment of neurocognitive impairment after off-pump and on-pump techniques for coronary artery bypass graft surgery: prospective randomised controlled trial. *BMJ,* 2002;325:1268-1272.
[109] Lee JD, Lee SJ, Tsushima WT, et al. Benefits of off-pump bypass on neurologic and clinical morbidity: a prospective randomized trial. *Ann. Thorac. Surg.,* 2003;76:18-25.
[110] Selnes OA, McKhann GM. Neurocognitive complications after coronary artery bypass surgery. *Ann. Neurol.,* 2005;57:615-621.
[111] van Dijk D, Jansen EW, Hijman R, et al. Octopus Study Group. Cognitive outcome after off-pump and on-pump coronary artery bypass graft surgery: a randomized trial. *JAMA,* 2002;287:1405-1412.
[112] van Dijk D, Spoor M, Hijman R, et al. Octopus Study Group. Cognitive and cardiac outcomes 5 years after off-pump vs on-pump coronary artery bypass graft surgery. *JAMA,* 2007;297:701-708.
[113] Rasmussen LS, Larsen K, Houx P, Skovgaard LT, Hanning CD, Moller JT. The assessment of postoperative cognitive function. *Acta. Anaesthesiol. Scand.,* 2001;45:275-289.
[114] Browne SM, Halligan PW, Wade DT, Taggart DP. Cognitive performance after cardiac operation: implications of regression toward the mean. *J. Thorac. Cardiovasc. Surg.,* 1999;117:481-485.
[115] Newman MF, Kirchner JL, Phillips-Bute B, et al. The Neurological Outcome Research Group and the Cardiothoracic Anesthesiology Research Endeavors Investigators. Longitudinal assessment of neurocognitive function after coronary-artery bypass surgery. *N. Eng. J. Med.,* 2001;344:395-402.
[116] Nierich AP, Diephuis J, Jansen EW, Borst C, Knape JT. Heart displacement during off-pump CABG: how well is it tolerated? *Ann. Thorac. Surg.,* 2000;70:466-472.
[117] Mariscalco G, Engström KG. Postoperative atrial fibrillation is associated with late mortality after coronary surgery, but not after valvular surgery. *Ann. Thorac. Surg.,* 2009;88:1871-6.
[118] Maisel WH, Rawn JD, Stevenson WG. Atrial fibrillation after cardiac surgery *Ann. Intern. Med.,* 2001;135:1061-1073.
[119] Mathew JP, Fontes ML, Tudor IC, et al. A multicenter risk index for atrial fibrillation after cardiac surgery *JAMA,* 2004;291:1720-1729.
[120] Athanasiou T, Aziz O, Mangoush O, et al. Does off-pump coronary artery bypass reduce the incidence of postoperative atrial fibrillation? A question revisited. *Eur. J. Cardiothorac. Surg.,* 2004;26:701-710.
[121] Maitra G, Ahmed A, Rudra A, Wankhede R, Sengupta S, Das T. Renal dysfunction after off-pump coronary artery bypass surgery- risk factors and preventive strategies. *Indian. J. Anaesth.,* 2009;53:401-7.
[122] Weerasinghe A, Athanasiou T, Al-Ruzzeh S, et al. Functional renal outcome in on-pump and off-pump coronary revascularization: a propensity-based analysis. *Ann. Thorac. Surg.,* 2005;79:1577-1583.
[123] Nigwekar SU, Kandula P, Hix JK, Thakar CV. Off-pump coronary artery bypass surgery and acute kidney injury: a meta-analysis of randomized and observational studies. *Am. J. Kidney Dis.,* 2009;54:413-23.

[124] Rothenhausler HB, Grieser B, Nollert G, Reichart B, Schelling G, Kapfhammer HP. Psychiatric and psychosocial outcome of cardiac surgery with cardiopulmonary bypass: a prospective 12-month follow-up study. *Gen. Hosp. Psychiatry.*, 2005;27:18-28.
[125] Newman MF, Grocott HP, Mathew JP, et al. Report of the substudy assessing the impact of neurocognitive function on quality of life 5 years after cardiac surgery. *Stroke*, 2001;32:2874-2881.
[126] Mortensen OS, Madsen JK, Haghfelt T, et al, DANAMI study group. Health related quality of life after conservative or invasive treatment of inducible postinfarction ischaemia. *Heart*, 2000;84:535-540.
[127] Duits AA, Boeke S, Taams MA, Passchier J, Erdman RA. Prediction of quality of life after coronary artery bypass graft surgery: a review and evaluation of multiple, recent studies. *Psychosom. Med.*, 1997;59:257-268.

In: Off-Pump Coronary Artery Bypass Grafting
Editors: S.G. Raja and M. Amrani
ISBN 978-1-62081-575-5

Chapter 11

OUTCOMES OF OFF-PUMP CORONARY ARTERY BYPASS GRAFTING IN THE PRESENCE OF ATHEROSCLEROTIC AORTA

Sotiris C. Stamou[1], Robert C. Hagberg[2] and Kevin W. Lobdell[3]
[1]Division of Thoracic and Cardiovascular Surgery,
Fred and Lena Meijer Heart Center Grand Rapids, MI, US
[2]Division of Cardiovascular Surgery, Beth Israel Deaconess Medical Center,
Harvard Medical School, Boston, MA, US
[3]Sanger Heart and Vascular Institute, Carolinas Medical Center, Charlotte, NC, US

ABSTRACT

Atherosclerotic disease of the ascending aorta has been thought to contribute significantly to the release of emboli during aortic manipulation and clamp application during conventional coronary artery bypass grafting (CABG) and has been identified as an independent predictor of both mortality and stroke after cardiac surgery. Different modalities have been suggested to diagnose atheromatous disease of the ascending aorta including preoperative computed tomography of the chest, intraoperative transesophageal echocardiography, manual digital palpation and epiaortic ultrasound. Different operative strategies have been described to manage atherosclerotic aorta, including a "no-touch" technique, replacement of the ascending aorta under hypothermic circulatory arrest, aortic arch endarterectomy, endoaortic occlusion balloon, modification in sites of cannulation and proximal anastomoses, CABG under hypothermic fibrillatory arrest or pump assist on-pump CABG. Off-pump coronary artery bypass (OPCAB) grafting decreases or can eliminate aortic manipulation. The differences in the degree of aortic manipulation, with the elimination of total aortic occlusion, may be responsible for the reduction in the postoperative rate of stroke observed with OPCAB over conventional CABG. Total arterial revascularization with the use of in situ or composite arterial grafts obviates the need to attach grafts to the aorta, thus allowing clampless OPCAB. Alternatively, when total arterial revascularization is not possible, epiaortic ultrasound is a useful tool to identify atherosclerosis-free areas of the anterior wall of the ascending aorta and create proximal clampless vein graft anastomoses using the heartstring proximal anastomotic system. Hybrid revascularization is another approach that may be indicated in patients with atheromatous aortas and depressed left ventricular function who may not tolerate manipulation of the heart during revascularization of the circumflex system. Multiple studies have demonstrated the benefits of "no-touch" OPCAB including a lower risk of stroke and mortality as well as an improved mid-term survival. Future prospective randomized studies to compare on-pump CABG with OPCAB, in the specific subset of patients with atheromatous aortic disease are needed to validate the results of the retrospective studies. This chapter provides an overview of the issues associated with atherosclerotic aorta, briefly discusses diagnostic modalities and therapeutic options for this subset of patients and focuses on the outcomes of OPCAB grafting in this situation.

Introduction

Despite refinements in cardiopulmonary bypass (CPB) technology such as improved arterial filtration and membrane oxygenators, the incidence of stroke after surgical coronary revascularization remains significant, ranging from 1.0% to 2.5%. [1,2,3] Although numerous pathophysiologic mechanisms for stroke after coronary artery bypass grafting (CABG) have been suggested, the most probable cause is cerebral embolization of atherosclerotic plaque debris from the ascending aorta, released during the maneuvers of cannulation and occlusion [4,5]. Atherosclerotic disease of the ascending aorta has been thought to contribute significantly to the release of emboli during aortic manipulation and clamp application during conventional cardiac operations [6]. Atheromatous disease of the ascending aorta has been identified as an independent predictor of both mortality and stroke after cardiac surgery [7,8]and maybe associated with an operative mortality as high as 14%[9].

Different approaches have been described to address the issue including a "no-touch" technique to handle the ascending aorta, replacement of the ascending aorta [10] under hypothermic circulatory arrest [11], aortic arch endarterectomy [12,13], endoaortic occlusion balloon [14], modification in sites of cannulation and proximal anastomoses [15], coronary artery bypass (CABG) under hypothermic fibrillatory arrest or pump assist on-pump CABG. Intra-aortic filtration has been recently reported to reduce adverse neurologic events [16]. However, the application of these approaches and other surgical techniques in this subset of high-risk patients has yielded unpredictable and disappointing results [17] .

Previous studies have demonstrated decreased risk of stroke and mortality with off-pump coronary artery bypass (OPCAB) grafting compared to on-pump CABG [18,19,20], while others have not [21]. Off-pump CABG decreases or can eliminate aortic manipulation during surgery [22]. The differences in the degree of aortic manipulation, with the elimination of total aortic occlusion, may be responsible for the reduction in the postoperative rate of stroke observed with OPCAB over conventional CABG.

Diagnosis of Aortic Atherosclerosis

Different modalities have been suggested to diagnose atheromatous disease of the ascending aorta including preoperative computed tomography (CT) of the chest, intraoperative transesophageal echocardiography (TEE), manual digital palpation and epiaortic ultrasound. Preoperative CT chest may add to the total cost of the operation and cannot be recommended as a routine preoperative work-up. However, for certain high-risk patients such as the elderly, patients with carotid artery disease, left main stenosis, chronic renal failure, poorly controlled hypertension or severe peripheral vascular disease, preoperative CT chest is a useful tool to identify aortic atherosclerosis (Figure 1).

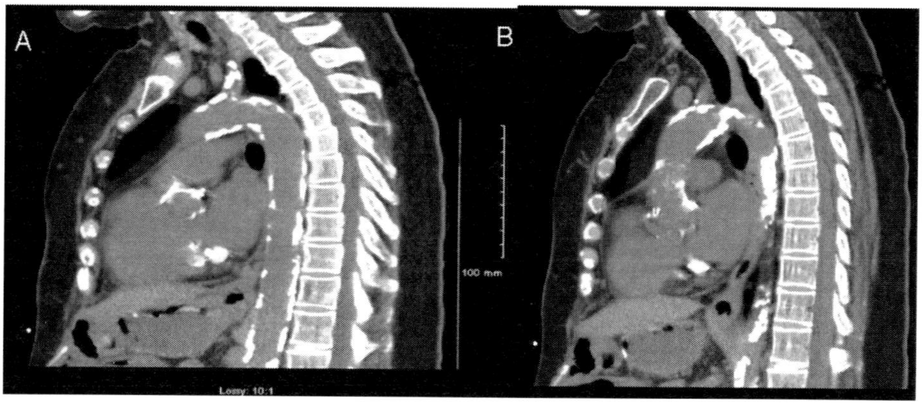

Figure 1. Computed tomography of the chest demonstrates severe calcification of the arch, descending aorta (panel A) and proximal ascending aorta (panel B).

Intraoperative TEE may underestimate the prevalence and severity of aortic atherosclerosis in the ascending aorta because of the interposition of the trachea and the main stem bronchus [23]. Epiaortic ultrasound is more accurate than TEE for identification of atherosclerosis of the ascending aorta but both techniques are superior to palpation [23]. Palpation can be misleading particularly in the instance of diffuse soft intramural plaque material. The severity of atherosclerosis is graded on a four-point scale as normal, mild, moderate or severe [23]. A *normal aorta* is defined as that having no identifiable intimal thickening; *mild atherosclerosis* is defined as $\leq$ 3 mm intimal thickening without intimal irregularities; *moderate atherosclerosis* is >3.0 mm intimal thickening with diffuse irregularities or calcification, or both; and *severe atherosclerosis as* >5.0 mm intimal thickening in addition to one or more of the following: large protruding atheromatous debris or thrombus, extensive calcification or ulcerated plaques [23].

Operative Strategies to Manage Aortic Atherosclerosis

There are many perioperative strategies that have been proposed and implemented in an attempt to reduce the neurologic cognitive and encephalopathic changes associated with atherosclerotic aorta. Aortic cannulation has repeatedly been the cause of cerebral emboli, as confirmed with transcranial Doppler imaging. The type of arterial cannula during on-pump CABG have been advocated to affect the incidence of stroke. Use of dispersion cannula and intraaortic filtration have been suggested as ways to decrease or avoid the embolic load in patients with mild or moderate atherosclerosis of the ascending aorta. Innominate artery or subclavian artery cannulation has been advocated as a neuroprotective strategy in patients with advanced aortic pathology. On the contrary, femoral arterial cannulation with the “sand blast” effect may increase the risk of embolic events. Endovascular balloon-like clamps offer an additional spectrum of safety in minimizing or preventing aortic manipulation. The complete avoidance of aortic clamping, cannulation and manipulation of the aorta, the so called "no-touch technique" have been shown to be effective [24].

The single-clamp technique, when feasible has been shown to prevent stroke in patients with advanced aortic atherosclerosis. Previous reports of attempts at replacing the diseased aorta or perform limited or extensive aortic endarterectomies, although initially promising in limited series, long-term follow up and larger series have yielded stroke rates that equal or surpass those of conventional cardiac surgery [24]. Aortic resection should be reserved for highly selected cases. Avoidance of cross-clamping of the ascending aorta using hypothermic fibrillatory arrest and creation of the proximal anastomoses using sealing devices, such as the heartstring proximal anastomotic system is another useful option.

Pump-Assist Beating Heart Surgery

Conventional on-pump CABG may be an option when aortic clamping may be performed in areas free of atheroma, usually in the more proximal ascending aorta. However, in most instances, severely calcified posterior aorta precludes aortic clamping. The tendency to incomplete revascularization and technical difficulties in constructing coronary anastomoses remain the principal limitation to the OPCAB technique, while pump-assist beating heart CABG allows coronary revascularization even in patients with cardiomegaly or significant left main stenoses. OPCAB in these patients may result in hemodynamic collapse during revascularization of the circumflex system, while pump-assist beating heart CABG allows complete revascularization on a decompressed heart without the deleterious effects on heart geometry and systemic hemodynamics [25].

Pump-assist beating heart CABG is also indicated in patients with severely depressed ejection fraction, because the procedure can be performed without major changes in ventricular geometry, valvular competence and heart retraction. Moreover, patients taken to the operating suite who are unstable secondary to an acute myocardial infarction, severely reduced left ventricular ejection fraction, acute coronary artery closure or dissection, or other catheterization laboratory misadventure represent a difficult population for traditional OPCAB.

Heart displacement by positioning and epicardial stabilization may result in hemodynamic compromise during OPCAB [25] that is more prominent during revascularization of the circumflex system. Gründeman and colleagues reported that ninety-degree anterior displacement of the beating heart caused primarily right ventricular dysfunction as a result of mechanical interference with diastolic expansion without concurring valvular incompetence [26]. Pump-assist beating heart surgery normalized stroke volume and mean arterial pressure by increasing left ventricular preload[26].

Manipulation of the aorta during construction of the proximal anastomoses has been shown to be associated with postoperative neurologic events, when the aorta is diseased. The heartstring proximal anastomotic system is a device that allows the surgeon to perform standard proximal clampless anastomoses [27]. Epiaortic ultrasonography is a useful tool to identify atherosclerosis-free areas of the anterior wall of the ascending aorta to create the proximal anastomoses. In selected high-risk patients, pump-assist beating-heart CABG may be an acceptable trade-off between conventional cardioplegia and OPCAB. It is still associated with the potentially detrimental effects of CPB but eliminates intraoperative global myocardial ischemia.

TOTAL ARTERIAL REVASCULARIZATION WITHOUT CARDIOPULMONARY BYPASS

OPCAB obviates the need for aortic cannulation and cross clamping and offsets untoward effects of CPB. Nevertheless, the use of partial aortic clamps is still necessary to construct proximal aortic anastomoses. A significant association for postoperative stroke correspondingly increasing with the extent of aortic manipulation was demonstrated by some studies (stroke incidence respectively increasing from 0.8% to 1.6% to a maximum of 2.2%, $p < 0.01$). Patients who had a full and a tangential aortic clamp applied were 1.8 times more likely to have a stroke versus those without any aortic manipulation (95% confidence interval: 1.15 to 2.74, $p < 0.01$) and 1.7 times more likely to develop a postoperative stroke than those with only a tangential aortic clamp applied (95% confidence interval: 1.11 to 2.48, $p < 0.01$). Because of this, albeit few exceptions, to date, only modest neurological benefit has been observed following OPCAB in comparison to on-pump CABG. Consistent benefits in major neurologic outcome was not evident [16,28,29].

Total arterial revascularization with the use of in situ or composite arterial grafts obviates the need to attach grafts to the aorta, thus allowing clampless (untouched aorta) OPCAB [30]. The technique includes using pedicled right internal mammary or radial artery as a "Y" graft from the left internal mammary artery (LIMA). These conduit configurations as a "Y" or ∏ graft, although technically challenging prevent manipulation of the aorta and may decrease the risk of major neurologic events [31] . In diabetic patients use of both internal mammary arteries may increase the risk of sternal wound infection [32] and other options such as use of one or both radial arteries as pedicled LIMA to LAD with T-graft radial coming off the LIMA to the obtuse marginal branches may be valid alternatives. Alternatively, when total arterial revascularization is not possible, epiaortic ultrasound is a useful tool to identify atherosclerosis-free areas of the anterior wall of the ascending aorta and create proximal clampless vein graft anastomoses using the heartstring proximal anastomotic system (Guidant, Indianapolis, IN) [33].

THE ROLE OF HYBRID REVASCULARIZATION IN PATIENTS WITH ATHEROSCLEROTIC AORTA

Hybrid revascularization combines OPCAB or MIDCAB (minimally invasive direct coronary artery bypass via a left anterior thoracotomy approach) with concomitant percutaneous coronary interventions to achieve complete revascularization for high-risk patients with coronary artery disease and atherosclerotic aortas. This approach may be indicated in patients with atheromatous aortas and depressed left ventricular function who may not tolerate manipulation of the heart during revascularization of the circumflex system. As a first step, patients have minimally invasive surgery with left-internal-thoracic-artery grafting to the left anterior descending artery on the beating heart without the use of CPB. In a second step (within two days), percutaneous intervention is performed in the right coronary or the circumflex artery [34]. However, this approach is more expensive, cannot be performed at all hospitals, and the long-term benefits are not proven [35,36].

Outcomes of OPCAB in Patients with Aortic Atherosclerosis

Early Mortality

OPCAB surgery has been associated with lower risk of death in patients with atheromatous aortic disease [37,38] . In a retrospective study on 125 patients older than 80 years of age with atheromatous aortic disease, who were operated for isolated myocardial revascularization (63 using CPB and 62 with OPCAB), Sharony and associates showed that the type of surgery (CPB or OPCAB) was an independent predictor of operative mortality and stroke (P = 0.0375) [37]. The odds ratio (OR) indicated that operative mortality and stroke occurred 4 times (OR = 4.171) more often in on-pump patients than in OPCAB patients.

In a similar study, propensity matched pair analysis was used to match patients undergoing off-pump CABG (n = 3,000) with 3,000 patients undergoing on-pump CABG [39]. Multivariate analysis revealed that increased mortality was associated with conventional coronary artery bypass grafting compared to OPCAB. Other authors have showed comparable mortality between OPCAB and on-pump CABG. [40]

Late Mortality

Some studies have showed improved mid-term survival after OPCAB than on-pump CABG in patients with atheromatous aortic disease [37]. Sharony et al. demonstrated that at 36 month follow-up, multivariate analysis revealed that increased mortality was associated with age (P = 0.001), previous MI (P = 0.03), and renal disease (P = 0.04), whereas increased survival was associated with increased number of grafts (P = 0.001) and OPCAB (P = 0.01) [37]. Other studies have not shown any difference in the late mortality between the two techniques [38].

Neurocognitive Outcomes

Djaiani et al. showed that patients with aortic atheroma > 2mm have a lower risk of new ischemic brain lesions as identified by diffusion weighted magnetic resonance imaging (MRI) after OPCAB compared with on-pump CABG [41]. The prevalence of new ischemic brain lesions on DW-MRI was 0% in the OPCAB group and 61% in the ONCAB group (P = 0.001). Patients in the OPCAB group were less confused during the first two postoperative days [41].

Avoiding aortic manipulation during OPCAB reduces the risk for atheroembolic complications and may, thus, benefit elderly patients who are prone to atherosclerotic aortic involvement. Lev-Ran and associates compared 103 undergoing clampless OPCAB were compared to 57 patients in whom side clamps were applied [40].

The incidence of major neurological complications (0% vs 5.3%, p = 0.044) and the combined outcome of stroke or mortality (3% vs 12%, p = 0.035) were lower in the clampless group. Multivariate analysis identified side clamping as a predictor for the occurrence of stroke or mortality (OR, 6.28, CL 1.39 –28.4, p = 0.017), increasing this risk by sixfold[40]. Other studies using propensity score matching to compare OPCAB with on-pump CABG in patients with atheromatous aortic disease have demonstrated lower risk of stroke with OPCAB compared with on-pump CABG [37, 38, 39, 40].

Avoiding partial aortic clamping during off-pump CABG was associated with a further decrease in the incidence of stroke compared to OPCAB with partial clamping of the aorta [42,40,43,44]. In another report, Halbersma and coworkers recently suggested OPCAB no-touch with total arterial Y grafts as the best treatment option [45]. They presented 4-year data of 400 consecutive patients that were compared with the surgical arm of the SYNTAX trial with regard to neurologic outcome. The authors identified a clear trend toward a reduction of stroke (0.8%) compared with the surgical arm of the syntax trial (2.2%) [45].

Perioperative Morbidity

Many studies have demonstrated a significant reduction in perioperative morbidity after OPCAB than on-pump CABG in patients with atheromatous aortic disease. In a study by Emmert and associates [44], the authors evaluated the incidence of stroke, mortality, major adverse cardiac and cerebrovascular events (MACCE), and a non-cardiac composite end point including respiratory failure, renal failure, and bleeding between OPCAB and on-pump CABG. The mortality rate (1.6% vs 2.4%; propensity-adjusted odds ratio [PAOR] = 0.51; CI 95%, 0.26-0.99; P = .047), MACCE (7.9% vs 17.1%; PAOR = 0.67; CI 95%, 0.52-0.84; P = .001) including myocardial infarction (1.1% vs 2.2%; PAOR = 0.50; CI 95%, 0.26-0.98; P = .044) and stroke (1.1% vs 2.4%; PAOR = 0.35; CI 95%, 0.17-0.72; P = .005) as well as the non-cardiac composite (PAOR = 0.46; CI 95%, 0.35-0.91; P < .001) were significantly lower for OPCAB when compared with on-pump CABG. In comparison with partial clamping of the aorta, OPCAB patients using the heartstring anastomotic device for creation of proximal anastomoses had significantly lower rates of stroke (0.7% vs 2.3%; PAOR = 0.39; CI 95%, 0.16-0.90; P = .04) and MACCE (6.7% vs 10.8%; PAOR = 0.55; CI 95%, 0.38-0.79; P = .001) than on-pump CABG[44]. Other studies have reported similar results [37, 38, 39, 43].

Completeness of Revascularization and Graft Patency

Despite the benefits of OPCAB in patients with atheromatous aortic disease concern has been raised as to whether potential benefits of OPCAB have come at a cost of less complete revascularization and lower graft patency compared with conventional CABG. A meta-analysis of randomized trials has consistently shown a lower number of grafts per patient in off-pump versus on-pump CABG (2.6 versus 2.8, p < .0001) [46]. Graft patency has been evaluated in many randomized trials from in-hospital to 1 year postoperatively. Puskas demonstrated no difference in graft patency at discharge [47], whereas Khan showed a decreased graft patency in the off-pump group at 3 months [48]. Other authors showed no difference in graft patency at 1 year [49]. A meta-analysis at 1 year confirmed that there is no significant difference between off-pump and on-pump revascularization [46].

Conclusion

OPCAB is a useful tool for myocardial revascularization in patients with atheromatous aortic disease. However, it is important to remember that off-pump surgery does not eliminate the danger of atherosclerotic embolization, as long as partial occluding clamps are still used on the ascending aorta. Increased experience with aortic connectors for proximal anastomoses and complex internal mammary artery grafting offer the possibility of further decreasing the aortic trauma and embolization risk associated with off-pump surgery in retrospective studies.

Future prospective randomized studies to compare on-pump CABG with OPCAB, in the specific subset of patients with atheromatous aortic disease are needed to validate the results of the retrospective studies. Both on-pump and off-pump surgical strategies are in evolution. Combinations of perfusion (either partial or total CPB) and beating-heart surgery are being explored and employed in patients with atheromatous aorta. As Dr. Lytle points out "the one size fits all era is over, and multiple strategies for performing surgical revascularization are available and effective. The mission of coronary surgeons in the future will be to apply the approaches available to different subsets of patients in a way that maximizes long-term benefit and minimizes short-term risk" [50].

References

[1] Calafiore AM, Di Mauro M, Teodori G, et al. Impact of aortic manipulation on incidence of cerebrovascular accidents after surgical myocardial revascularization. *Ann. Thorac. Surg.*, 2002;73:1387-1393.

[2] Puskas JD, Winston AD, Wright CE, et al. Stroke after coronary artery operations, incidence, correlates outcomes and cost. *Ann. Thorac. Surg.*, 2000;69:1053-1056.

[3] Fearn SJ, Pole R, Burgess SG, Ray TL, Hooper CN, McCollum CN. Cerebral embolization during modern cardiopulmonary bypass. *Eur. J. Cardiothorac. Surg.*, 2001;20:1163-1167.

[4] Barbut D, Hinton RB, Statrowski TP, et al. Cerebral emboli detected during bypass surgery are associated with clamp removal. *Stroke,* 1994;25:2398 -2402.

[5] Wareing TH, Davila-Roman VG, Barzilai B, Murphy SF, Kouchoukos NT. Management of the severely atherosclerotic ascending aorta during cardiac operations. *J. Thorac. Cardiovasc. Surg.*, 1992;103:453-462.

[6] van der Linden J, Casimir-Ahr H. When do cerebral emboli appear during opean heart operations? A transcranial Doppler study. *Ann. Thorac. Surg.*, 1991;51:237–241.

[7] Roach GW, Kanchuger M, Mangano CM, et al. Adverse cerebral outcomes after coronary bypass surgery. Multicenter Study of Perioperative Ischemia Research Group

and the Ischemia Research and Education Foundation Investigators. *N. Engl. J. Med.*, 1996;335:1857-1863.

[8] Gardner TJ, Horneffer PJ, Manolio TA, et al. Stroke following coronary artery bypass grafting: a ten-year study. *Ann. Thorac. Surg.*, 1985;40:574-581.

[9] Wareing TH, Davila-Roman VG, Daily BB, et al. Strategy for the reduction of stroke incidence in cardiac surgical patients. *Ann. Thorac. Surg.*, 1993;55:1400-1408.

[10] Mills NL, Everson CT. Atherosclerosis of the ascending aorta and coronary artery bypass. Pathology, clinical correlates, and operative management. *J. Thorac. Cardiovasc. Surg.*, 1991;102:546-553.

[11] Meharwal ZS, Mishra YK, Kohli V, Bapna R, Singh S, Trehan N. Off-pump multivessel coronary artery surgery in high-risk patients. *Ann. Thorac. Surg.*, 2002;74:S1353-S1357.

[12] Hart JC, Puskas JD, Sabik JF, 3rd. Off-pump coronary revascularization: current state of the art. *Semin. Thorac. Cardiovasc. Surg.*, 2002;14:70- 81.

[13] Hernandez F, Cohn WE, Baribeau YR, et al; Northern New England. In-hospital outcomes of off-pump versus on-pump coronary artery bypass procedures: a multicenter experience. *Ann. Thorac. Surg.*, 2001;72:1528-1534.

[14] Cosgrove DM. Management of the calcified aorta: an alternative method of occlusion. *Ann. Thorac. Surg.*, 1983;36:718-719.

[15] Stern A, Tunick PA, Culliford AT, et al. Protruding aortic arch atheromas: risk of stroke during heart surgery with and without aortic arch endarterectomy. *Am. Heart. J.*, 1999;138:746 -752.

[16] Arom KV, Flavin TF, Emery RW, Kshettry VR, Petersen RJ, Janey PA. Is low ejection fraction safe for off-pump coronary bypass operation? *Ann. Thorac. Surg.*, 2000;70:1021-1025.

[17] Grossi EA, Kanchuger MS, Schwartz DS, et al. Effect of cannula length on aortic arch flow: protection of the atheromatous aortic arch . *Ann. Thorac. Surg.*, 1995;59:710-712.

[18] Stamou SC, Jablonski KA, Garcia JM, Boyce SW, Bafi AS, Corso PJ. Operative mortality after conventional versus coronary revascularization without cardiopulmonary bypass. *Eur. J. Cardiothorac. Surg.*, 2004;26:549-553.

[19] Magee MJ, Jablonski KA, Stamou SC, et al. Elimination of cardiopulmonary bypass improves early survival for multivessel coronary artery bypass patients. *Ann. Thorac. Surg.*, 2002;73:1196-203.

[20] Stamou SC, Jablonski KA, Pfister AJ, et al. Stroke after conventional versus minimally invasive coronary artery bypass. *Ann. Thorac. Surg.*, 2002;74:394-399.

[21] van Dijk D, Nierich AP, Jansen EW, et al; Octopus Study Group. Early outcome after off-pump versus on-pump coronary bypass surgery: results from a randomized study. *Circulation*, 2001;104:1761-1766.

[22] Patel NC, Pullan MD, Fabri BM. Does off-pump total arterial revascularization without aortic manipulation influence neurological outcome? A study of 226 consecutive, unselected cases. *Heart Surg. Forum*, 2001;5:28-32.

[23] Dávila-Román, VG, Phillips KJ, Daily BB, et al. Intraoperative transesophageal echocardiography and epiaortic ultrasound for assessment of atherosclerosis of the thoracic aorta. *J. Am. Coll. Cardiol.*, 1996;28:942-947.

[24] Franco Kl, Verrier ED. Advanced therapy in Cardiac Surgery. Hamilton, Ontario, B.C. Decker Inc. 1999: 51-61.

[25] Mathison M, Edgerton JR, Horswell JL, Akin JJ, Mack MJ. Analysis of hemodynamic changes during beating heart surgical procedures. *Ann. Thorac. Surg.,* 2000;70:1355-1361.
[26] Gründeman PF, Borst C, Verlaan CW, Meijburg H, Mouës CM, Jansen EW. Exposure of circumflex branches in the tilted, beating porcine heart: echocardiographic evidence of right ventricular deformation and the effect of right or left heart bypass. *J. Thorac. Cardiovasc. Surg.,* 1999;118:316-323.
[27] Medalion B, Meirson D, Hauptman E, Sasson L, Schachner A. Initial experience with the Heartstring proximal anastomotic system. *J. Thorac. Cardiovasc. Surg.,* 2004;128:273-277.
[28] Puskas JD, Williams WH, Duke PG, et al. Off-pump coronary artery bypass grafting provides complete revascularization with reduced myocardial injury, transfusion requirements and length of stay: a prospective randomized comparison of two hundred unselected patients undergoing off-pump versus conventional coronary artery bypass grafting. *J. Thorac. Cardiovasc. Surg.,* 2003;125:797-808.
[29] Angelini GD, Taylor FC, Reeves BC, Ascione R. Early and mid-term outcome after off-pump and on-pump surgery in Beating Heart Against Cardioplegic Arrest Studies (BHACAS 1 and 2): a pooled analysis of two randomised controlled trials. *Lancet,* 2002;359:1194-9.
[30] Lev-Ran O, Paz Y, Pevni D, et al. Bilateral internal thoracic artery grafting: midterm results of composite versus in situ crossover graft. *Ann. Thorac. Surg.,* 2002;74:704-11.
[31] Prapas SN, Panagiotopoulos IA, Ayyad MA, et al. Female risk using OPCAB, pi-circuit, and aorta no-touch coronary revascularization. *Heart Surg. Forum,* 2009;12:E344-348.
[32] Grossi EA, Esposito R, Harris LJ, et al. Sternal wound infections and use of internal mammary artery grafts. *J. Thorac. Cardiovasc. Surg.,* 1991;102:342-347.
[33] Medalion B, Meirson D, Hauptman E, Sasson L, Schachner A. Initial experience with the Heartstring proximal anastomotic system. *J. Thorac. Cardiovasc. Surg.,* 2004;128:273-277.
[34] Friedrich GJ, Bonatti J, Dapunt OE. Preliminary experience with minimally invasive coronary-artery bypass surgery combined with coronary angioplasty. *N. Engl. J. Med.,* 1997;336:1454-1455.
[35] Murphy GJ, Bryan AJ, Angelini GD. Hybrid coronary revascularization in the era of drug-eluting stents. *Ann. Thorac. Surg.,* 2004;78:1861-1867.
[36] Vassiliades TA Jr, Douglas JS, Morris DC, et al. Integrated coronary revascularization with drug-eluting stents: immediate and seven-month outcome. *J. Thorac. Cardiovasc. Surg.,* 2006;131:956-962.
[37] Sharony R, Bizekis CS, Kanchuger M, et al. Off-pump coronary artery bypass grafting reduces mortality and stroke in patients with atheromatous aortas: a case control study. *Circulation,* 2003;108 Suppl 1:II15-20.
[38] Sharony R, Grossi EA, Saunders PC, et al. Propensity case-matched analysis of off-pump coronary artery bypass grafting in patients with atheromatous aortic disease. *J. Thorac. Cardiovasc. Surg.,* 2004;127:406-413.
[39] Mishra M, Malhotra R, Karlekar A, Mishra Y, Trehan N. opensity case-matched analysis of off-pump versus on-pump coronary artery bypass grafting in patients with atheromatous aorta. *Ann. Thorac. Surg.,* 2006;82:608-614.

[40] Lev-Ran O, Loberman D, Matsa M, Pevni D, Nesher N, Mohr R, Uretzky G. Reduced strokes in the elderly: the benefits of untouched aorta off-pump coronary surgery. *Ann. Thorac. Surg.,* 2004;77:102-107.
[41] Djaiani G, Fedorko L, Cusimano RJ, et al. Off-pump coronary bypass surgery: risk of ischemic brain lesions in patients with atheromatous thoracic aorta. *Can. J. Anaesth.,* 2006;53:795-801.
[42] Lev-Ran O, Braunstein R, Sharony R, Kramer A, Paz Y, Mohr R, Uretzky G. No-touch aorta off-pump coronary surgery: the effect on stroke. *J. Thorac. Cardiovasc. Surg.,* 2005;129:307-313.
[43] Kapetanakis EI, Stamou SC, Dullum MK, et al. The impact of aortic manipulation on neurologic outcomes after coronary artery bypass surgery: a risk-adjusted study. *Ann. Thorac. Surg.,* 2004;78:1564-1571.
[44] Emmert MY, Seifert B, Wilhelm M, Grünenfelder J, Falk V, Salzberg SP. Aortic no-touch technique makes the difference in off-pump coronary artery bypass graft *J. Thorac. Cardiovasc. Surg.,* 2011;142:1499-506.
[45] Halbersma WB, Arrigoni SC, Mecozzi G, et al. Four-year outcome of OPCAB no-touch with total arterial Y-graft: making the best treatment a daily practice. *Ann. Thorac. Surg.,* 2009;88:796-801.
[46] Puskas J, Cheng D, Knight J, et al. Off-pump versus conventional coronary artery bypass grafting: A meta-analysis and consensus statement from the 2004 ISMICS consensus conference. *Innovations,* 2005; 1:3.
[47] Puskas JD, Williams WH, Mahoney EM, et al. Off-pump vs conventional coronary artery bypass grafting: Early and 1-year graft patency, cost, and quality-of-life outcomes. A randomized trial. *JAMA*, 2004; 291:1841-9.
[48] Khan NE, De Souza A, Mister R, et al. A randomized comparison of off-pump and on-pump multivessel coronary-artery bypass surgery. *N. Engl. J. Med.,* 2004; 350:21-8.
[49] Nathoe HM, van Dijk D, Jansen EWL, et al. A comparison of on-pump and off-pump coronary bypass surgery in low-risk patients. *N. Engl. J. Med.,* 2003; 348:394-402.
[50] Lytle BW, Sabik JF. On-pump and off-pump bypass surgery: Tools for revascularization. *Circulation,* 2004; 109:810-2.

In: Off-Pump Coronary Artery Bypass Grafting
Editors: S.G. Raja and M. Amrani ISBN 978-1-62081-575-5

Chapter 12

OUTCOMES OF SEQUENTIAL OFF-PUMP CORONARY ARTERY BYPASS GRAFTING

Robert L. Quigley
Regional Medical Director, Americas Region, International SOS Assistance, Inc.
Trevose, PA, US

ABSTRACT

Techniques in coronary revascularization have evolved over the last fifty years to accommodate the increasing medical needs of an aging population. Traditionally coronary artery disease (CAD) was addressed through a sternotomy with cardiopulmonary bypass (CPB) using venous bypass conduits on the arrested heart. Such an invasive approach is no longer realistic or even practical today where, at least in Western countries, people are living longer with increasing co-morbidities. Consequently less invasive strategies, to accomplish similar objectives, are becoming the standard of care. Resurgence of off-pump coronary artery bypass (OPCAB) grafting is one such less invasive strategy that has positively impacted the incidence of complications associated with CPB. Similarly, sequential grafting technique is reported to offer the hemodynamic advantage of increased total graft flow through improved distal runoff and, by extension, increased graft patency rates. Additional benefits include greater conservation of conduit, reduced aortic manipulation and last but not least more complete revascularization by allowing anastomoses to smaller coronary arteries, which theoretically should translate into improved clinical outcomes. Interestingly, combination of OPCAB with sequential grafting to provide the maximum benefit is still regarded as a high-risk strategy owing to concerns regarding the quality and completeness of revascularization during OPCAB and dependence of multiple grafts on a common inflow in sequential grafting with the possibility of catastrophic consequences in the event of a proximal occlusion. This perceived threat of the large myocardium at risk coupled with the disadvantages of increased conduit manipulation, suboptimal conduit configuration and the complexity of certain side-to-side anastomoses are predominant concerns preventing universal adoption of sequential grafting. In this chapter the author presents his experience of this strategy focusing in particular on the merits and efficacy of the sequential grafting technique.

Introduction

The landscape of coronary artery revascularization has changed coincident with the continued success of percutaneous transluminal coronary angioplasty (PTCA) and the drug eluting stents. The BARI (Bypass Angioplasty Revascularization Investigation) randomized trial was designed to compare the results of PTCA vs. coronary artery bypass grafting (CABG) in the management of multivessel coronary artery disease (CAD) [1]. The 5-year survival was similar for both cohorts at least in non-diabetic patients. Consequently clinicians and patients alike have generally opted for PTCA over CABG for their initial treatment of CAD. With increasing life span of Western population, the impact on the cardiac surgical community has been significant such that in 2011 the patients presenting for surgical revascularization typically are elderly with multiple co-morbidities, and limited targets with compromised ventricular function. Surgeons have therefore needed to modify their techniques to accommodate this challenging patient population. The adaptation has included expertise in the application of beating heart surgery techniques as well as the application of shorter conduits. The former to avoid the deleterious effects of invasive cardiopulmonary bypass (CPB) and the latter for complete revascularization where conduit is limited (i.e. peripheral vasculopathies or previous surgery).

Experience with Sequential Grafting on the Arrested Heart

Our initial exposure, and routine utilization of the sequential reversed saphenous vein graft (rSVG), dates back to the early 1970s. In fact this sequential technique was used exclusively for 15 years to surgically revascularize the myocardium using CPB until the introduction of the left internal mammary artery (LIMA) graft to our armamentarium. The configuration of our original sequential rSVG, prior to the use of the LIMA, referred to as the "snake" graft, was very deliberate. The typical case was a quadruple bypass, beginning at the aortic root then side-side anastomoses to the diagonal, to the left anterior descending (LAD), to the posterior descending artery (PDA), and ending with an end-to-side anastomosis to an obtuse marginal (OM) branch of the circumflex artery [2](Figure 1A).

The aforementioned deliberate configuration of the "snake" graft differed from the conventional rSVG sequential graft [3,4] in that it lay parallel, yet more caudad, to the native coronary artery ring ("crown"): the right and circumflex arteries encircle the heart in the atrioventricular groove. Sewell, one of the original pioneers of the sequential vein graft, hypothesized that the left ventricle, the model of which is a thick-walled ellipsoid of revolution, "strips" the "snake" graft with each systole [2]. Such "stripping" is created by ventricular wall stress that acts in 3 directions: radial, circumferential, and meridional [5].

Once the LIMA graft was clearly established as the standard of care for revascularization of the anterior myocardium (LAD) we altered the configuration of our snake to exclude bypassing the LAD with this rSVG (Figure 1B). Many of the controversies regarding the safety and efficacy of our "snake" graft were addressed in a retrospective review of the results of one surgeon [6]. We noted firstly, that the revascularization is more complete since anastomoses can be made to smaller (<2.0mm) coronaries. Secondly long-term angiography revealed that proximal graft closure, contrary to popular belief, does not result in diffuse myocardial ischemia since the "snake" graft can and does function as a large intercoronary epicardial collateral vessel. At the time we believed that these 2 observations were dependent upon the anastomosis of the terminal end of the snake to a "large" coronary artery with a robust vascular bed (runoff).

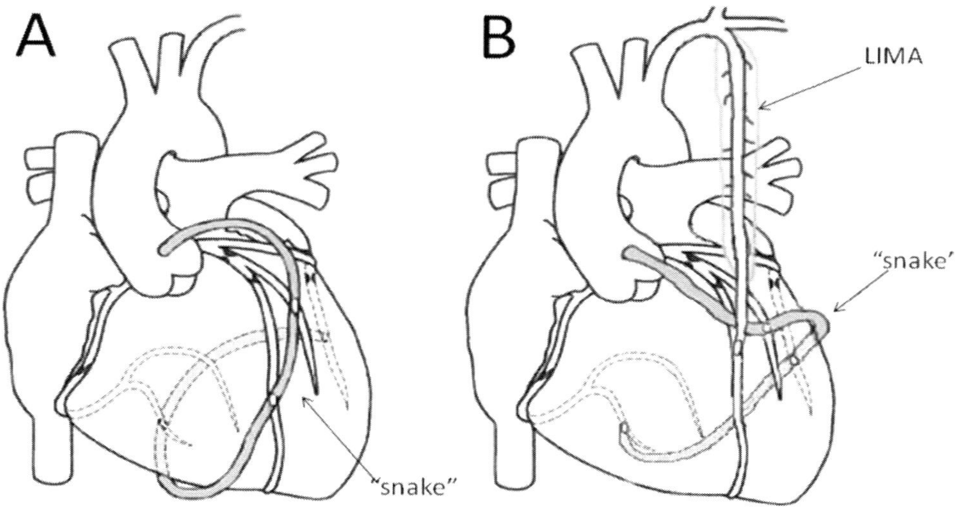

Figure 1. Sequential rSVG ("snake"). A) Without LIMA graft; B) With LIMA graft.

The 15 year results of our retrospective study revealed a 67% survival and 4% incidence of redo CABG, using CPB, in those patients bypassed with a "snake" graft. This was competitive with the outcome of the LIMA graft to the LAD: 72% survival and 5.6% reoperation rates [7].

EXPERIENCE WITH SEQUENTIAL GRAFTING ON THE BEATING HEART

As the surgical population became older, with more co-morbidities, it was inevitable that the conventional surgical revascularization approach: LIMA/rSVG on CPB would need to be modified to accommodate these new clinical challenges. To that end beating heart surgery, also termed off-pump coronary artery bypass (OPCAB) grafting, was introduced with the intention of achieving the same morbidity/mortality results without CPB. Success was dependent on cooperation between the surgeon and the anesthesiologist and adequate exposure. The LAD was routinely grafted first, not only because it was the most accessible coronary, but because it supplies up to 70% of the myocardial blood flow. The creative use of intravenous fluid, stabilizers, pericardiotomies, and surgical tapes facilitated exposure of the lateral and inferior walls.

We extrapolated from the success we had experienced with the sequential "snake" graft, where CPB was used, to the OPCAB arena. In fact once the technique of beating heart surgery was mastered we preferentially performed all of our coronary revascularizations, including our redo operations, on the beating heart with a LIMA graft and a rSVG "snake". The ischemic myocardium however was the one exception where CPB was routinely utilized. Many of our patients had coincidental peripheral vascular disease, diabetes, and/or venous insufficiency. Since the length of a "snake" graft rarely exceeds 40cm we were able to harvest one segment, usually from one thigh. The endoscopic approach limited any morbidity previously encountered using the open technique of vein harvesting.

We soon began to explore the use of alternative conduits during OBCAB surgery. We reported our series of total arterial revascularization procedures where composite and/or creative grafting was utilized [8]. The predominant composite graft was a T-graft (where the radial artery (RA) was anastomosed to the LIMA). The LIMA and/or the RA could be sequenced with the resultant surgery labeled as an OPCAB x 2, OPCAB x 3, or even a OPCAB x 4. We reserved this all arterial approach for our younger patients and maintained the LIMA/rSVG ("snake") technique for our aged patients.

To further demonstrate that there are few, if any, contraindications to OPCAB surgery, with the exception of the ischemic myocardium, we evaluated a series of patients with compromised left ventricular function who underwent OPCAB *[9]* . There were 40 cases with a mean ejection fraction of 29% (range = 20-40%). Interestingly in all cases we used exclusively arterial conduits in either sequential or composite configuration. The observed 30-day mortality was 2.5% (1/40) while the Society of Thoracic Surgeons (STS) predicted rate for this cohort was 3.8%.

Technical Aspects

Despite an excellent 30-day observed mortality rate for both our on-pump "snake" series (1%)[1] and our total off-pump arterial series (3.1%)[2] there remained physiologic issues that needed to be addressed: Are flow rates compromised by the number of bypasses in a sequential graft and does the final, end-to-side, anastomosis on a sequential graft need to be to the largest diameter coronary artery? Prior to our report (see below) it had been published by others, that the combination of sequential coronary grafting and OPCABG surgery is feasible and safe [10]. In fact 10 of the 45 patients outlined in this study by Al-Ruzzeh et al underwent early postoperative coronary angiography. All sequential grafts were patent. There were no mortalities. Furthermore with the use of flow values and pulsatility indexes, grafting of a rSVG proximally to a larger coronary bed does not appear to have a significant effect on blood flow in the distal segment of a sequential bypass [11]. This study by Gwozdziewicz et al. was unique in that their intraoperative flow model allowed for the transformation of an individual graft to a sequential one in the same coronary territory simply by the strategic placement of a bulldog clamp.

Over a 24 month period we reviewed a consecutive series of 175 patients all of whom underwent OPCAB, performed by a single surgeon (RLQ) with 1 LIMA graft and 1 sequential rSVG ("snake") *[12]*. Flow rates were measured in each segment of the "snake" using a Transonic Flowmeter (HT314, Transonic Systems Inc., Ithaca, NY). We quantified blood flow in the proximal segment(s) with and without distal limb clamp occlusion. In this

[1] STS did not have a database nor a mortality risk analysis in 1981.
[2] The STS predicted rate was 3.82% for this same population.

fashion, similar pathophysiologic conditions, in relation to vascular resistance, were maintained, which was necessary for quantifying and comparing regional blood flow.

The mean flow through the distal segment of the "snake" was 36ml/min and this value was not significantly influenced by the number of proximal coronary anastomoses nor the size of the proximal coronary bed noted during preoperative angiography. Flow <27ml/min, in any segment, was interpreted as unacceptable. Under these circumstances the "snake" was evaluated for spasms/twists/kinks. Simultaneously other potential causes were considered such as a small target coronary (<1.5mm), a decrease in diastolic pressure, and the existence of diffuse and/or distal CAD. Based on this strategy anastomoses were redone particularly when the systolic peak dominated the flow profile, and/or in the context of negative diastolic flow (n=6).

The 30-day mortality and stroke rate was 0% (0/175). The incidence of post-operative atrial fibrillation, in those patients with a baseline of normal sinus rhythm, was 29% (49/169). Regardless of the choice of conduit (artery or rSVG) we have noted, in all of our published reports, that the incidence of postoperative atrial fibrillation, in our patients who underwent OPCAB, was similar and in some cases higher than that predicted by the STS. The aforementioned predicted value is based on a similar population of patients where CPB was instituted. If postoperative atrial fibrillation is merely a result of myocardial/pericardial trauma and resultant inflammation one would have expected the incidence of postoperative atrial fibrillation to be markedly less in the OPCAB cohort where instrumentation is minimal. Clearly the etiology of postoperative atrial fibrillation must be multifactorial [13].

There were neither postoperative myocardial infarctions (using enzyme/EKG criteria) nor incidents of renal failure requiring dialysis.

It was noteworthy that in this off-pump series we did not adhere to the requirement, previously published, that the distal (end-side) anastomosis should be completed to the largest coronary with the largest runoff [6]. In fact in this more recent series the diameter of the distal coronary artery and/or the number of branches of the target coronary artery (runoff) were not even considered in the configuration of each "snake" graft. Furthermore the "snake" in this series, where the LIMA was always anastomosed to the LAD, rather than the "snake," did not even crown the ventricles (compare Figure 1A to Figure 1B) as originally proposed by Sewell. This fundamental principle was originally thought to be a requirement to the patency success of the "snake" graft [6].

Upon successful and complete conversion of our cardiac program to a predominately beating heart practice we noticed a slight increase in the incidence of thromboembolic events such as deep venous thrombosis (DVT) and pulmonary embolus (PE). Traditionally it was assumed that following open-heart surgery, where CPB and hypothermia were instituted, the coagulation, complement, and Kallikrein/Kinin cascades were activated. This resultant relative state of hypocoagulation was further enhanced by the extracorporeal passage/consumption of platelets and factor dilution [14]. We hypothesized that in the absence of such activation(s) the risk of a thrombotic event would be similar to that seen with major orthopedic surgery or general surgery where post-operative anticoagulation regimes define the standard of care.

Using thrombelastography (TEG) we prospectively studied 17 patients undergoing OPCAB, and 6 patients undergoing conventional CABG with hypothermia and CPB [15]. Each patient served as its own control where blood samples were analyzed preoperatively, intraoperatively, and postoperatively. The study demonstrated that OPCAB surgery indeed produces a relative state of procoagulation when compared to on-pump surgery, as indicated by TEG, at least inclusive of postoperative day 3 (data beyond postoperative day 3 was not collected due to patient discharge).

Based on these results, and in the clinical context of a slight increase in thromboembolic events, we altered our postoperative protocol, for the management of OPCAB patients, to include the administration of a once daily Clopidogrel tablet (Plavix) 75mg beginning postoperatively day 1 for a total of 6 weeks [16].

More recently we have noted that there is an increasing subset of CAD patients with diffuse/distal disease that are refractory to conventional surgical and/or percutaneous revascularization due to unsuitable targets. Typically these patients have undergone multiple percutaneous procedures where numerous stents have been deployed and are on maximal medical therapies. Sadly most of these patients, who still have viable anterior myocardial muscle, have crippling unstable angina.

Again, extrapolating from our decades of using the sequential rSVG ("snake"), we designed a procedure to address these unfortunate individuals. We began by selecting patients who had viable anterior walls (based on thallium imaging studies) and took them to the operating theatre where, off-pump, we revascularized their lateral and inferior walls with the sequential rSVG ("snake") and their anterior wall with a Vineberg implant plus transmyocardial laser channels [17]. In our series of 21 OPCAB patients all had relief of their angina and postoperative thallium imaging revealed significantly improved perfusion.

In this case the "snake" was an ideal conduit in that it could be used in the context of small targets and could serve as an intercoronary epicardial collateral in the case of an occluded segment. Despite our hypothesis that the benefits of this procedure were the result of angiogenesis (secondary to the additive effect of the Vineberg and the laser channels) we still could not scientifically rule out the fact that the reperfusion of the anterior wall was actually a result of intramyocardial collaterals fed by the epicardial sequential "snake".

Conclusion

The sequential coronary bypass grafting (artery or rSVG) has always been our preferred technique to revascularize diseased coronary arteries. We have published our flow dynamic studies to confirm the efficacy of the sequential graft. The fact that typically only 40cm of rSVG and only one aortotomy are required represent obvious added merits of the sequential grafting strategy.

Acknowledgement

The author would like to acknowledge the pioneer work of William (Bill) H. Sewell, MD and Karlene V. Sewell, BA without whom many of these sequential techniques would never have been made possible.

REFERENCES

[1] The BARI Investigators. The final 10-year follow-up results from the BARI randomized trial. *J Am Coll Cardiol* 2007;49:1600-1606.

[2] Sewell WH, Swell KV. Technique for the coronary snake graft operation. *Ann Thor Surg* 1976;22:58-65.

[3] O'Neill MJ Jr, Wolf PD, O'Neill TK, Montesano RM, Waldhausen JA. A rationale for the use of sequential coronary artery bypass grafts. *J Thorac Cardiovasc* Surg 1981;81:686-690.

[4] Christenson JT, Schmuziger M. Sequential venous bypass grafts: Results 10 years later. *Ann Thorac Surg* 1997;63:371-376.

[5] Yin FCP. Ventricular wall stress. *Circ Res* 1981;49:829-842.

[6] Quigley RL, Dienhart KJ, Pelkowski DJ, Evans, LC. Coronary artery bypass with "snake" grafts: 15 year follow-up. *J Card Surg* 1998,13:18-23.

[7] Cameron A, Kemp HG Jr, Green GE. Bypass surgery with the internal mammary artery graft: 15 year follow-up. *Circulation* 1986;74(Suppl III):30-36.

[8] Quigley RL, Weiss SJ, Highbloom RY, Pym J. Creative arterial bypass grafting can be performed on the beating heart. *Ann Thorac Surg* 2001;72:793-797.

[9] Quigley RL, Weiss, SJ, Highbloom RY, Pym J. A low ejection fraction does not preclude total arterial revascularization on the beating heart. *J Card Failure* 2000;6(3 Suppl.):41.

[10] Al-Ruzzeh S, Bustami M, Khan S, Amrani M. The early clinical and angiographic outcome of sequential coronary artery bypass grafting with the off-pump technique. *J Thorac Cardiovasc Surg* 2002;123:525-530.

[11] Gwozdziewicz M, Nemee P, Simek M, Hajek R, Troubil M. Sequential bypass grafting on the beating heart: blood flow characteristics. *Ann Thorac. Surg* 2006;82:620-623.

[12] Quigley RL. Sequential bypass on the beating heart can be achieved without compromising patient safety or regional myocardial blood flow. *Inter Surg* 2010;95:257-260.

[13] Katariya K, DeMarchena E, Bolooki H. Oral amiodarone reduces incidence of postoperative atrial fibrillation. *Ann. Thorac. Surg.* 1999;68:1599-1604

[14] Shammas NW. Pulmonary embolus after coronary artery bypass surgery: a review of the literature. *Clin Cardiol* 2000;23:637-644.

[15] Quigley RL, Fried DW, Salenger R, Pym J, Highbloom RY. Thrombelastographic Changes in OPCAB Surgical Patients. *Perfusion* 2002;17:363-367.

[16] Quigley, RL. Symmetry aortic connector system. *J Thorac Cardiovasc Surg* 2003;125:1173-1174.

[17] Quigley RL. Synergy of old and new technology results in successful revascularization of the anterior myocardium with relief of angina in the absence of suitable targets. *Heart Surg Forum* 2004;7:409-413.

In: Off-Pump Coronary Artery Bypass Grafting
Editors: S.G. Raja and M. Amrani
ISBN 978-1-62081-575-5

Chapter 13

OUTCOMES OF TOTAL ARTERIAL OFF-PUMP CORONARY ARTERY BYPASS GRAFTING

***Jan G. Grandjean*[1] *and Massimo A. Mariani*[2]**
[1]Consultant Cardiothoracic Surgeon, Department of Cardiothoracic Surgery
Thoraxcenter Twente, Enschede, The Netherlands
[2]Professor and Head, Department of Cardiothoracic Surgery,
Thoraxcenter University Medical Center of Groningen,
Groningen, The Netherlands

ABSTRACT

The success of coronary artery bypass grafting, the gold standard for the treatment of multivessel coronary artery disease, is limited by poor long-term vein-graft patency. By contrast, the left internal mammary artery has been demonstrated to have a superior graft patency rate and has provided excellent clinical results. This suggests that the use of arterial conduits for coronary artery bypass grafting may be beneficial for long-term results. Recently, there has been an upsurge in the use of arterial grafts for myocardial revascularization based on the clinical advantage of the use of the left internal mammary artery as a bypass conduit. Many retrospective studies have supported the safety and the effectiveness of arterial grafting. At the same time, abundant evidence to verify the safety and efficacy of off-pump coronary artery bypass (OPCAB) grafting exists. Despite increasing recognition that off-pump coronary artery bypass surgery and total arterial revascularization individually are associated with improved outcomes, concerns persist regarding the safety of combining these two techniques. This chapter presents in detail the authors' experience of total arterial off-pump coronary artery bypass grafting.

INTRODUCTION

Coronary artery bypass grafting (CABG) is the most widespread cardiac procedure and represents the gold standard for the treatment for three-vessel and left main coronary artery disease. Addressing the issue of long-term outcome of total arterial off-pump coronary artery bypass is somewhat difficult because most of the published studies are single-center and include insufficient numbers to draw conclusion that can lead to guidelines. Therefore, we focused on our own experience that goes back to beginning of the 1990s, with the use of multiple arterial grafting. This experience with complete arterial revascularization was initially performed on-pump and evolved during the Nineties with the introduction and the growth of off-pump techniques [1]. The development of the off-pump coronary artery bypass grafting (OPCAB) technique aimed to avoid some of the adverse effects associated with the use of cardiopulmonary bypass [2]: cardioplegic arrest of the heart, manipulation of the aorta, stimulation of the inflammatory cascade related to the blood-air and blood-circuit contact, and clotting disorders. Over the past two decades several studies have shown that OPCAB surgery is superior to conventional CABG owing to a decreased incidence of cerebrovascular accidents, blood loss and transfusion, reoperation for bleeding, ventilation time, and resource utilization [3-5].The "no-touch technique" is a surgical strategy aiming to avoid aortic manipulation by using either pedicled or composite arterial grafts combined with OPCAB. Some recent studies demonstrated that the aortic no-touch technique is safe and effective [6-8]. Even in high-risk patients this strategy results in fewer neurologic events [9-11].

Several years ago we choose to adopt the use of the off-pump no-touch technique with the left internal mammary artery and the radial Artery (RA) as standard clinical care, after having evaluated the good results of the total arterial revascularization with on-pump techniques.

The RA was first used in CABG by Carpentier in 1971. Due to the 35% incidence of hyperspasticity and high occurrence of intimal hyperplasia, the RA was quickly abandoned as bypass conduit for CABG [12]. Over the last two decades however, early and late patency of the RA as a bypass conduit has improved significantly thanks to the introduction of novel harvesting techniques, perioperative use of anti-spasm agents like papaverine and postoperative treatment with calcium-channel blockers [12]. Prevention of spasm has proven to be beneficial in the acute period following CABG. As a result of this new evidence, the RA is regaining popularity as bypass conduit and is replacing the saphenous vein in complementing the left internal mammary artery in CABG [13-14]. Nevertheless, one of the major limitations of the RA is still its higher susceptibility to spasm compared to the left internal mammary artery and the saphenous vein. This tendency to spasm, occurring in 5%-10% of the patients, has been correlated to a significant proportion of early RA graft failures [12]. The vasoactive properties of a bypass conduit are crucial since the spasm may significantly increase the chance of angina and myocardial infarction during the peri- and post-operative period [15-16]. The role of the adventitia in vascular function of the RA is not entirely established yet. It is generally accepted that the adventitia provides structural support to the vessel and contibutes to vascular tone through perivascular innervations. Recent studies have indicated that the adventitia has an active role in vasomotor tone, which implies that adventitia may negatively influence vasomotor tone [17-18]. It can be assumed that mechanical unloading by opening the adventitia, may play a role in the vascular reactivity of the RA as a bypass graft, when vasomotor tone is no longer controlled by innervations.

The peri-operative vasodilator regimen may not sufficiently protect the RA graft from postoperative spasm [15-16]. In addition to the treatment with pharmacological agents, the method of RA harvesting and handling can play a central role in the development of spasm. Therefore, since the Nineties we harvest the RA with subfascial dissection as standard clinical care. Subfascial dissection is performed in attempt to reduce vasospasm of the graft, potentially related to the vasomotor tone of adventitia and to allow the RA to reach its maximal diameter. The clinical impact of different RA harvesting techniques has been investigated [19-20]. Conventional RA harvesting consists of an incision from about 2 centimeters from the wrist extended until about 3 centimeters from the elbow, along the medial margin of the brachialis muscle. A recent review showed the lack of comparative studies about RA complications related to the harvesting technique [19]. Another interesting issue is the incidence of peripheral neurological complications after RA harvesting. The incidence oscillates between 30% [21] and 67% [22] after conventional harvesting and between 2% [23] and 84% [24] for endoscopic harvesting. This extreme variability is most probably due to the small sample-size of these studies and to the lack of uniformity of the harvesting techniques. However, there are up to now few studies which investigate the degree of patients' satisfaction after RA harvesting. In this chapter we report patients' satisfaction and the incidence of wound-site complications after RA harvesting with open technique.

AUTHORS' EXPERIENCE OF TOTAL ARTERIAL OFF-PUMP CORONARY ARTERY BYPASS GRAFTING

We performed a clinical, anatomic and pharmacologic study to assess the outcomes of off-pump coronary surgery using the aortic no-touch technique and composite arterial grafting with the left internal mammary artery (LIMA), right internal mammary artery (RIMA) and RA. The study was approved by the Institutional Ethics Committee.

Inclusion Criteria

The study cohort consisted of 407 consecutive patients enrolled as "all-comers," irrespective of emergent or urgent status. Seven patients were excluded from the study because of intraoperative conversion to on-pump surgery owing to hemodynamic instability (n = 5) and because total arterial revascularization was not possible as a result of the unsuitability of the radial artery (n = 2).

End Points

The primary end point was defined as in-hospital and 12-month major adverse cardiovascular or cerebrovascular event rate (MACCE), defined as all-cause death, stroke, myocardial infarction (MI), and any repeat revascularization [25]. Myocardial infarction was defined according to the definition by the Academic Research Consortium [25]. Secondary end points were defined as 12-month MACCE compared with the randomized arms of the SYNTAX trial, MACCE at 4-year and 6-year follow-up. The assessment of vasoreactivity of the RA and Quality of Life (QoL) at 6-year follow- up were also defined as secondary end-points.

Data Collection

Preoperative, operative, and postoperative data were retrospectively collected from our institutional custom-made database (Medical Computer Support, version 5.10.0, Wilp, The Netherlands). Four hundred consecutive `all-comers´ operated on at the TCT between September 2004 and May 2008 were selected. They underwent OPCAB no-touch coronary surgery, with a Y-graft of the LIMA and the RA. The operations were performed by 4 surgeons. Preoperative patients' demographics are listed in Table 1. In-hospital mortality was defined as 30-day and or in-hospital mortality (whatever condition occurred). In 94 patients there was a left main stenosis of more than 50%.

Table 1. Preoperative patient characteristics

Age, y (range)	63.9 ± 9.1 (28–85)
Male/female (%)	327/73 (81.8%/18.2%)
Body mass index, kg/m^2	27.6 ± 3.8
EuroSCORE	3.8 ± 4.3
3-Vessel disease	346
Left main stenosis >50%	94

Surgical Technique

All procedures were performed through a median sternotomy [1]. The internal mammary arteries were harvested as pedicles, both for free and in-situ grafting. All arterial conduits were distally divided after heparinization of the patient and were irrigated with 1% saline solution of papaverine.

Heparinization was achieved by giving heparin 150 IU/kg to obtain a target activated clotting time longer than 400 seconds [26]. Protamine sulfate was used to reverse the heparin dose at the completion of the procedure. To obtain a better visualization of the target coronary arteries a suction stabilizer (Axius Vacuum 2 Stabilizer System; Guidant, Santa Clara, CA, or Octopus 3; Medtronic, Minneapolis, MN) was used to stabilize the target coronary artery. Intracoronary shunt occluders were used in all grafted vessels, unless the coronary anatomy made the insertion impossible.

The RA was harvested as a pedicle, together with surrounding tissue and veins. All RAs were distally divided after systemic heparinization and irrigated with 1% saline solution of papaverine, as previously described [27]. After irrigation with papaverine 1%, subfascial dissection of RA was performed, intended as a surgical cutdown of the fascia along the entire vessel length, leaving nearly half of the subfascial area exposed (Figure 1). This was followed by the cleavage of the subfascial lining, leaving the media exposed.

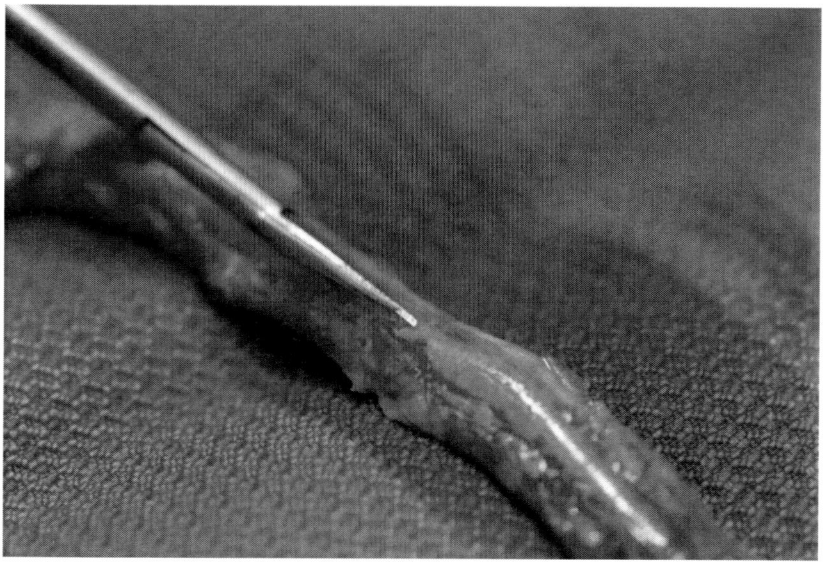

Figure 1. Subfascial dissection of radial artery.

Postoperative Medication

All patients received postoperative low-molecular-weight heparin 3,000 IU twice daily until discharge. Acetylsalicylic acid was given intravenously (500 mg) once, 6 hours after admission on the intensive care unit, and continued lifelong at a dose of 100 mg daily orally, starting from postoperative day 1.

Follow-Up

Out of the 400 patients from the institutional custom-made database (Medical Computer Support, version 5.10.0, Wilp, The Netherlands), 306 patients were consecutively telephonically contacted. Through a Quality of Life questionnaire these patients were asked to report their postoperative pain, mobility, neurological disorders, and degree of satisfaction about the aesthetic result after RA harvesting. This Quality of Life questionnaire was performed telephonic, by using the Likert scale in order to define the degree of patients' satisfaction. The Likert scale is a psychometric scale commonly used in questionnaires and is the most widely used scale in survey research [28,29]. The Likert scale is the sum of responses on several Likert items. Likert items are accompanied by an analog scale: a horizontal line, on which a subject indicates his or her response. The format implies specific metric relations among the response levels. Likert scaling is a bipolar scaling method, measuring attitude in terms of level of agreement/disagreement to a target statement, according to any kind of subjective or objective criteria. Verbal labels are symmetrical about a neutral middle. We used five ordered response level. After the questionnaire was completed, each item was analyzed separately.

Radial Artery Histological Analysis

Surplus material of RA (n = 13), which would have otherwise been discarded, was collected. Written informed consent was obtained from patients prior to surgery. This study was intended as an all-comers study. No selection criteria for the use of the radial artery were applied. Thirteen consecutive patients undergoing off-pump coronary surgery were included in the study, according to the standard practice of the two participating centers.

Organ Bath Technique

The organ bath technique was used in the functional analysis of RA vasoreactivity. While performing subfascial dissection, the most distal RA graft segments were left unharvested, without subfascial dissection, for comparison. Therefore, vasoreactivity of the RA with and without subfascial dissection could be tested within each single patient. Following retrieval, segments of RA were kept in 4ºC Krebs-Henseleit buffer solution and functional analysis was performed within 24 hours following RA harvesting. For functional analysis, the RAs were carefully dissected from their surrounding fat tissue and divided into vascular rings of approximately 3 mm in length. Distal segments were discarded in order to avoid potential influence of harvesting manipulations. Two wire stirrups were placed through each ring and attached to a force transducer for isometric tension measurements. The upper wire was attached to a transducer measuring the detection and the lower stirrup is fixed. The rings were lowered into separate organ chambers, filled with 15mL of Krebs-Henseleit buffer (pH 7.4, 37ºC) continuously bubbled with 95% O_2 and 5% CO_2. Experiments were performed in duplo representing an average response for the same patient.

Data Management and Statistical Analysis

All clinical data were entered in an Excel spreadsheet (Microsoft Corp, Redmond, WA). Statistical analysis was performed using SPSS 15.0 (SPSS Inc, Chicago, IL). Values are reported as mean ± standard deviation or as percentages. A probability value less than 0.05 was considered significant. For statistical analysis Kaplan-Meier plots were constructed and Fisher's exact test was used to compare differences in complication rates between the SYNTAX trial and the TCT data. Estimates of the cumulative event rates of MI, stroke, repeat revascularization, symptomatic graft occlusion, and death were calculated by the Kaplan–Meier method. Statistical analysis of the pharmacologic study was performed using PASW Statistics 18.0.3 (SPSS Inc.). Experiments in organ bath studies were performed in duplo and the mean value used to represent the patient's average response. The baseline characteristics of the patients are reported as mean ± standard deviation or as percentages.All data of the QoL assessment were entered in an Excel spreadsheet. Statistical analysis was performed using SPSS 15.0 (SPSS Inc., Chicago, IL). Values are reported as mean ± standard deviation or as percentage. Modal score and median value were calculated for each Likert item. The data are expressed as scores, therefore the sample mode is known as the modal score.

Clinical Results

Intraoperative data are listed in Table 2. Mean operating time was 187 ± 33 minutes. The number of distal anastomoses per patient was 3.5 ± 0.8 (range, 2 to 6). The composite graft was made with the left internal mammary artery and the radial artery in 94.3% of patients. In other cases the right internal mammary artery was used as a free graft to construct a composite Y-graft with the left internal mammary artery. In-hospital outcomes are listed in Table 3.

The mean hospital stay was 7.5 ± 5.5 days. One patient died in the hospital. This patient died of multiorgan failure on the second postoperative day. Reoperation for bleeding was required in 17 patients (4.2%).

Table 2. Intraoperative data

Operation time, min	187 ± 33
Distal anastomoses (range)	3.5 ± 0.8 (2–6)
LIMA-RA (%)	377 (94.3)
LIMA-FRIMA (%)	22 (5.5)
RIMA-RA (%)	1 (0.3)
LIMA-RA-GEA (%)	2 (0.5)

FRIMA = free right internal mammary artery; GEA = gastroepiploic artery; LIMA = left internal mammary artery; RA = radial artery; RIMA = right internal mammary artery.

Table 3. In-hospital data

All-cause mortality (%)	1 (0.2)
Myocardial infarction (%)	5 (1.2)
Stroke (%)	1 (0.2)
Repeat revascularization (%)	1 (0.2)
Symptomatic graft occlusion (%)	1 (0.2)
MACCE (%)	7 (1.7)
Reoperation for bleeding (%)	17 (4.2)

MACCE = major adverse cardiovascular or cerebrovascular event rate.

Overall results are plotted in Figure 2. Cumulative 6-year survival and freedom from MACCE were 90.2±1.9% and 91.4±2.4%, respectively. Cumulative 6-year freedom from repeat revascularization, symptomatic graft occlusion and cerebrovascular accidents (CVA) were 94.9±1.2%, 97.5%, 96.6%±1%, respectively.

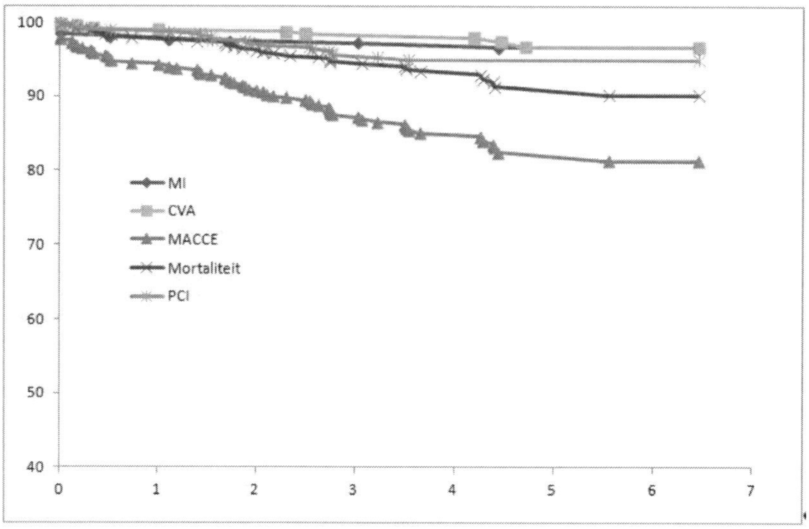

(MI = myocardial infarction; CVA = cerebrovascular accident; MACCE = major adverse cardiovascular or cerebrovascular event; Mortaliteit = mortality; PCI = repeat revascularization).

Figure 2. Kaplan-Meier curves for 6-year survival.

Anatomical Study

When studying the RA morphology from the subfascial aspect with spectral electron microscopy (SEM), collagen fibers are shown to form large bundels of fibrils which increase in size from its innermost component, closest to the media, to its outermost aspect.

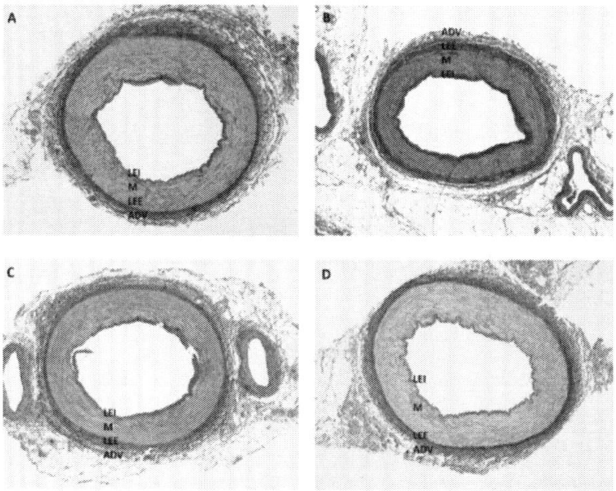

Figure 3. Histological and morphological examination demonstrate that only the adventitial lining, composed of large, polymerized collagen bundles, is dissected by the subfascial dissection technique and that adventitial volume is left unchanged.

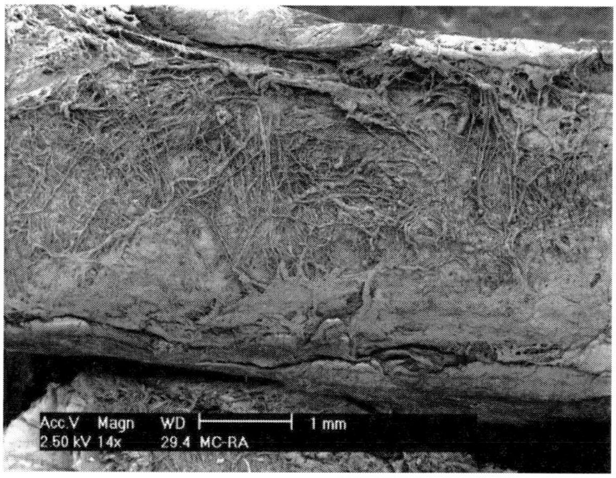

Figure 4. As confirmed by light microscopy, SEM images reveal that adventitial stripping of the RA is associated with a higher degree of tissue manipulation. In some areas of the samples, the media is exposed as a result of pulling away the connective tissue layers with forceps, as smooth muscle cells are now forming the outermost layer.

This is in agreement with the observations made by light microscopy (Figure 3). In the majority of subfascial dissected samples, large collagen bundels have been dissected and a dense connective tissue consisting of small collagen fibrils (diameter 5-10 um) forms the outermost layer. One sample shows segments where large (100-200 um) and middle-sized (20-50 um) collagen bundles cross the vessel circumference, covering smaller collagen fibrils of the adventitia just below the fascia. Strenghtening the light microscopy observations, we conclude that only the outer adventitial lining is manipulated during subfascial dissection, as the media is never exposed on SEM images (Figure 4).

Pharmacologic Results

Endothelium-dependent relaxation of RA rings with subfascial dissection was significantly increased compared to RA rings without subfascial dissection (Figure 5).

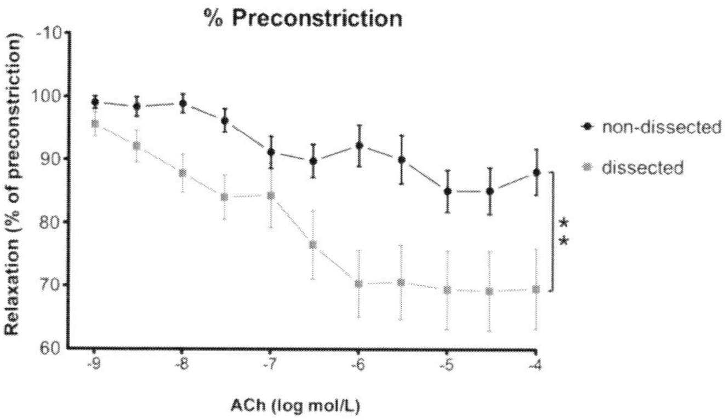

Figure 5. Phramacologic response of dissected and non-dissected radial artery rings.

Quality of Life Results

The median values and the modal scores achieved the maximal value (5) of satisfaction for all site-related complications. The mean score for all site-related complications confirmed the satisfactory median and modal values, remaining > 4. The median value and the modal score which expressed patients' general health state were 4. The mean value was slightly inferior at 3.96.

Six patients complained of constant postoperative pain. Two hundred thirty-four patients (76%) never suffered from postoperative pain. Five patients considered extremely poor the aesthetic result of the wound. Three hundred patients (98%) considered the aesthetic result of the wound as at least acceptable. Three patients described daily problems in performing simple normal handlings. Fifteen patients (4.9%) complained of constant sensation or neurological disturbances. Fifty-one patients complained about frequent sensitive or neurological disturbances. Therefore, the recorded incidence of invalidating peripheral neurological complications was 16.7%. Twenty-one patients defined their general health state poor or extremely poor. However, the mean scores of the remaining four Likert items of these patients were ≥ 4.

COMMENT

The aim of this study was to analyze the clinical midterm follow-up of patients who underwent OPCAB using total arterial grafting and no-touch technique.

The cumulative 6-year survival and freedom from MACCE confirmed the safety and efficacy of OPCAB no-touch technique at long-term follow-up. The results of the 3-year SYNTAX trial have been recently published [30] and represent the contemporary results of revascularization treatment in patients with three-vessel disease or left main stenosis. Even though the results in the surgical arm of the SYNTAX trial were superior to those of the PCI arm, the high incidence of stroke and repeat revascularization in the SYNTAX trial needs to be addressed. Aortic manipulation and derangements related to cardiopulmonary bypass are the most significant determinants of stroke after coronary surgery. The release of emboli in the case of atherosclerotic walls of the ascending aorta and macro and micro cerebral embolization related to cardiopulmonary bypass are the mechanisms responsible for the cerebral injuries. Strokes are potentially fatal and invalidating complications that negatively influence the outcome of patients who undergo surgical revascularization.

In our study population we aimed to improve the neurologic outcome of coronary surgery by avoiding manipulation of the ascending aorta. At the same time, we intended to improve the surgical results in term of MI, repeat revascularization, and death, by using only arterial grafts. The results of the off-pump no-touch technique showed a clear trend toward a reduction in these complications.

The low percentage of stroke for the off-pump no-touch technique group (2.3%) observed at 6 years' follow-up proves the additional value of the neurologic protection offered by the off-pump no-touch technique.

Some authors have raised concerns about the patency of multiple anastomoses with composite grafts, assuming that competitive flow may jeopardize the results especially in cases of moderate stenosis of the native vessels [31,32]. Other concerns were whether the interactions between coronary branches and the graft arrangement can influence flow distribution.

However, other studies demonstrated that the flow reserve of the internal mammary artery was adequate for multiple coronary anastomoses, irrespective of the choice of the second arterial graft, and the results of graft flow in sequential internal mammary artery grafting were comparable with those in single grafting [33]. Finally, recent studies on the adaptability of the internal mammary artery to flow dynamics concluded that Y-grafts were able to regulate flow capacity to myocardial demand, probably through the release of endothelial vasoactive mediators [34]. The observed low percentage of graft occlusion in our study population (2.1%) at follow-up confirmed the satisfactory patency of composite grafts using total arterial conduits.

The anatomical and pharmacological study highlights the importance of tissue handling in determining the long-term patency. Besides the LIMA, the RA plays a prominent role in the off-pump no-touch technique. Therefore utmost care should be taken in optimizing surgical harvesting of the RA, which is known to be more sensitive to spasm than other arterial grafts. Failure to comply with a standardized and specific harvesting technique for the RA may lead to disappointing results. The use of specific pharmacologic agents, both locally as papaverin and systemically as calcium-antagonists, plays also a key role in optimizing the performance of arterial grafts. This fact is especially of paramount importance for the RA.

Another secondary end point of this study was to establish the feasibility of off-pump no-touch technique. The low percentage of cases (1.7%; 7 patients) in whom this surgical technique could not be performed owing to intraoperative circumstances, such as unsuitable anatomy or hemodynamic instability, clearly showed its high feasibility. In addition, since we did not record MACCE at follow-up in these 7 patients, we can conclude that we did not overestimate the outcome in the study population by removing these patients from the analysis.

Another aim of this study was to assess the vasoreactivity of the RA, in relationship with the technique of harvesting. It is generally accepted that the adventitia is involved in the modulation of vasomotor tone. Changes in vasoreactivity are most likely due to a change in mechanical properties of the vessel. We showed that subfascial dissection of RA could reduce the mechanical barrier of adventitia and the vascular tone of its smooth muscle cells.

Moreover, we compared RA rings with and without subfascial dissection by means of a Scanning Electron Microscope analysis to investigate which tissue layer was harvested during subfascial dissection of RAs. In the samples of RA rings with subfascial dissection, large collagen bundles have been cut open and small collagen fibrils form the outermost layer. We hypothesize that the dissection of the outer bundles can at least partially disconnect the sympathetic and parasympathetic nerves contained in the adventitia which end on the smooth muscle cells of the media modulating their spasm.

As far as the technique concerns, subfascial dissection of RA during CABG surgery is relatively easy to perform and requires minimal tissue handling.

RAs with subfascial dissection are more prone to vasorelaxation and less susceptible to vasoconstriction *in vitro*. Furthermore, from the technical standpoint, relaxation of the RA leads to an enlargement of the diameter and this facilitates the surgeon in performing the anastomoses, thus optimizing the whole surgical procedure.

The last issue addressed in this study is the QoL at 6-year follow-up, in general and specifically referred to the use of the RA. Considering the high mean scores obtained for all Likert items, patients' degree of satisfaction after off-pump no-touch technique with the use of RA can be considered more than satisfactory. The median values and the modal scores reached the maximal value for all the site-related complications thereby confirming the minimal impact on patients' quality of life related to the surgical site of RA harvesting.

As far as arm cosmestic result is concerned, 98% of patients considered the cosmetic result of the wound at least acceptable. As far as arm mobility concerns, less than 1% of patients mentioned persistent disability in performing simple handlings. We consider this result mainly important for old patients that could have a collateral decrease of age-related self-government. In the study cohort 93 patients were older than 75 years.

As far as invalidating peripheral sensory and neurological complications is concerned, the incidence is lower than those showed in previous studies (16.7%) [21-22]. A recent study of Dick et al. [34] investigated patients in whom both the radial artery and the saphenous vein had been harvested and showed that harvest-site discomfort affected arms and legs equally (39%). However, the study did not describe the technique of conduits' harvesting. We believe that the standardization of harvesting technique permits to optimize the quality of the conduit and to minimize the damage of the harvest-site. In fact, we hypothesize that the daily practice of a standard RA harvesting technique strongly contributed to the lower incidence of neurological complications in our study. As far as general health state concerns, twenty-one patients defined their general health state poor or extremely poor. However, the mean scores of these patients were ≥ 4 for all the other Likert items. Therefore, we could presume that the reasons responsible of the poor health state were not strictly related to RA harvesting.

We believe that the standardized harvesting technique of RA mainly concurred in the satisfactory results of this study. In conclusion, the degree of patients' satisfaction after off-pump no-touch technique with the use of the RA can be defined more than satisfactory and the incidence of wound-site complications acceptable.

Conclusion

This study shows that use of a state-of-the-art surgical technique such as the off-pump no-touch technique with the use of the RA can further improve the advantage of surgical treatment with respect to PCI, as shown by the 3-year SYNTAX trial. In addition, this study shows that neurologic complications by using off-pump no-touch technique are not different from the PCI arm of the SYNTAX trial. Therefore, we can conclude that the off-pump no-touch technique can be reasonably seen as the treatment of choice for patients with three-vessel disease and left main stenosis and can be used as daily practice, irrespective of the anatomic variability of the patients.

Acknowledgements

We acknowledge Dr. J.H. Buikema for the anatomic and pharmacologic study. This study will be submitted in extended version for peer-reviewed publication. We also acknowledge

Dr. S.C. Arrigoni for the Quality of Life study. This study too has been submitted in extended version for peer-reviewed publication.

References

[1] Bergsma TM, Grandjean JG, Voors AA, et al. Low recurrence of angina pectoris after coronary artery bypass graft surgery with bilateral internal thoracic and right gastroepiploic arteries. *Circulation*, 1998;97:2402-5.

[2] Mariani MA, D'Alfonso A, Grandjean JG. Total arterial off-pump coronary surgery: time to change our habits? *Ann. Thorac. Surg.*, 2004;78:1591-7.

[3] Reber D, Fritz M, Germing A, Marks P, Laczkovics. Early outcome after off pump coronary artery bypass grafting:effect on mortality and stroke. *Rev. Bras. Cir. Cardiovasc.*, 2008;3:23-8.

[4] Puskas JD, Kilgo PD, Lattouf OM et al. Off-pump coronary bypass provides reduced mortality and morbidity and equivalent 10-years survival. *Ann. Thorac. Surg.*, 2008; 86:1139-46.

[5] Lattouf OM, Vinod HT, Kilgo PD, et al. Influence of on-pump versus off-pump techniques and completeness of revascularization on long-term survival after coronary artery bypass. *Ann. Thorac. Surg.*, 2008; 86:797-805.

[6] Navia D, Vrancic M, Vaccarino G, et al. Total arterial off-pump coronary revascularization using bilateral internal thoracic arteries in triple vessel disease: surgical technique and clinical outcomes. *Ann. Thorac. Surg.*, 2008; 86: 524-31.

[7] Kim WS, Lee J, Lee YT, et al. Total arterial revascularization in triple vessel disease with off-pump and aortic no-touch technique. *Ann. Thorac. Surg.*, 2008;86:1861-5.

[8] Tanaka K, Naruse Y, Sato K. Off-pump coronary artery bypass grafting using in-situ right internal thoracic artery extended with radial artery as I-composite graft. *Kyobu. Geka*, 2008; 61:175-9.

[9] Bolotin G, Shapira Y, Gotler Y, et al. The potential advantage of "no-touch" aortic technique in off-pump complete arterial revascularization. *Int. J. Cardiol.*, 2007;114:11-5.

[10] Vallely MP, Potger K, McMillan D, et al. Anaortic techniques reduce neurological morbidity after off-pump coronary artery bypass surgery. *Heart Lung Circ.*, 2008 ;17:299-304.

[11] Motallebzadeh R, Martin Bland J, Markus HS, et al. Neurocognitive function and cerebral emboli: randomized study of on-pump versus off-pump coronary artery bypass surgery. *Ann. Thorac. Surg.*, 2007;83:475-82.

[12] Kobayashi J. Radial Artery as a graft for coronary artery bypass grafting. *Circ. J.*, 2009;73:1178-83.

[13] Manabe S, Sunamori M. Radial artery graft for coronary artery bypass surgery: biological characteristics and clinical outcome. *J. Card. Surg.*, 2006; 21:102-15.

[14] Murakami E, Iwata H, Imaizumi M, Takemura H. Prevention of arterial graft spasm by botulinum toxin: an in-vitro experiment. *Interact. Cardiovasc. Thorac. Surg.*, 2009;9:395-8.

[15] Rukosujew A, Reichelt R, Fabricius AM, et al. Skeletonization versus pedicle preparation of the radial artery with and without the ultrasonic scalpel. *Ann. Thorac. Surg.,* 2004;77:120-5.

[16] Kun X, Lefeng W, Rongjing D, Xincun Y. RhoA/ROK pathway related to the mechanism of higher susceptibility to spasm in RA than in IMA. *J. Card. Surg.,* 2009;24:766-71.

[17] Laflamme K, Roberge CJ, Grenier G, et al. Adventitia contribution in vascular tone: insights from adventitia-derived cells in a tissue-engineered human blood vessel. *FASEB J.,* 2006; 20:1245-7.

[18] Auger FA, D'Orléans-Juste P, Germain L. Adventitia contribution to vascular contraction: Hints provided by tissue-engineered substitutes. *Cardiovasc. Res.,* 2007;65:669-78.

[19] Aziz O, Athanasiou T, Darzi A. Minimally invasive conduit harvesting: a systematic review. *Eur. J. Cardiothorac. Surg.,* 2006;29:324-33.

[20] Medalion B, Tobar A, Yosibash Z, et al. Vasoreactivity and histology of the radial artery: comparison of open versus endoscopic approaches. *Eur. J. Cardiothorac. Surg.,* 2008;34:845-9.

[21] Denton TA, Trento L, Cohen M, Kass RM, Blanche C, Raissi S, Cheng W, Fontana GP, Trento A. Radial artery harvesting for coronary bypass operations: neurologic complications and their potential mechanisms. *J. Thorac. Cardiovasc. Surg.,* 2001;121:951-6.

[22] Saeed I, Anyanwu AC, Yacoub MH, Amrani M. Subjective patient outcomes following coronary artery bypass using the radial artery: results of a crosssectional survey of harvest site complications and quality of life. *Eur. J. Cardiothorac. Surg.,* 2001;20:1142-6.

[23] Galajda Z, Jagamos E, Maros T, Peterffy A. Radial artery grafts: surgical anatomy and harvesting techniques. *Cardiovasc. Surg.,* 2002;10:476-80.

[24] Shapira OM, Eskenazi B, Murphy R, Anter E, Bao Y, Lazar HL, Shemin RJ, Hunter CT. Endoscopic radial artery harvest for coronary artery bypass grafting: initial clinical experience. *Heart Surg. Forum,* 2004;7:E411-5.

[25] Cutlip DE, Windecker S, Mehran R, et al. Clinical end points in coronary stent trials: a case of standardized definitions. *Circulation,* 2007; 115: 2344-51.

[26] Mariani MA, Guy J, Boonstra PW, Grandjean JG, Van Oeveren W, Ebels T. Procoagulant activity after off-pump coronary operation: is the current anticoagulation adequate? *Ann. Thorac. Surg.,* 1999;67:1370-5.

[27] Halbersma, W.B., Arrigoni, S.C., Mecozzi, et al. Four-year outcome of OPCAB no-touch with total arterial Y-graft: making the best treatment a daily practice. *Ann. Thorac. Surg.,* 2009;88:796-801.

[28] Kiaii B, Moon BC, Massel D, et al. A prospective randomized trial of endoscopic versus conventional harvesting of the saphenous vein in coronary artery bypass surgery. *J. Thorac. Cardiovasc. Surg.,* 2002;123:204-12.

[29] Kappetein AP, Feldman TE, Mack MJ, et al. Comparison of coronary bypass surgery with drug-eluting stenting for the treatment of left main and/or three-vessel disease: 3-year follow-up of the SYNTAX trial. *Eur. Heart J.,* 2011;32:2125-34.

[30] Pevni D, Hertz I, Medalion B, et al. Angiographic evidence for reduced graft patency due to competitive flow in composite arterial T-grafts. *J. Thorac. Cardiovasc. Surg.*, 2007;133:1220-5.

[31] Nakajima H, Kobayashi J, Tagusari O, Bando K, Niwaya K, Kitamura S. Competitive flow in arterial composite grafts and effect of graft arrangement in Off-Pump coronary revascularization. *Ann. Thorac. Surg.*, 2004;78:481-6.

[32] Nakajima H, Kobayashi J, Funatsu T, et al. Predictive factors for the intermediate-term patency of arterial grafts in aorta no-touch off-pump coronary revascularization. *Eur. J. Cardiothorac. Surg.*, 2007;32:711-7.

[33] Lemma M, Innorta A, Pettinari M, et al. Flow dynamics and wall shear stress in the left internal thoracic artery: composite arterial graft versus single graft. *Eur. J. Cardiothorac. Surg.*, 2006;29:473-8.

[34] Dick F, Hristic A, Roost-Krähenbühl E, et al. Persistent sensitivity disorders at the radial artery and saphenous vein graft harvest sites: a neglected side effect of coronary artery bypass grafting procedures. *Eur. J. Cardiothorac. Surg.*, 2011;40:221-6.

In: Off-Pump Coronary Artery Bypass Grafting
Editors: S.G. Raja and M. Amrani
ISBN 978-1-62081-575-5

Chapter 14

QUALITY OF LIFE OUTCOMES AFTER OFF-PUMP CORONARY ARTERY BYPASS GRAFTING

Christian H. Møller[1] and Daniel A. Steinbrüchel[2]
[1]Senior Resident, PhD, Department of Cardiothoracic Surgery, Rigshospitalet, Copenhagen University Hospital, Copenhagen, Denmark
[2]Professor of Cardiothoracic Surgery, Department of Cardiothoracic Surgery, Rigshospitalet, Copenhagen University Hospital, Copenhagen, Denmark

ABSTRACT

Quality of life and health related quality of life (HRQoL) both refer to the physical, psychological and social domains of health, which are seen as distinct areas that are influenced by a person´s experiences, beliefs, expectations and perceptions. Objective outcome measures (i.e., survival, mortality, morbidity, complication rate, symptom recurrence, and need for re-interventions) have long been used as benchmarks for successful cardiac surgery, including coronary artery bypass grafting (CABG). Along with these objectively measurable outcome indicators, acquired improvement by cardiac surgery in subjectively experienced HRQoL has gained importance during the last decade in cardiac surgical research. If an increasing proportion of adult patients referred for CABG are elderly, octogenarians or even nonagenarians, the acquired HRQoL benefit from bypass surgery should be considered to be at least as important an outcome measure as potentially marginal improvement in life expectancy or longevity alone. This chapter discusses the impact of on-pump and off-pump CABG on quality of life outcomes.

INTRODUCTION

The beneficial effect of coronary artery bypass grafting (CABG) for multivessel and left main coronary artery disease is well documented. It relieves angina effectively and improves survival compared to both medical treatment and percutaneous coronary intervention (PCI) [1,2]. However, CABG is associated with the risk of postoperative morbidity and mortality. Cerebral morbidity is a devastating complication of CABG and has largely been attributed to the use of cardiopulmonary bypass (CPB) [3,4]. The manipulation of the aorta during cannulation and cross clamping may increase the risk of postoperative stroke and the extracorporeal circulation generates microemboli, which may affect cognitive function. Decline in cognitive dysfunction can diminish the improvement in quality of life afforded by CABG [5]. In an attempt to reduce the postoperative morbidity and mortality seen after CABG performed with CPB (on-pump CABG) interest in coronary artery bypass surgery performed without CPB on the beating heart (off-pump CABG or OPCAB) increased during the 1990s [6]. Systematic reviews of randomized trials comparing coronary artery bypass surgery performed with versus without CPB have so far not been able to demonstrate superiority of one technique over the other as regard mortality, myocardial infarction, or stroke [7,8]. Operating on the beating heart is technically more challenging and concern about the quality of anastomosis has been raised [9]. Furthermore, as the population of patients with advanced age referred for CABG is increasing the improvement in life expectancy may be minor and therefore, the improvement in relief of symptoms and quality of life may play a more important role in the choice surgical strategy.

Health Related Quality of Life

Quality of life and health related quality of life (HRQoL) both refer to the physical, psychological and social domains of health, which are seen as distinct areas that are influenced by a person´s experiences, beliefs, expectations and perceptions [10]. Each of the domains of health has many components and translating the various domains and components of health into a quantitative value indicating quality of life is a complex task [10].

In randomized trials comparing off-pump versus on-pump CABG the most used instrument to assess quality of life is the Short Form 36 [11]. This is a generic instrument for scoring physical and mental health status. The instruments measures 8 health domains including physical functioning, role limitation due to physical health problems, bodily pain, general health perceptions, vitality, social functioning, role limitation due to emotional problems, and mental health. Furthermore the 8 domains can be summarized into a physical health component and mental health component. Other types of generic instruments to assess quality of life are the Euro quality of life (EuroQoL) and WHOQoL.

Some trials also report more disease-specific measurements such as the Seattle Angina Questionnaire (SAQ) and Coronary Revascularization Outcome Questionnaire (CROQ).

Comparison of HRQoL after Off-Pump Versus On-Pump CABG

HRQoL has been reported in 12 randomized controlled trials (RCTs) comparing off-pump versus on-pump CABG (Table 1). In seven of these trials quality of life was assessed preoperatively [12-18]. In general, both off-pump and on-pump CABG resulted in improved quality of life.

In five trials quality of life was assessed between 3 weeks to 3 month postoperatively [12,14,16,18,19]. In a trial including 168 patients, Al-Ruzzeh et al. [12], reported a trend toward improved quality of life after off-pump CABG based on the WHO quality of life questionnaire as well as a better preservation of neurocognitive function compared with on-pump CABG. In contrast none of the other 4 trials were able to show any significant difference in quality of life based on the SF-36 instrument between off-pump and on-pump CABG. In the OCTOPUS trial 281 patients were included. After 1 month significant improvement was seen in the following SF-36 domains: physical functioning, general health perception, vitality and mental health. The improvement was independent of the surgical technique used [18]. In a sub-study of the Best Bypass Surgery Trial, quality of life and cognitive dysfunction was assessed in 120 moderate-to-high risk patients (EuroSCORE ≥5). Three month after CABG improvement in quality of life in all 8 SF-36 domains was observed and without clinically relevant differences between the off-pump and on-pump groups [13]. Neither was there any significant difference in cognitive dysfunction between the two groups [20].

Similar improvements in quality of life after 3 months were reported by Mathisen et al., who randomized 120 patients to off-pump versus on-pump CABG [14]. Angina relief was significant in both groups at 3 months after surgery. Likewise, Puskas et al. [16] have reported similar quality of life 4-6 weeks after off-pump and on-pump CABG in the SMART trial, in which 200 patients were included.

Quality of life six to twelve month after off-pump versus on-pump CABG has been assessed in 9 randomized trials. In a small Australian trial including 36 patients, a general increase in all SF-36 domains was seen from baseline to 6 months without difference between off-pump and on-pump CABG. At 6 month follow-up in the PROMISS trial quality of life was assessed by the Euro quality of life visual analog scale [21]. One hundred and fifty patients were enrolled in the trial. Although, this trial showed reduced graft patency in the off-pump group no significant difference was observed in quality of life.

In the trial by Mathisen et al. quality of life was assessed again at 12 months. In the SF-36 domains 'bodily pain' and 'role limitation caused by physical problems' improvement was observed between 3 and 12 months postoperatively without difference between groups [14]. Similar findings have been reported from the OCTOPUS trial in which 'bodily pain' and 'general health perceptions' improved further from 3 to 12 months, but without significant difference between groups in any of the 8 SF-36 domains [19]. In the SMART trial no significant difference between groups were found for any of the 8 domains or summary component scores of the SF-36 or the EuroQol at 12 months. A trend towards better social functioning in the off-pump group was observed at 12 month [16]. In a trial including 212 patients Motallebzadeh et al. assessed quality of life at 6 and 18 month postoperatively using the SF-36. No significant difference between off-pump and on-pump CABG was found [22]. Quality of life was measured using SF-36 in 202 patients included in the MASS III trial [15]. After six and 12 months quality of life had improved compared to baseline values, but without differences between off-pump and on-pump CABG. In a Canadian trial, Légaré et al. [23] measured quality of life in 300 patients 12 months after bypass surgery using the Seattle Angina Questionnaire.

Table 1. Randomized controlled trials comparing HRQoL outcomes after on-pump and off-pump CABG

Trial/investigator	Country	Inclusion period	HRQoL instrument	Patient population	Response rate	Follow-up	Findings	Notes
BHACAS I +II(24,25)	United Kingdom	March 1997 - November 1999	SF-36, CROQ, SAQ, EuroQoL	200 OPCAB 201 CABG	82% (2-4 years)	2-4 years and 6-8 years	At 2-4 as well as 6-8 years follow-up patients undergoing off-pump and on-pump CABG had similar symptoms, generic and disease-specific QoL.	Patients were blinded for their intervention Single surgeon trial
BBS(13)	Denmark	July 2002 - December 2004	SF-36	61 OPCAB 59 CABG	96%	Baseline and 3 months	HRQoL improved in both group at 3 months. No significant difference between groups.	Moderate to high risk patients
Légaré et al.(23)	Canada	August 1999 - March 2003	SAQ	150 OPCAB 150 CABG	88%	12 months	No significant differences in the 5 domains.	
Al-Ruzzeh et al.(12)	United Kingdom	Not reported, published 2006	WHOQoL	84 OPCAB 84 CABG	Unclear	Baseline, 6 weeks, and 6 months	Overall no significant difference over 6 month.	Single surgeon trial Patients were blinded to the procedure
Mathisen et al.(14)	Norway	March 1999 - March 2002	SF-36, QOLS-N	60 OPCAB 60 CABG	Unclear	Baseline, three, six and 12 months postoperative	No significant differences between groups were demonstrated in the cross-sectional or longitudinal cross co-variance analysis.	Both groups improved significantly on all SF-36 subscales from baseline to 3 moths postoperatively
OCTOPUS(18,19,26)	Netherlands	March 1998 - August 2000	EuroQoL, SF-36	142 OPCAB 139 CABG	88% (3 months) 85% (5 years)	Baseline, 1,3, and 12 months as well as 5 years postoperative	Marked improvement in overall QoL after 3 months and each of the 8 subdomains in both groups. Only bodily pain and general health perception improved further from 3 to 12 months, but no significant differences between groups. After 5 years , the on-pump group did significantly better in the domain of role limitation due to physical health problems.	Multicenter trial
PROMISS(21)	Portugal	April 2005 - July 2007	EQ 5D	75 OPCAB 75 CABG	Unclear	1 year	QoL assessed by EQ-VAS at 6 months showed no difference between groups.	Low graft patency was observed In the OPCAB group

Trial/investigator	Country	Inclusion period	HRQoL instrument	Patient population	Response rate	Follow-up	Findings	Notes
SMART(16)	United States	March 2000 - August 2001	EuroQoL, SF-36	100 OPCAB 100 CABG	79% (12months)	Baseline, 6 weeks, 6 months, and 12 months postoperative	No significant differences between groups were found for any of the subscale or summary component scores of the SF-36 or the EuroQoL at any of the follow-up time points.	Single surgeon trial
MASS III(15)	Brazil	January 2002 - December 2006	SF-36	105 OPCAB 97 CABG	80%	Baseline, 6 and 12 months postoperative	Improved QoL compared with baseline in both groups, but no significant differences between groups.	SF-36 questionnaire administered in interview
Motallebzadeh et al.(22)	United Kingdom	August 2002 - March 2004	SF-36	108 OPCAB 104 CABG	73% (6 months) 46% (18 month)	6 and 18 months	No differences in QoL between patients undergoing off-pump and on-pump CANG at both 6 and 18 months after surgery.	
Tully et al.(17)	Australian	June 1999 - July 2003	SF-36	30 OPCAB 36 CABG	90%	Baseline and 6 months	General increase in all domains from baseline to the 6-month assessment. No significant differences between groups in QoL.	

None of the 5 domains: physical limitation, angina stability, angina frequency, treatment satisfaction, or disease perception showed any significant difference between patients operated off-pump versus on-pump.

Quality of life was assessed after 2-4 years and again 6-8 years in the BHACAS trials [24,25]. The BHACAS I and II included 401 patients randomized to off-pump versus on-pump CABG. Quality of life was assessed with 4 instruments (SF-36, EuroQol, Seattle Angina questionnaire and Coronary Revascularization Outcome Questionnaire). After 2-4 years of follow-up there was no difference in self-reported symptoms and quality of life in patient who underwent off-pump and on-pump CABG [24]. Similar findings were reported with extended follow-up in the same cohort after 6-8 years of follow-up [25]. In both the physical and mental components summary scores of the SF-36 instrument the mean value was above 50, which represents the mean for the reference 'normal' population. The OCTOPUS trial has also published long-term follow-up of heath related quality of life. In accordance with the BHACAS trials no significant differences were demonstrated between off-pump and on-pump CABG in angina status or the overall measure of quality of life assessed by SF-36. Only in the domain of role limitations due to health problems the on-pump group did slightly better than the off-pump group [26]. However, both off-pump and on-pump CABG patients had significantly better quality of life compared with their preoperative status.

COMMENT

It seems convincing, that on-pump and off-pump CABG result in a clearly improved HRQoL when comparing baseline levels. However, without performing a regular meta-analysis, the evidence from randomized controlled trials on HRQoL after off- pump versus on-pump CABG is quite unambiguous: there is no difference between the two procedures with respect to HRQoL, independently of which instrument has been used to quantify self reported quality of life. This conclusion is not surprising, since there is no difference between the 2 procedures with respect to the factors which do have major impact on quality of life. Sofar, no difference has been demonstrated in survival, stroke, myocardial infarction and other serious side effects, as well as need for permanent dialysis or major impairment of cognitive function, which do jeopardize quality of life and the events are found in an equal low frequency after both procedures [7,8]. At the same time both procedures seem to be equally efficient with respect to symptom relief.

Most patients included in these trials were in stable conditions and had a normal left ventricle ejection fraction, however the same beneficial outcome could be shown as well in moderate to high risk, elderly, and less stable patients [13].

Only two RCTs report long term (>5 years) outcome [25,26] and the improvement of HRQoL seems to be consistent over time without apparent difference between the two different revascularization strategies. This seems to confirm the simple assumption that an equal improvement in quality of life at 3 and 12 months after surgery is unlikely to deteriorate specifically in one of the groups over time, especially if long term survival and graft patency at 1 year were identical in both groups.

The fact that the primary indication for revascularization in the majority of patients was symptom relief in terms of freedom from angina and not an expected prognostic improval of long term survival, underlines the importance of the outcome measure "HRQoL", which often is regarded as secondary or tertiary. None of the RCTs was really powered to demonstrate small and subtle differences with respect to conventional cardiovascular outcome measures as death, stroke and reinfarction. That an equal improvement of HRQoL both longitudinal and cross sectional is demonstrated after off-pump and on-pump CABG does increase the probability, that an eventual difference between the two procedures, as far as long term survival may be small

Conclusion

Currently, evidence from RCTs reporting the treatment results of CABG and acquired health benefits in terms of HRQoL suggest that neither traditional on-pump CABG nor redefined OPCAB technique is superior to other. Although it seems that patients who have undergone bypass surgery by using the OPCAB technique present with fewer neurocognitive deficits during short-term follow-up, the achieved advantage in terms of ameliorated neurocognition evened out during long-term follow-up. Relentless use of only the OPCAB technique therefore cannot be rationalized by HRQoL-related factors. The premises are more dependent on the preference and experience of the surgeon, and ultimately patient-related characteristics that may have an effect on selected techniques.

References

[1] Yusuf, S., Zucker, D., Peduzzi, P., et al. Effect of coronary artery bypass graft surgery on survival: overview of 10-year results from randomised trials by the Coronary Artery Bypass Graft Surgery Trialists Collaboration. *Lancet* 1994; 344:563-570.

[2] Kappetein, A. P., Feldman, T. E., Mack, M. J., et al. Comparison of coronary bypass surgery with drug-eluting stenting for the treatment of left main and/or three-vessel disease: 3-year follow-up of the SYNTAX trial. *Eur. Heart J.* 2011.

[3] Likosky, D. S., Marrin, C. A., Caplan, L. R., et al. Determination of etiologic mechanisms of strokes secondary to coronary artery bypass graft surgery. *Stroke* 2003;34:2830-2834.

[4] Roach, G. W., Kanchuger, M., Mangano, C. M., et al. Adverse cerebral outcomes after coronary bypass surgery. Multicenter Study of Perioperative Ischemia Research Group and the Ischemia Research and Education Foundation Investigators. *N Engl. J. Med.* 1996; 335:1857-1863.

[5] Phillips-Bute, B., Mathew, J. P., Blumenthal, J. A., et al. Association of neurocognitive function and quality of life 1 year after coronary artery bypass graft (CABG) surgery. *Psychosom. Med.* 2006; 68:369-375.

[6] Borst, C., Jansen, E. W., Tulleken, C. A., Grundeman, P. F., et al. Coronary artery bypass grafting without cardiopulmonary bypass and without interruption of native coronary flow using a novel anastomosis site restraining device ("Octopus"). *J. Am. Coll. Cardiol.* 1996; 27:1356-1364.

[7] Wijeysundera, D. N., Beattie, W. S., Djaiani, G., et al. Off-pump coronary artery surgery for reducing mortality and morbidity: meta-analysis of randomized and observational studies. *J. Am. Coll. Cardiol.* 2005;46:872-882.

[8] Møller, C. H., Penninga, L., Wetterslev, J., Steinbruchel, D. A., Gluud, C. Clinical outcomes in randomized trials of off- vs. on-pump coronary artery bypass surgery: systematic review with meta-analyses and trial sequential analyses. *Eur. Heart J.* 2008;29:2601-2616.

[9] Takagi, H., Tanabashi, T., Kawai, N., Kato, T., Umemoto, T. Off-pump coronary artery bypass sacrifices graft patency: meta-analysis of randomized trials. *J. Thorac. Cardiovasc. Surg.* 2007;133:e2-e3.

[10] Testa, M. A., Simonson, D. C. Assesment of quality-of-life outcomes. *N Engl. J. Med.* 1996; 334:835-840.

[11] Ware, J. E., Jr., Kosinski, M., Gandek, B., et al. The factor structure of the SF-36 Health Survey in 10 countries: results from the IQOLA Project. International Quality of Life Assessment. *J. Clin. Epidemiol.* 1998;51:1159-1165.

[12] Al Ruzzeh, S., George, S., Bustami, M., et al. Effect of off-pump coronary artery bypass surgery on clinical, angiographic, neurocognitive, and quality of life outcomes: randomised controlled trial. *BMJ* 2006;332:1365.

[13] Jensen, B. O., Hughes, P., Rasmussen, L. S., Pedersen, P. U., Steinbruchel, D. A. Health-related quality of life following off-pump versus on-pump coronary artery bypass grafting in elderly moderate to high-risk patients: a randomized trial. *Eur. J. Cardiothorac. Surg.* 2006;30:294-299.

[14] Mathisen, L., Andersen, M. H., Hol, P. K., et al. Patient-reported outcome after randomization to on-pump versus off-pump coronary artery surgery. *Ann. Thorac. Surg.* 2005;79:1584-1589.

[15] Nogueira, C. R., Hueb, W., Takiuti, M. E., et al. Quality of life after on-pump and off-pump coronary artery bypass grafting surgery. *Arq. Bras. Cardiol.* 2008;91:217-244.

[16] Puskas, J. D., Williams, W. H., Mahoney, E. M., et al. Off-pump vs conventional coronary artery bypass grafting: early and 1-year graft patency, cost, and quality-of-life outcomes: a randomized trial. *JAMA* 2004;291:1841-1849.

[17] Tully, P. J., Baker, R. A., Kneebone, A. C., Knight, J. L. Neuropsychologic and quality-of-life outcomes after coronary artery bypass surgery with and without cardiopulmonary bypass: a prospective randomized trial. *J. Cardiothorac. Vasc. Anesth.* 2008;22:515-521.

[18] Van Dijk, D., Nierich, A. P., Jansen, E. W., et al. Early outcome after off-pump versus on-pump coronary bypass surgery: results from a randomized study. *Circulation* 2001;104:1761-1766.

[19] Van Dijk, D., Jansen, E. W., Hijman, R., et al. Cognitive outcome after off-pump and on-pump coronary artery bypass graft surgery: a randomized trial. *JAMA* 2002;287:1405-1412.

[20] Jensen, B. O., Hughes, P., Rasmussen, L. S., Pedersen, P. U., Steinbruchel, D. A. Cognitive outcomes in elderly high-risk patients after off-pump versus conventional coronary artery bypass grafting: a randomized trial. *Circulation* 2006;113:2790-2795.

[21] Sousa, U. M., Cavaco, S., Oliveira, A. G., et al. Early graft patency after off-pump and on-pump coronary bypass surgery: a prospective randomized study. *Eur. Heart J.* 2010;31:2492-2499.

[22] Motallebzadeh, R., Bland, J. M., Markus, H. S., Kaski, J. C., Jahangiri, M. Health-related quality of life outcome after on-pump versus off-pump coronary artery bypass graft surgery: a prospective randomized study. *Ann. Thorac. Surg*. 2006;82:615-619.

[23] Karolak, W., Hirsch, G., Buth, K., Legare, J. F. Medium-term outcomes of coronary artery bypass graft surgery on pump versus off pump: results from a randomized controlled trial. *Am. Heart J.* 2007;153:689-695.

[24] Ascione, R., Reeves, B. C., Taylor, F. C., Seehra, H. K., Angelini, G. D. Beating heart against cardioplegic arrest studies (BHACAS 1 and 2): quality of life at mid-term follow-up in two randomised controlled trials. *Eur. Heart J.* 2004;25:765-770.

[25] Angelini, G. D., Culliford, L., Smith, D. K., et al. Effects of on- and off-pump coronary artery surgery on graft patency, survival, and health-related quality of life: long-term follow-up of 2 randomized controlled trials. *J. Thorac. Cardiovasc. Surg.* 2009;137:295-303.

[26] Van Dijk, D., Spoor, M., Hijman, R., et al. Cognitive and cardiac outcomes 5 years after off-pump vs on-pump coronary artery bypass graft surgery. *JAMA* 2007;297:701-708.

In: Off-Pump Coronary Artery Bypass Grafting
Editors: S.G. Raja and M. Amrani
ISBN 978-1-62081-575-5

Chapter 15

ECONOMIC OUTCOMES OF OFF-PUMP CORONARY ARTERY BYPASS GRAFTING

Dinesh Kurian,[1] Michael Simmons,[2] Soroosh Kiani,[3] and Robert S. Poston[4]

[1]Research Associate, Boston University, Boston, MA, US
[2]Research Associate, University of Arizona
College of Medicine, Tucson, AZ, US
[3]Vascular Medicine Research Fellow, Whitaker Cardiovascular Institute,
Boston Medical Center, Boston, MA, US
Research Associate, Division of Cardiac and Thoracic Surgery,
University of Arizona College of Medicine, Tucson, AZ, US
Boston Medical Center, Division of Cardiology, Boston, MA, US
[4]Chief Division of Cardiothoracic Surgery,
Jack G. Copeland Endowed Chair of Cardiovascular Surgery,
Michael Drummond Distinguished Professor of Cardiovascular and Thoracic Surgery,
University of Arizona, Tucson, AZ, US

ABSTRACT

With the percentage of gross national product allocated to healthcare continuing to rise in the Western world, resource allocation has become an issue. Percutaneous coronary intervention for coronary artery disease continues to be a viable option for many patients, with lower initial costs. However, long-term angina-free results often require further interventions or eventual surgery. Once coronary artery revascularization therapy is selected, it is worthwhile to evaluate the cost considerations inherent to various techniques. Off-pump coronary artery bypass graft surgery has seen a resurgence, with improved technology and lower hospital costs than on-pump bypass surgery. Numerous factors contributing to cost in coronary surgery have been studied and several are documented here, including the potential benefits of early extubation and the use of standardized optimal care pathways. A wide range of hospital-level cost variation has been noted, and standardization issues remain. With the advent of advanced computer-assisted robotic techniques, a push toward totally endoscopic bypass surgery has begun, with the eventual hope of reducing hospital stays to a minimum while maximizing outcomes, thus reducing intensive care unit and stepdown care times, which contribute a great deal toward overall cost. At the present time, these techniques add a significant premium to hospital charges, outweighing any potential length-of-stay benefits from a cost standpoint. This chapter aims to discuss the economic value of coronary revascularization, with a focus on coronary artery bypass grafting and its alternatives.

INTRODUCTION

Coronary revascularization, among the most common major surgical procedures performed worldwide, is both high cost and high revenue for hospitals. In 2010, total health care costs for major cardiovascular disease were $503.2 billion [1]. Attempts to reign in the high cost of health care have proven to be difficult. Perhaps one of the most significant shortcomings in this task is that hospitals tend to have poor cost calculating measures [2]. Without a thorough understanding of the resources required to perform coronary revascularization, the medical community cannot determine where and how to best control cost. Understanding how resources are utilized to offer desired patient outcomes is an important step in creating an understanding of the costs and benefits of various therapeutic options.

The objective of this chapter is to discuss the economic value of coronary revascularization, with a focus on coronary artery bypass grafting (CABG) and its alternatives.

UNDERSTANDING COST

A "value framework" is required for understanding costs associated with CABG. This refers to understanding patient outcomes in comparison to the costs of this procedure. Most often, variable costs are included in such an analysis and include the price of the materials and supplies used during hospitalization (operating room [OR] supplies, blood products), cost of hospital stay (intensive care unit [ICU] time, ward time), and outpatient appointments, in addition to any costs to manage complications or revise unwanted outcomes. However, there are additional cost considerations for this procedure that are not often considered, including lost productivity during convalescence, such as leave from work, lost salary or utilization of sick pay. There are also less tangible, though significant, issues such as ongoing underemployment for patients that return to work after a lengthy recuperation (Figure 1).

DIFFERENCES IN COST BETWEEN PERCUTANEOUS INTERVENTION AND CABG

There are two main options that provide coronary artery revascularization: CABG and percutaneous coronary artery intervention (PCI) using angioplasty and stenting. In a cost analysis of the largest prospective randomized comparison of CABG vs. PCI performed to date (i.e. SYNTAX trial), the index cost for PCI was found to be just over $31,000 while the index cost of CABG was more than twice that, at just over $63,000 [3]. The main drivers of increased cost for CABG are the additional resources required for the operating room, including increased staffing costs, and increased length of stay in the hospital [4]. Although cost of materials for the index procedure is higher with PCI by over $6,000, the total cost of index hospitalization is higher with CABG after taking into consideration physician fees and length of stay [4].

At one year following index hospitalization, PCI patients have a higher incidence of requiring revascularization procedures [4]. Follow-up for PCI was associated with increased costs for repeat hospitalization, medication costs, and physician costs (though CABG was associated with higher rehabilitation costs) [4]. While the follow-up costs for PCI patients are higher at one year by over $2000 (e.g. costs of repeat revascularization, additional medications and clinic visits, etc.), this does not offset the high cost of the index hospitalization for CABG. As a result, the total one-year cost of CABG is just over $3,000 higher than PCI [4]. However, the cost differences between these two modalities vary depending on the complexity of the coronary anatomy. In comparison to those with coronary artery lesions of mild to moderate complexity, patients judged to have the most severe complexity (i.e. SYNTAX scores above 32) showed a significant improvement in cost per quality-adjusted-life-years (QALY) gained at 1 year when treated with CABG [4].

Provider Costs	PCI	CCABG	OPCAB	RCAB
Materials for Initial Procedure	Guide wires, Stents, Contrast	Surgical supplies, cardiopulmonary bypass supplies	Surgical supplies, cardiac stabilization device	Robotic supplies, surgical supplies, cardiac stabilization device
Staffing cost for procedure	Assistants, technicians	Nursing	Nursing	Nursing
ICU cost	Lower LOS than CABG	Higher LOS than PCI	Lower LOS than CCAB	Lower LOS than Sternotomy CABG
Ward cost	Lower LOS than CABG	Higher LOS than PCI	Lower LOS than CCAB	Lower LOS than Sternotomy CABG
Cost of re-intervention	Higher than CABG	Lower than PCI	Same as CCABG	Same as Sternotomy CABG
Social Costs				
Hospital fees	Lower than CABG	Higher than PCI	Same as CCABG	Same as Sternotomy CABG
Professional fees	Lower than CABG	Higher than PCI	Same as CCABG	Same as Sternotomy CABG
Time lost to hospitalization	Lowest	Highest	High	Low
Cost of rehabilitation	Lowest	Highest	High	Low
Productivity lost to recovery	Lowest	High	High	Lower
Long term consequences	Restenosis	Neurocognitive changes (rare)	Neurocognitive changes (rare)	Fewer than Sternotomy CABG

Figure 1. Sources of cost. Although prices and reimbursements will change based on individual contracts or government policy changes, a conceptual understanding of cost will help providers calculate individual cost to benefit ratios of each option.

From the perspective of the costs to society for treating coronary artery disease, PCI has been considered as a classic example of a "disruptive innovation" that results in similar clinical outcomes for selected candidates with dramatic improvement in costs during and after hospitalization. In addition to greater reimbursement costs of CABG, it has been demonstrated that the longer recovery period associated with CABG results in disability costs that were $8,114 higher than PCI. For patients actively employed at the time of their procedure, absenteeism costs were $5,500 higher for CABG vs. PCI [3].

This lost worker productivity has further downstream effects on employers and therefore society including the need to hire and train replacement workers, the risk of underemployment when the patient returns to work and the financial impact on family caregivers.

Differences in Cost between Off-Pump Coronary Artery Bypass Grafting and On-Pump CABG

The largest prospective comparison of on-pump vs. off-pump CABG (i.e. ROOBY trial) demonstrated that on-pump CABG had a higher resource requirement than off-pump coronary artery bypass (OPCAB) grafting. Patients undergoing on-pump CABG spent longer time in the OR (approx. 42 minutes) and required more blood products. Length of stay in the ICU was higher as well, though ward time was comparable [5]. Overall, this resulted in an additional $2,284 in costs over OPCAB [5]. Numerous other trials corroborate comparable improvements in cost effectiveness for OPCAB [5,6]. Each of these studies show that cost is saved through efficient resource utilization by avoiding the disposable parts required to use cardiopulmonary bypass and the need for additional blood products. Many of the studies also show improved turnover time in the OR and ICU with fewer ICU re-admissions. In almost every study performed to date, health outcomes at one year have been equivalent between these techniques for the return of symptoms, survival, and quality of life. As a result, OPCAB has consistently demonstrated an improved cost per QALY over conventional CABG.

Differences in Cost between Robot-Assisted and Sternotomy CABG

CABG can also be performed with less invasive surgical incisions using robotic assistance (RCAB). This appears to be a promising alternative to sternotomy CABG, although the wide-spread adoption of this technique has been limited. In an analysis performed by our group, the up-front costs of RCAB were found to be higher due to increased OR time and the higher price of operative supplies and robotic instruments. However, the postoperative costs were considerably lower than CABG via sternotomy [7]. Cost savings were the result of a number of differences, most notably decreased length of stay, reduced requirement for blood products, and reduced lengths of stay in the ICU and hospital. These savings partially offset the intraoperative costs, resulting in only $1,000 more total costs per case for RCAB than sternotomy CABG (Figure 2).

A conceptual tool for comparing outcomes between various healthcare options, called an Outcome Measures Hierarchy, can be used to define other potential economic advantages of RCAB over the alternatives [8]. The most important question regarding these three options is whether RCAB offers similar short- and long-term mortality. The few available studies suggest identical graft patency between the two options [9,10], despite a learning curve associated with initiating an RCAB program that has been documented to be as many as 100 cases [11]. One-year results demonstrate improved patient satisfaction and a lower risk of major adverse cardiac and cerebrovascular events for RCAB vs. conventional CABG [12].

Most, but not all studies [13], have shown that RCAB has no difference in 3-year survival. Some surgeons believe that the robot assisted technique requires less anatomic and physiologic manipulation. As a result, long-term outcomes may be improved due to less neurocognitive and inflammatory changes in the perioperative period [14].

RCAB demonstrates its strengths over sternotomy based CABG among the dimensions of quality of life in the early postoperative period and time to return to normal functional status. Both of these parameters have been found to be considerably shorter amongst RCAB patients[12].

RCAB	**Sternotomy CABG**
Survival	
Identical graft patency to Sternotomy CABG	Identical graft patency to RCAB
Degree of Recovery	
Shorter time to recovery (2 to 3 weeks)	Typically, 1-2 months to return of normal activities
Time to recovery	
Improved cosmesis No risk of mediastinitis (except those requiring conversion to sternotomy) Reduced physiological and anatomical manipulation	Midline sternal scarring 1-2 % risk for mediastinitis
Sustainability of recovery	
No difference in three-year survival	No three-year survival advantage
Long-term consequences of care	
Potential for improved patient compliance with healthcare if decision for RCAB was part of a shared decision making strategy	Unclear long-term consequences on such issues as neurocognitive changes, higher inflammation during surgery, postoperative depression, etc.

Figure 2. A comparative outcomes measures framework comparing RCAB to Sternotomy CABG.

Of note, patients who required conversion to sternotomy CABG did not show any difference in outcomes to patients in the sternotomy group. One study quantifying RCAB outcomes noted no morbidity and a markedly decreased length of stay [9]. Given that RCAB outperforms conventional CABG in time to recovery and disutility of care, it represents a very attractive option for patients and may be cost effective in terms of QALY gained. However, further analysis is required.

ADDITIONAL FINANCIAL BENEFITS OF RCAB

RCAB has the potential to offer additional benefits to health care providers, which may be more difficult to measure directly [15]. The designation of sternal infections as a "never event" by Medicare offers a strong incentive for procedures such as RCAB, which spare the sternum. Many patients eligible for CABG often have risk factors for sternal infection and mediastinitis, including patients who are obese, active smokers, or who have diabetes. Avoiding sternal incisions on these patients avoids the risk of being hit with the unreimbursed cost of managing mediastinitis, estimated at roughly $50,000 per case. If avoiding sternotomy for half of CABG procedures can prevent two cases of mediastinitis per year, this would help hospitals forgo a cost of roughly $100,000 per year.

Furthermore, stroke and mediastinits are the two most costly complications for patients undergoing CABG. By avoiding aortic manipulation, RCAB offers an additional advantage by reducing the risk of stroke. Both of these complications factor into the STS composite quality rating, which is publically reported and used by Medicare to drive pay for performance incentives. Currently, plans offer a 2% bonus payment for centers that are rated at "three stars". For an institution that receives $5 million in Medicare reimbursement, this would yield an additional bonus of $100,000.

Shorter recovery time allows providers to leverage operational efficiencies as well. Efficient bed utilization helps offset the higher intraoperative cost. The ability to discharge RCAB patients 2-3 days earlier than sternotomy CABG patients allows hospitals to capture a larger share of DRG reimbursements as revenue, while also being able to use the available beds to treat other patients.

CONCLUSION

CABG is more resource intensive than PCI, but offers greater benefits in certain patient subsections. For patients that benefit from surgical revascularization, OPCAB uses resources more efficiently than conventional CABG. RCAB offers a promising alternative. While the intraoperative costs of RCAB are higher, postoperative costs are lower, and benefits to patients may be greater. Understanding cost and resource utilization is important, especially given the recent stress on efficient use of resources.

REFERENCES

[1] Mintel. (2010, December). *Heart Disease Statistics and Trends.* Retrieved from http://academic.mintel.com/.

[2] Kaplan and Porter. How to solve the cost crisis in health care. *Harvard Business Review* 2011;89: 46-64

[3] Zhao, Z., Winget, M. Economic burden of illness of acute coronary syndromes: medical and productivity costs. *BMC Health Serv. Res.* 2011;11:35.

[4] Cohen, D. J., et al. Economic outcomes of percutaneous coronary intervention with drug-eluting stents versus bypass surgery for patients with left main or 3-vessel coronary artery disease: One-year results from the SYNTAX trial. *Catheter. Cardiovasc. Interv.* 2011 May 3. doi: 10.1002/ccd.23147. [Epub ahead of print]

[5] Al-Ruzzeh, S., et al. Economic evaluation of coronary artery bypass grafting surgery with and without cardiopulmonary bypass: cost-effectiveness and quality-adjusted life years in a randomized controlled trial. *Artif. Organs* 2008;32:891-897.

[6] Nathoe, H. M., et al. A comparison of on-pump and off-pump coronary bypass surgery in low-risk patients. *N Engl. J. Med.* 2003;348:394-402.

[7] Poston, R. S., et al. Comparison of economic and patient outcomes with minimally invasive versus traditional off-pump coronary artery bypass grafting techniques. *Ann. Surg.* 2008;126:281-289.

[8] Porter, M. E. What is value in health care?. *N Engl. J. Med.* 2010; 363:2477-81.

[9] Atluri, P., et al. Off-pump, minimally invasive and robotic coronary revascularization yield improved outcomes over traditional on-pump CABG. *Int. J. Med. Robot* 2009;5:1-12.

[10] Argenziano, M., et al. Results of the prospective multicenter trial of robotically assisted totally endoscopic coronary artery bypass grafting. *Ann. Thorac. Surg.* 2006;81:666-74.

[11] Oehlinger, A., et al. Robotic endoscopic left internal mammary artery harvesting: what have we learned after 100 cases?. *Ann. Thorac. Surg.* 2007;83:1030-4.

[12] Bonaros, N., Schachner, T., Wiedemann, D., et al. Quality of life improvement after robotically assisted coronary artery bypass grafting. *Cardiology* 2009;114:59-66

[13] Jegaden, O., et al. Is there an optimal minimally invasive technique for left anterior descending coronary artery bypass?. *J. Cardiothorac. Surg.* 2011;6:37.

[14] Gottesman, R. F., et al. Early postoperative cognitive dysfunction and blood pressure during coronary artery bypass graft operation. *Arch. Neurol.* 2007;64:1111-4.

[15] Kurian, D., et al. Change management during the implementation of an innovative approach to heart bypass surgery. *Physician Exec.* (2011) In press.

SECTION 2: CONCERNS

In: Off-Pump Coronary Artery Bypass Grafting
Editors: S.G. Raja and M. Amrani
ISBN 978-1-62081-575-5

Chapter 16

GRAFT PATENCY AND QUALITY OF ANASTOMOSIS IN OFF-PUMP CORONARY BYPASS GRAFTING

Mark D. Pullan
Consultant Cardiac Surgeon, Liverpool Heart and Chest Hospital NHS Trust, Liverpool, UK

ABSTRACT

For over forty years cardiac surgeons have been constructing delicate coronary anastomoses on cardiopulmonary bypass (CPB). However, the price of a still and bloodless field is ultimately paid by the patients in the form of sequelae of negative effects of CPB including blood trauma, activation of a series of inflammatory responses, nonpulsatile flow, and possible embolization of air or debris. In an attempt to avoid these deleterious effects of CPB, off-pump coronary artery bypass (OPCAB) surgery has been rediscovered and refined. Although abundant evidence is available to suggest that excellent results can be achieved when CPB is avoided, concerns have been raised about quality of anastomosis and graft patency rates after OPCAB surgery. This chapter discusses in detail these concerns.

INTRODUCTION

There is evidence that performing coronary artery bypass grafting (CABG) without cardiopulmonary bypass (CPB) decreases the incidence of post-operative adverse events. [1] Large databases have reported that off-pump CABG reduces operative mortality in high-risk patients and provides similar long-term survival. [2-4] Despite reassuring data showing no statistically significant difference in graft patency between the two techniques, [5-9] concerns have been persistently raised about quality of anastomosis and graft patency after off-pump CABG. [10] This chapter discusses in detail the issue of quality of anastomosis and graft patency, regarded universally as the Holy Grail of coronary artery bypass surgery, in light of the current best available evidence.

Graft Patency and Anastomotic Quality Concerns

Technical shortcomings affecting construction of coronary anastomoses make the on- or off-pump debate irrelevant as the quality of the end result will be compromised irrespective of the revascularization strategy. On the other hand, watching expert off-pump surgeons construct perfect anastomosis to any coronary territory at a leisured pace, without the use of volume loading or inotropic support, with minimal or no hemodynamic compromise makes one question the legitimacy of concerns about quality of anastomoses during off-pump coronary artery bypass (OPCAB) grafting. This section analyzes the current evidence raising concerns about graft patency following OPCAB.

Evidence Questioning Quality of Anastomosis and Graft Patency in Off-Pump Grafting

Khan et al. [10] in 2004 published a study in the New England Journal of Medicine that attracted much attention and was frequently referenced by the popular press. The main conclusion of the study was that the graft patency rate was lower at three months in the off-pump group than in the on-pump group. This study was heavily criticized as the surgeons had a total experience of 98 cases prior to embarking on this trial.

In 2006 Lim et al. [11] published a systematic review of the randomized trials comparing revascularization rate and graft patency of off-pump and conventional coronary surgery. These investigators demonstrated the relative risk of graft patency in off-pump CABG compared with conventional CABG was 0.959 (95% confidence interval 0.936-0.983; p = .001). The analysis was repeated after excluding one specific trial because of clinical and statistical heterogeneity ($chi^2(6) = 27.78$; $p < .001$). The resultant relative risk of 0.953 (95% confidence interval 0.927-0.980; p = .001) was obtained with no further evidence of heterogeneity ($chi^2(5) = 5.35$; $p = .374$). In 5 trials, that included the mean number of grafts performed per arm, the standardized mean difference in revascularization comparing off-pump with conventional surgery was -0.164 (-0.286 to -0.043; $p = .008$).

Recently the concerns regarding graft patency were heightened by two meta-analyses by Takagi et al. [12,13]. The latest of these meta-analyses identified 8 prospective randomized controlled clinical trials that compared graft patency of 3 or more months after off-pump and on-pump CABG. In total, this meta-analysis included data on 6898 grafts. Pooled analysis demonstrated a statistically significant 32% increase in overall graft occlusion in off-pump compared with on-pump CABG (fixed-effects RR, 1.32; 95% CI, 1.18–1.48; $p < .00001$; p for heterogeneity = .20).

This alarming statistic is derived by taking into account the findings of the 2009 publication of Shroyer and associates, ROOBY trial. [14] They demonstrated in follow-up angiograms in 1371 patients, who underwent 4093 grafts, that the overall rate of graft patency was lower in the off-pump group than in the on-pump group (82.6% vs. 87.8%, P<0.01). This clearly isn't 32%, as reported by Takagi et al. [13]!

The findings of the ROOBY trial [14] have been questioned by several leaders in the field of off- pump surgery [15,16]. Puskas [16] commented "*In a majority of patients, CABG was performed by surgical trainees under the supervision of attending surgeons who were remarkably inexperienced in the off-pump procedure and much more experienced in the on-pump procedure. The reported 12.4% rate of intraoperative conversion from planned off-pump CABG to on-pump CABG was five times the rate reported in the national database of the Society of Thoracic Surgeons and is an explicit indictment of the off-pump inexperience of surgeons, trainees, and anesthesia–nursing teams participating in the ROOBY trial. It is illogical to conduct a randomized trial comparing patient outcomes with alternative surgical techniques among surgical operators who have grossly asymmetric experience and expertise with the two procedures that are being compared. This is the "fatal flaw" of the ROOBY trial."*

Also Taggart [15] pointed out that "*the inexperience of the surgeons with respect to this more demanding surgical technique was particularly notable, since the 53 participating surgeons enrolled on average only eight patients per year during a 5-year period and had unacceptably high conversion rates to on-pump surgery (12%) and incomplete revascularization (18%). It is likely that their inexperience contributed to other less favorable clinical outcomes as well.*"

When analyzing the studies that compare off-pump versus on-pump outcomes it is very easy to loose sight of major confounding factors. In the above examples the very limited experience of the surgeons would have a serious impact on the results. Other confounders include combination of multiple technologies such as anastomotic connectors or endoscopic vein harvest with OPCAB grafting. For example in the PREVENT IV trial [17] what appeared to be a marked difference in vein graft patency was largely accounted for by the greater use of endoscopic vein harvest in the off-pump cohort. Interestingly the observed saphenous vein failure rate was 25% in both groups. One-year clinical outcomes (MACCE) were better with off-pump than with on-pump CABG, suggesting benefits not related to vein graft patency.

With the limitations of the various randomized controlled trials in assessing graft patency on- versus off-pump, one could conclude that the quality and size of randomized controlled trials leave a lot to be desired! Similar conclusion was drawn by Farrokhyar [18] et al. in their paper published in the Canadian Journal of Surgery.

Evidence Supporting Similar Graft Patency after Off- and On-Pump Grafting

Clearly, the important question remains: Are there any good quality randomized controlled trials that have reasonable numbers, conducted by surgeons that are well versed in both off- and on-pump techniques and what are their outcomes? A good example would be the trial conducted by Puskas and associates [6]. In this randomized single-surgeon trial recruiting unselected patients with angiographic follow-up, OPCAB achieved similar graft patency in the hospital and at 1 year. Cardiac outcomes and health-related quality of life at 30 days and 1 year were similar and patients incurred a lower cost.

A follow-up of this study at a minimum of 6.8 years (maximum, 8.4 years; mean, 7.5 years) confirmed that off-pump and on-pump CABG were associated with similar early and late graft patency, incidence of recurrent or residual myocardial ischemia, need for reintervention, and long-term survival. [19]

Al-Ruzzeh and colleagues [8] in 2006 carried out a randomized controlled trial of 168 patients looking at graft patency as well as other outcomes. A total of 151 patients had their grafts evaluated by angiography and graft patency was similar between on-pump and off-pump groups (risk difference - 1%, 95% confidence interval - 5% to 4%), with the off-pump group considered the treatment group. Again this was a single surgeon with an extensive experience of both off- and on-pump grafting.

Assessment of graft patency can be difficult from a practical standpoint as the average asymptomatic postoperative patient does not wish to undergo angiography. With the advent of higher resolution computed tomography (CT) scanning, CT angiography is offering a more palatable solution. Angelini et al. [20] in 2009 published their long-term follow up (6-8 years) of the patients enrolled into their two randomized control trials. Patency was studied in 199 of 349 survivors. There was no evidence of attrition bias. The likelihood of graft occlusion was no different between off-pump (10.6%) and on-pump (11.0%) groups (odds ratio, 1.00; 95% confidence interval, 0.55-1.81; $p > .99$).

Off-pump CABG requires a unique skill set and a different conduct of operation compared with on-pump CABG. Not only must the surgeon perform anastomoses on the beating heart, but he/she must understand the hemodynamic consequences of cardiac positioning and stabilization, the effects of regional ischemia on hemodynamic function, contractility, and arrhythmias, and the importance of anesthesia and grafting sequence given variants of anatomy and clinical conditions. Given these differences, the ability to teach off-pump CABG to residents and surgeons places unique demands on the teaching surgeon. [21] With good off-pump training, the learning curve can be shortened resulting in acquisition of skills that can enable capable trainees to perform off pump CABG effectively and safely with acceptable results.

Assessment of Anastomotic Quality

A logical approach to determine the differences in anastomotic quality after on- and off-pump CABG will necessitate evaluation of published scientific evidence. A caveat when looking at data in the literature is already hinted at previously in this chapter. Early results were marred by incomplete revascularization as the circumflex territory was considered a challenge during the initial resurgence period for OPCAB grafting. The circumflex territory was either left ungrafted or grafts were more likely to be rushed through before the hemodynamic collapse occurred. In addition, tight vascular slings, coronary artery bulldogs, non-humidified carbon dioxide blowers and stiff shunts all have damaging influences on the intima of the coronary [22] and are bound to affect the quality of anastomosis and durability of any graft.

Intraoperative Assessment of Anastomotic Quality

When trying to assess anastomotic quality at the operating table, there are two modalities currently in use: transit time flow measurement (TTFM) and the intraoperative fluorescence imaging (IFI). Added to this there are a whole host of surrogates such as postoperative ischemia and infarct, cardiac enzyme release, inotrope use, ventilator times etc. The list of surrogates is almost endless but all fail to provide the operator with a direct knowledge of the anastomotic quality.

The Novadaq Spy system was first used in 2004 [23] as a method of subjectively assessing the quality of anastomoses. Indocyanin green (ICG) dye is injected into the patient, and when illuminated with 806-nm light, ICG fluoresces and emits light at 830 nm. This fluorescent light is captured by a charged couple device video camera at 30 frames per second and displayed on a computer monitor. This can then be checked to see if there are constrictions or other defects at the anastomotic site. There is also the opportunity to qualitatively assess the run-off into the distal vessel. Reuthebuch and colleagues [23] published on its utility in off-pump surgery demonstrating less than 4% of grafts needed revision on table.

The other method that is currently being used is the Transit Time Doppler (TTD) to gain TTFM as an assessment of grafts. Newer versions of this hardware can also give 2D images of anastomoses but these are currently qualitative. TTFM can give qualitative numbers for the pulsatility index and the graft flow. This requires the right size probe to be placed on the graft and a good contact to be made for accurate analysis.

Several publications have reported on the utility of TTFM and tried to ascertain a difference between on-and off-pump grafting. Hassanein and associates [24] in 2005 carried out a good sized study of 445 off-pump patients with an equal number of matched on-pump cases and looked at the TTD data from each group. The average pulsatile index in OPCAB was 2.09 +/- 1.03 (mean flow, 39 +/- 22.63 mL/min), whereas with on-pump coronary artery bypass grafting it was 1.9 +/- 0.98 (mean flow, 44.19 +/- 23.58 mL/min); $p = 0.005$. Subgroup analysis showed significantly lower mean flows and higher pulsatile index with OPCAB grafts to the obtuse marginal, diagonal, and right coronary artery, but not to the left anterior descending territory. This higher pulsatility index was well below the index of five which is deemed as the upper limit of acceptable. The most plausible conclusion based on these findings will be that grafting on-pump was better than in off-pump. However there is a predictable confounder that was not dealt with in this study. Guden et al. [25] in 2003 demonstrated how fallible TTFM was to hemodilution. They had three cohorts, off-pump, on-pump and off-pump with hemodilution. The degree of hemodilution in the off-pump group was equivalent to that seen with CPB. All three groups had equivalent pulsatility indices but the on-pump and off-pump hemodiluted groups had equal and higher graft flows than the off-pump group.

Balacumaraswami and colleagues [26] in 2005 and Desai et al. [27] in 2006 looked at comparing the results of TTFM with IFI. Both groups found deficits in TTFM with grafts that appeared normal with IFI. Balacumaraswami and associates [26] showed that 10% of patients may get their grafts revised unnecessarily if using TTFM. Desai et al. [27] showed the sensitivity and specificity of indocyanine green angiography to detect greater than 50% stenosis or occlusion was 83.3% and 100%, respectively. The sensitivity and specificity of transit-time ultrasonic flow measurement to detect greater than 50% stenosis or occlusion was 25% and 98.4%, respectively. These figures were generated in the presence of standard x-ray angiography at post-operative day 4.

Gao et al. [28] have used 64 slice gated computed tomography (CT) for assessment of graft patency. This clearly does not give an on table assessment but they carried out the CT scans at one month, 1 year, 2 years, 3 years and 4 years. They demonstrated that patency of left internal mammary artery (LIMA) was higher than that of saphenous vein grafts (SVG) in both on-pump and off-pump patients; no significant difference was seen in LIMA patency and SVG patency between the two groups. They concluded that 64-slice CT indicates that OPCAB grafting provides similar patency to conventional surgery with CPB.

Impact of High Volume Off-Pump Practice on Graft Patency

The evidence for concerns regarding graft patency with OPCAB surgery is certainly present. Hannan and associates [4] showed from the New York Registry that there was a 4% lower freedom from repeat revascularization in the off-pump patients. Despite the quality of data it is difficult to state whether this reflects under grafting at the time of the index operation or a true reduction in the number of patent grafts. When looking at the evidence there are many confounding and interlinked factors. These include the experience of the surgeons, the other technologies used in conjunction with the grafting, the markers of quality and how sensitive or specific they are, and the list is almost endless.

In high volume practices with good follow up, there would be a clear difference in survival rates and freedom from revascularization between off-pump and on-pump surgery if there was a true anastomotic and graft quality concern. Interestingly, this is not seen in Puskas' series [19]. There were 26 deaths from all causes among OPCAB patients and 31 among CPB patients. Graft patency was similar between groups among 622 grafts assessed by angiography before hospital discharge (99% OPCAB versus 97.7% CPB; $p = 0.22$, Fisher's exact test), among 511 grafts assessed by angiography at 1 year (93.6% OPCAB versus 95.8% CPB; $p = 0.33$), and among 190 grafts assessed by computed tomographic angiography at late follow-up (76% OPCAB versus 83.5% CPB; p = 0.44). Twelve of 34 OPCAB (35.3%) and 16 of 39 CPB patients (41.0%) had any ischemia on positron emission tomography scanning (p = 0.62). Four OPCAB patients (11.8%) and 9 CPB patients (23.1%) had an ischemic region in excess of 10% of myocardium (p = 0.21). At late follow-up, recurrent angina had occurred in 11 of 43 (25.6%) OPCAB patients and 5 of 44 (11.4%) CPB patients (p = 0.09). Percutaneous reintervention had been performed at the discretion of blinded local cardiologists in 1 of 43 (2.3%) OPCAB patients and 1 of 44 (2.3%) CPB patients (p = 1.0). No patient in either group has undergone repeat CABG. They concluded that in this randomized trial, off-pump and on-pump CABG were associated with similar early and late graft patency, incidence of recurrent or residual myocardial ischemia, need for reintervention, and long-term survival.

In our own unit (Liverpool Heart and Chest Hospital) the experience is similar. At a median follow-up of 4 years there was no difference in re-intervention rates, either by percutaneous coronary intervention (on-pump 1.6%, off-pump 2.0%; $p = 0.2$) or redo surgery (on-pump 0.3%, off-pump 0.3%; $p = 0.68$) for two groups of propensity matched cohorts of 3096 patients, indicating similar revascularization completeness and quality. There was also no difference in mid–term survival ($p = 0.83$) (Figure 1), which is again what you would expect from similar revascularization completeness and quality. The long term data is very favorable when off-pump grafting is done as a routine in a centre with a high volume of experience and a good teaching programme.

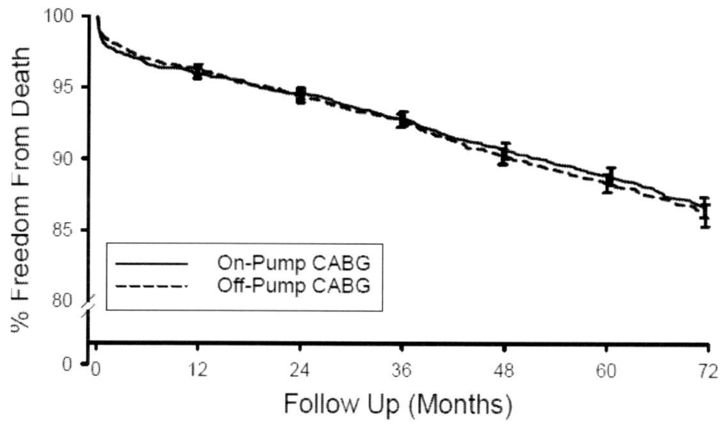

Figure 1. Impact of on-pump and off-pump CABG on mid-term survival at Liverpool Heart and Chest Hospital.

CONCLUSION

Current best available evidence regarding graft patency after off-pump CABG is dominated by trials with conflicting results. These conflicting results may be due to differences in patient selection, surgical expertise, technique, antithrombotic protocols, and timing of patency control. It can be hypothesized that with uniform standardized techniques and large experience in off-pump CABG, there would be no difference in graft patency in patients undergoing CABG with or without CPB.

Finally, technical precision, anastomotic quality, and completeness of revascularization in OPCAB grafting can be achieved universally by methodically adopting the strategy and negotiating learning curve through careful patient selection.

REFERENCES

[1] Cheng, D. C., Bainbridge, D., Martin, J. E., Novick, R. J.; The Evidence-Based Perioperative Clinical Outcomes Research Group. Does off-pump coronary artery bypass reduce mortality, morbidity and resource utilization when compared with conventional coronary artery bypass? A meta-analysis of randomized trials. *Anesthesiology* 2005;102:188-203.

[2] Sellke, F. W., Michael DiMaio, J., et al. Comparing on-pump and off-pump coronary artery bypass grafting: numerous studies but few conclusions: a scientific statement from the American Heart Association council on cardiovascular surgery and anesthesia in collaboration with the interdisciplinary working group on quality of care and outcomes research. *Circulation* 2005;111:2858-2864.

[3] Puskas, J. D., Kilgo, P. D., et al. Off-pump techniques disproportionately benefit women and narrow the gender disparity in outcomes after coronary artery bypass surgery. *Circulation* 2007;116:I-192-I-199.

[4] Hannan, E. L., Chuntao, W., et al. Off-pump versus on-pump coronary artery bypass graft surgery. Differences in short-term outcomes and in long-term mortality and need for subsequent revascularization. *Circulation* 2007;116:1145-1152.

[5] Nathoe, H.M., Van Dijk, D., et al.; Octopus Study Group. A comparison of on-pump and off-pump coronary bypass surgery in low-risk patients. *N Engl. J. Med.* 2003;348:394-402.

[6] Puskas, J., Williams, W. H., et al. Off-pump versus conventional coronary artery bypass grafting: Early and 1-year graft patency, cost and quality of life outcomes. *JAMA* 2004;291:1841-1849.

[7] Kobayashi, J., Tashiro, T., et al.; for the Japanese Off-Pump Coronary Revascularisation Investigation (JOCRI) Study Group. Early outcome of a randomized comparison of off-pump and on-pump multiple arterial coronary revascularization. *Circulation* 2005;112(Suppl. I):I-338-I-343.

[8] Al-Ruzeh, S., George, S., et al. Effect of off-pump coronary artery bypass surgery on clinical, angiographic, neurocognitive and quality of life outcomes: randomized controlled trial. *Br. Med. J.* 2006;332:1365-1368.

[9] Lingas, P. S., Hol, P. K., et al. Clinical and radiologic outcome of Off-Pump coronary surgery at 12 month follow-up: a prospective randomized trial. *Ann. Thorac. Surg.* 2006;81:2089-2096.

[10] Khan, N. E., De Souza, A., Mister, R., et al. A randomized comparison of off-pump and on-pump multivessel coronary-artery bypass surgery. *N Engl. J. Med.* 2004;350:21-8.

[11] Lim, E., Drain, A., Davies, W., Edmonds, L., Rosengard, B. R. A systematic review of randomized trials comparing revascularization rate and graft patency of off-pump and conventional coronary surgery. *J. Thorac. Cardiovasc. Surg.* 2006;132:1409-13.

[12] Takagi, H., Tanabashi, T., Kawai, N., Kato, T., Umemoto, T. Off-pump coronary artery bypass sacrifices graft patency: meta-analysis of randomized trials. *J. Thorac. Cardiovasc. Surg.* 2007;133:e2-3.

[13] Takagi, H., Matsui, M., Umemoto, T. Lower graft patency after off-pump than on-pump coronary artery bypass grafting: an updated meta-analysis of randomized trials. *J. Thorac. Cardiovasc. Surg.* 2010;140:e45-7.

[14] Shroyer, A. L., Grover, F. L., Hattler, B., et al; Veterans Affairs Randomized On/Off Bypass (ROOBY) Study Group. On-pump versus off-pump coronary-artery bypass surgery. *N Engl. J. Med.* 2009;361:1827-37.

[15] Taggart, D. P. On-pump versus off-pump CABG. *N Engl. J. Med.* 2010;362:852; author reply 853-4.

[16] Puskas, J. D., Mack, M. J., Smith, C. R. On-pump versus off-pump CABG. *N Engl. J. Med.* 2010;362:851; author reply 853-4.

[17] Mehta, R. H., Ferguson, T. B., Lopes, R. D., et al; Project of Ex-vivo Vein Graft Engineering via Transfection (PREVENT) IV Investigators. Saphenous vein grafts with multiple versus single distal targets in patients undergoing coronary artery bypass surgery: one-year graft failure and five-year outcomes from the Project of Ex-Vivo Vein Graft Engineering via Transfection (PREVENT) IV trial. *Circulation* 2011;124:280-8.

[18] Farrokhyar, F., Chu, R., Whitlock, R., Thabane, L. A systematic review of the quality of publications reporting coronary artery bypass grafting trials. *Can. J. Surg.* 2007;50:266-77.

[19] Puskas, J. D., Williams, W. H., O'Donnell, R., et al. Off-pump and on-pump coronary artery bypass grafting are associated with similar graft patency, myocardial ischemia, and freedom from reintervention: long-term follow-up of a randomized trial. *Ann. Thorac. Surg.* 2011;91:1836-42

[20] Angelini, G. D., Culliford, L., Smith, D. K., et al. Effects of on- and off-pump coronary artery surgery on graft patency, survival, and health-related quality of life: long-term follow-up of 2 randomized controlled trials. *J. Thorac. Cardiovasc. Surg.* 2009;137:295-303.

[21] Halkos, M. E., Puskas, J. D. Teaching off-pump coronary artery bypass surgery. *Semin. Thorac. Cardiovasc. Surg.* 2009;21:224-8.

[22] Manchio, J. V., Gu, J., Romar, L., et al. Disruption of graft endothelium correlates with early failure after off-pump coronary artery bypass surgery. *Ann. Thorac. Surg.* 2005;79:1991-8.

[23] Reuthebuch, O., Häussler, A., Genoni, M., et al. Novadaq SPY: intraoperative quality assessment in off-pump coronary artery bypass grafting. *Chest* 2004;125:418-24.

[24] Hassanein, W., Albert, A. A., Arnrich, B., et al. Intraoperative transit time flow measurement: off-pump versus on-pump coronary artery bypass. *Ann. Thorac. Surg.* 2005;80:2155-61.

[25] Güden, M., Sanisoglu, I., Sagbas, E., et al. Hemodilution during off-pump coronary artery bypass grafting: can we improve flow and reduce hypercoagulability? *Heart Surg. Forum* 2003;6:399-402.

[26] Balacumaraswami, L., Abu-Omar, Y., Choudhary, B., Pigott, D., Taggart, D. P. A comparison of transit-time flowmetry and intraoperative fluorescence imaging for assessing coronary artery bypass graft patency. *J. Thorac. Cardiovasc. Surg.* 2005;130:315-20.

[27] Desai, N. D., Miwa, S., Kodama, D., et al.A randomized comparison of intraoperative indocyanine green angiography and transit-time flow measurement to detect technical errors in coronary bypass grafts. *J. Thorac. Cardiovasc. Surg.* 2006;132:585-94.

[28] Gao, C., Liu, Z., Li, B., et al. Comparison of graft patency for off-pump and conventional coronary arterial bypass grafting using 64-slice multidetector spiral computed tomography angiography. *Interact. Cardiovasc. Thorac. Surg.* 2009;8:325-9.

In: Off-Pump Coronary Artery Bypass Grafting
Editors: S.G. Raja and M. Amrani
ISBN 978-1-62081-575-5

Chapter 17

Completeness of Revascularization in Off-Pump Coronary Artery Bypass Grafting

Nirav C. Patel[1] and Valavanur A. Subramanian[2]
[1]Vice Chairman, Department of Cardiothoracic Surgery,
Lenox Hill Hospital/North Shore –LIJ Health System, New York, NY, US
[2]Chairman, Department of Cardiothoracic Surgery,
Lenox Hill Hospital/North Shore –LIJ Health System, New York, NY, US

Abstract

Completeness of revascularization in patients with coronary artery disease leads to improved long term survival. The definition of completeness of revascularization is controversial. Majority of the randomized as well as case controlled studies have shown fewer number of grafts performed in off-pump patients compared to on-pump patients. Completeness of revascularization in off-pump patients is highly dependent on surgeon experience and patient selection. Similar completeness of revascularization to on-pump can be achieved in off-pump patients by an experienced surgeon using modern stabilization and cardiac positioning techniques. This chapter discusses the significance of completeness of revascularization, evaluates current evidence and analyzes factors affecting completeness of revascularization during off-pump coronary artery bypass grafting.

Introduction

Complete myocardial revascularization is the main advantage of coronary bypass grafting (CABG) as opposed to other modalities of treatment for coronary artery disease. The reports from coronary artery surgery registry and the Emory University in 1996 established the long-term survival benefit of complete coronary revascularization in cardiac surgical patients [1,2]. In BARI study investigators were unable to demonstrate survival benefits of complete revascularization compared to incomplete revascularization at 7 years follow-up [3]. However publications over the last decade have shown survival advantage with complete revascularization in CABG [4,5]. Recently the SYNTAX trial investigators in reporting their two- year outcomes on coronary surgery cohort concluded that incomplete revascularization rather than degree of coronary complexity adversely affects late-outcomes of coronary bypass [6]. In recent years, with advent of off-pump revascularization, to avoid the deleterious effect of cardiopulmonary bypass, the issue of completeness of revascularization has risen again.

Definition of Completeness of Revascularization

There has been inconsistency in defining completeness of revascularization. The traditional definition of completeness of revascularization assumes one graft for every significantly obstructed artery. This does not take in to consideration the size of the vessel and location of the obstruction. The functional definition of completeness of revascularization uses one graft each for all diseased primary arterial territories. The left anterior descending artery, the circumflex artery and the right coronary artery define the territories. The BARI study investigators compared the two definitions and found no significant difference in survival advantage for either compared to patients with incomplete revascularizations [3]. Some studies have used index of completeness of revascularization for each patient for comparing groups [7,9]. Index of completeness is defined as number of grafts constructed divided by number of diseased vessels on preoperative angiogram.

Majority of the retrospective cohort studies comparing off-pump versus on-pump revascularization use average number of grafts performed as a marker of comparing completeness of revascularization between groups [10-21]. However, in these studies factors influencing the decreased number of grafts seen in off-pump patients remain unclear.

Majority of prospective randomized trials comparing off-pump and on-pump revascularization addressed completeness of revascularization by defining number of grafts intended before surgery and number of grafts performed [22-25]. This is probably the most ideal method to define completeness of revascularization as it would take in to account the location of coronary lesions, extent of lesions and most importantly the size of the vessel.

Does Off-Pump Coronary Grafting Lead to Similar Completeness of Revascularization Compared to Conventional On-Pump Grafting?

Evidence from Randomized Trials

The ISMICS consensus statement performed meta-analysis of the randomized trials comparing off-pump versus on-pump bypass surgery [26]. This meta-analysis showed a lower number of grafts per patients in off-pump group compared to on-pump group. While there was statistical difference of 0.2 fewer grafts per patient, the clinical significance was difficult to assess. When the data were analyzed separately for earlier trials (i.e. prior to and including year 2000) and later trials (after year 2000), the number of grafts per patient in off-pump patient increased (2.1 to 2.7), but the difference remained significant of 0.2 grafts per patient less compared to on-pump patient. This could be explained on basis of selection of patients with more extensive disease in later trails.

Another systematic review done by Lim et al. [27] showed similar results with a statistically significant less number of grafts in off-pump patients compared to on-pump patients.

The large multicenter randomized trial (ROOBY trial) [25] comparing off-pump and on-pump bypass showed that the proportion of patients with fewer grafts than originally planned was higher in off-pump group than in on-pump group. Also there were statistically significant fewer grafts (0.1) per patient in off-pump group.

In conclusion the number of grafts performed and completeness of revascularization is slightly reduced in off-pump compared to off-pump in randomized controlled trials.

Evidence from Retrospective Cohort Studies

Majority of retrospective studies comparing off-pump and on-pump compare patients with historical or contemporary cohorts. All the studies show less number of grafts performed in off pump group [10-21]. Surgeons' experience with off-pump and patient selection has a large role to play in determining number of bypass grafts performed.

Factors Impacting Completeness of Revascularization

Surgeon Experience

Off-pump is a newer technique and issue of learning curve is an important one. It is only fair to acknowledge that off-pump requires a different skill set than on-pump bypass and that it is on the whole, a technically more demanding operation. This issue has been the main flaw of the ROOBY trial [25]. In that trial 53 surgeons performed on an average 8 off-pump cases per year in the previous 5 years. Also almost 50% percent of operations were performed by residents who have grossly unequal experience between off-pump and on-pump bypass surgery. This led to 12.5% conversion from off-pump to on-pump which is 5 times higher than that reported by STS database. This would have significant implications for completeness of revascularization.

The SMART trial investigators [24] showed that the number of grafts performed were equal between on-pump and off-pump group, likewise the index of completeness of revascularization between the groups as well as index of completeness of revascularization to the lateral wall was similar. In this study JD Puskas was the only operating surgeon and he had accumulated a personal experience in excess of 350 off-pump cases before undertaking the trial. Thus, the achievement of complete revascularization of lateral wall in unselected patients by an experienced off-pump surgeon was demonstrated.

Magee and colleagues in their study [9] did look at surgeon experience and index of completeness of revascularization. They looked at relationship between individual surgeon's practice mix of off-pump and on-pump bypass and the incidence of incomplete revascularization with each technique. They showed that the surgeons who use off-pump in greater than 25% of their CABG patients were equally likely to achieve complete revascularization regardless whether off-pump or on-pump was selected as technique. Conversely surgeons who use off-pump in fewer than 25% of their CABG patients were less likely to achieve complete revascularization in their off-pump patients compared with their on-pump patients.

Patient Selection

Impact of patient selection on completeness of revascularization was very well demonstrated by Lattouf et al. [8] and Magee et al. [9]. Lattouf and associates [8] divided patients into two categories based upon extent of revascularization: those requiring from 1-3 grafts and those requiring 4-7 bypass grafts. They demonstrated that surgeons tend to perform off-pump bypass in patients requiring 1-3 grafts than those requiring 4-7 grafts. Also some surgeons tend to perform off-pump in patients who have extensive aortic disease and peripheral vascular disease. In these patients fewer grafts is seen as less risky than using on-pump technique.

Role of Anastomotic Devices

Automated distal anastomotic devices have shown superior or equivalent short-term patency of bypass grafts [28-30]. It is easier and quicker to perform bypass to the lateral and posterior wall target vessels [28-30]. Use of these devices would reduce the learning curve of performing off-pump bypass grafts and have a positive impact on completeness of revascularization in off-pump coronary artery bypass grafting.

Conclusion

The ability to completely revascularize patients with multivessel coronary disease with off-pump CABG remains a major criticism among proponents of on-pump CABG, although the majority of evidence from randomized trials suggests equivalent completeness of revascularization. The evidence from retrospective studies in this regard may be the result of selection bias, since surgeons may choose to perform on-pump CABG on patients requiring more than three grafts. It is important that completeness of revascularization should not be compromised when deciding whether to use or avoid cardiopulmonary bypass unless the use of cardiopulmonary bypass poses obvious and significant risk for postoperative complications or mortality. At the same time, concerns regarding completeness of revascularization in off-pump CABG can be addressed through systematic training and appropriate patient selection.

REFERENCES

[1] Bell, M. R., Gersh, B. J., Schaff, H. V., et al. Effect of completeness of revascularization on long-term outcome of patients with three-vessel disease undergoing coronary bypass. A report from the Coronary Artery Surgery Study (CASS) registry. *Circulation* 1992;86:446-457.

[2] Jones, E. L., Weintraub, W. S. The importance of completeness of revascularization during long-term follow-up after coronary artery operations. *J. Thorac. Cardiovasc. Surg*. 1996;112:227-237.

[3] Vander Salm, T. J., Kip, K. E., Jones, R. H., et al. What constitutes optimal surgical revascularization? Answers from the Bypass Angioplasty Revascularization Investigation (BARI). *J. Am. Coll. Cardiol.* 2002;39:565-572.

[4] Kleisli, T., Cheng, W., Jacobs, M. J., et al. In the current era, complete revascularization improves survival after coronary artery surgery. *J. Thorac. Cardiovasc. Srug*. 2005;129:1283-1291.

[5] Synnergren, M. J., Ekroth, R., Oden, A., Rexius, H., Wiklund, L. Incomplete revascularization reduces survival benefit of Coronary artery bypass grafting: role of off-pump surgery. *J. Thorac. Cardiovasc. Surg*. 2008;136:29-36.

[6] Mohr, F. W., Rastan, A. J., Serruyus, P. W., et al. Complex coronary anatomy in coronary artery bypass graft surgery: impact of complex coronary anatomy in modern bypass surgery? Lessons learned from the SYNTAX trial after two years. *J. Thorac. Cardiovasc. Surg*. 2011;141:130-140.

[7] Lattouf, O. M., Thourani, V. H., Kilgo, P. D., et al. Influence of on-pump versus off-pump techniques and completeness of revascularization on long-term survival after coronary artery bypass. *Ann. Thorac. Surg*. 2008;86:797-805.

[8] Lattouf, O. M., Puskas, J. D., Thourani, V. H., et al. Does the number of grafts influence surgeons choice and patients benefits of off-pump over conventional on-pump coronary artery revascularization in multivessel coronary disease? *Ann. Thorac. Surg*. 2007;84:1485-1495.

[9] Magee, M. J., Hebert, E., Hebert, M. A., Prince, S. L., Dewey, T., Culica, D., and Mack, M. Fewer grafts in off-pump bypass surgery: Patient selection or incomplete revascularization? *Ann. Thorac. Surg*. 2009;87:1113-1118.

[10] Mack, M. J., Pfister, A., Bachand, D., et al. Comparison of coronary bypass surgery with and without cardiopulmonary bypass in patients with multivessel disease. *J. Thorac. Cardiovasc. Surg*. 2004;127:167-173.

[11] Arom, K. V., Flavin, T. F., Emery, R. W., et al. Safety and efficacy of off-pump coronary artery bypass grafting. *Ann. Thorac. Surg*. 2000;69:704-710.

[12] Czerny, M., Baumer, H., Kilo, J., et al. Complete revascularization in coronary artery bypass grafting with and without cardiopulmonary bypass. *Ann. Thorac. Surg*. 2001;71:165-169.

[13] Kim, K. B., Lim, C., Lee, C., et al. Off-pump coronary artery bypass may decrease the patency of saphenous vein grafts. *Ann. Thorac. Surg*. 2001;72(Suppl.):S1033-S1037.

[14] Sabik, J. F., Gillinov, A. M., Blackstone, E. H., et al. Does off-pump coronary surgery reduce morbidity and mortality? *J. Thorac. Cardiovasc. Surg*. 2002;124:698-707.

[15] Gerola, L. R., Buffolo, E., Jasbik, W., et al. Off-pump versus on-pump myocardial revascularization in low-risk patients with one or two vessel disease: perioperative results in a multicenter randomized controlled trial. *Ann. Thorac. Surg*. 2004;77:569-573.

[16] Straka, Z., Widimsky, P., Jirasek, K., et al. Off-pump versus on-pump coronary surgery: final results from a prospective randomized study PRAGUE-4. *Ann. Thorac. Surg*. 2004;77:789-793.

[17] Bucerius, J., Gummert, J. F., Walther, T., et al. Impact of off-pump coronary bypass grafting on the prevalence of adverse perioperative outcome in women undergoing coronary artery bypass grafting surgery. *Ann. Thorac. Surg*. 2005;79:807-813.

[18] Dewey, T. M., Herbert, M. A., Prince, S. L., et al. Does coronary artery bypass graft surgery improve survival among patients with end-stage renal disease? *Ann. Thorac. Surg*. 2006;81:591-598.

[19] Stamou, S. C., Hill, P. C., Haile, E., et al. Clinical outcomes of nonelective coronary revascularization with and without cardiopulmonary bypass. *J. Thorac. Cardiovasc. Surg*. 2006;131:28-33.

[20] Palmer, G., Herbert, M. A., Prince, S. L., et al. Coronary Artery Revascularization (CARE) registry: an observational study of on-pump and off-pump coronary artery revascularization. *Ann. Thorac. Surg*. 2007;83:986-992.

[21] Hannan, E. L., Wu, C., Smith, C. R., Higgins, R. S., et al. Off-pump versus on-pump coronary artery bypass graft surgery: differences in short-term outcomes and in long-term mortality and need for subsequent revascularization. *Circulation* 2007;116:1145-1152.

[22] Khan, N. E., De Souza, A., Mister, R., et al. A randomized comparison of off-pump and on-pump multivessel coronary-artery bypass surgery. *N Engl. J. Med*. 2004;350:21-28.

[23] Nathoe, H. M., Van Dijk, D., Jansen, E. W. L., et al.; Octopus Study Group. A comparison of on-pump and off-pump coronary bypass surgery in low-risk patients. *N Engl. J. Med*. 2003;348:394-402.

[24] Puskas, J. D., Williams, W. H., Duke, P. G., et al. Off-pump coronary artery bypass grafting provides complete revascularization with reduced myocardial injury, complete revascularization with reduced myocardial injury, transfusion requirements, and length of stay: A prospective randomized comparison of two hundred unselected patients undergoing off-pump versus conventional coronary artery bypass grafting. *J. Thorac. Cardiovasc. Surg*. 2003;125:797-808.

[25] Shroyer, A. L., Grover, F. L., Hattler, B., et al.; Veterans Affairs Randomized on/off bypass (ROOBY) study group. On-pump versus off-pump coronary-artery bypass surgery. *N Engl. J. Med.* 2009;361:1827-1837.

[26] Puskas, J., Cheng, D., Knight, J., et al. Off-pump versus conventional coronary artery bypass grafting: a meta-analysis and consensus statement from the 2004 ISMICS Consensus Conference. *Innovations: Technology and Techniques in Cardiothoracic and Vascular Surgery* 2005;1:3-27.

[27] Lim, E., Drain, A., Davies, W., Edmunds, L., Rosengard, B. R. A systematic review of randomized trials comparing revascularization rate and graft patency of off-pump and conventional coronary surgery. *J. Thorac. Cardiovas. Surg*. 2006;132:1409-1413.

[28] Klima, U., Falk, V., Maringka, M., et al. Magnetic vascular coupling for distal anastomosis in coronary artery bypass grafting: a multicenter trial. *J. Thorac. Cardiovasc. Surg*. 2003;126:1568-74.

[29] Carrel, T., Englberger, L., Keller, D., et al. Clinical and angiographic results after mechanical connection for distal anastomosis in coronary surgery. *J. Thorac. Cardiovasc. Surg*. 2004;127:1632-40.

[30] Kim, K. B., Cho, K. R., Choi, J. S., Ki, E. H. Initial experience of an automated anastomotic distal device in off-pump CABG. *Heart Surg. Forum*. 2004;7:E360-3.

In: Off-Pump Coronary Artery Bypass Grafting
Editors: S.G. Raja and M. Amrani
ISBN 978-1-62081-575-5

Chapter 18

LEARNING CURVE AND TRAINING IN OFF-PUMP CORONARY ARTERY BYPASS GRAFTING

Matteo Pettinari,[1] Valerie Dekoninck[2] and Paul Sergeant[3]
[1]Resident Cardiothoracic Surgery, University Hospital, Leuven, Belgium
[2]Medical Student, University Hospital, Leuven, Belgium
[3]Professor of Adult Cardiac Surgery, Consultant Cardiothoracic Surgeon, University Hospital, Leuven, Belgium

ABSTRACT

The technique of off-pump coronary artery bypass (OPCAB) surgery differs considerably from on-pump coronary artery bypass grafting (CABG). The differences in technique between conventional CABG and OPCAB demand that surgeons traverse a learning curve that includes new methods of heart and patient positioning and heart stabilization that permit adequate exposure of vessels, temporary occlusion of coronary arteries, use of intracoronary shunts, performing distal anastomoses on the stabilized heart, and possibly handling connector devices for proximal anastomoses. This chapter discusses the issues of learning curve and training in OPCAB surgery and focuses on strategies to successfully negotiate learning curve.

INTRODUCTION

The first description about learning and forgetting curves was made by Hermann Ebbinghaus in his memorable work " Über das Gedächtnis [1] " reporting the direct correlation between number of nonsense syllables and the time required for himself to memorize them. The largest gain in the learning curve is obtained at the first contact and this gain evens further down exponentially. Kjerstad [2] tested the factors or conditions defining the form of the learning curves. Arthur Bills [3] refined this into different types of learning curves: negative accelerations (convex curves), positive accelerations (concave curves), plateaus and finally ogive curves. In 1936 Theodore Paul Wright [4] reported that the unit labor costs in air-frame production declined with cumulative output. The underlying hypothesis of the Wright learning curve was that the man-hours necessary to complete a unit of production will decrease by a constant percentage each time the production quantity is doubled. This was further confirmed in different industrial production lines.

Learning curves in surgery could be measures of patient outcomes or measures of clinical process/task efficiency [5]. Outcome variables are early mortality and morbidity within an observation interval defined by hazard functions; process variables could be material and human resource consumption. Examples are the time taken and/or the number of procedures a surgeon need, to be able to perform a procedure independently with an acceptable outcome or process variable; or the graphic representation of the relationship between experience with a new procedure and an outcome or process variable.

Whatever the process involved, the effect of the experience is clearly cumulative and the improvements tend to be most rapid at first and then tail off. Therefore any learning curve should be described with three main features: the first point of the curve where the observation of the performance of an individual surgeon begins (first laparoscopic procedure for a general surgeon trainee, first skin suture for a medical student…); second the rate and the speed of learning expresses how fast a surgeon can learn a new procedure; third the asymptote that any surgeon reaches when his performance stabilizes. This chapter provides an overview of the learning curve associated with OPCAB surgery and discusses strategies to successfully negotiate the learning curve.

Definition of Learning Curve

A learning curve is the evolution of the performance in relation to the absence, presence and/or type of a learning process.

Factors Affecting Learning Curve

The determinants affecting the individual surgical learning and performance are multiple and hierarchical (Table 1). At the first level, there is the specialist community. In our domain this is the cardiac surgical and cardiological community creating knowledge in the form of manuscripts and distributing this knowledge as guidelines. The institution is the next level, impacting upon the learning curve through the availability of human and material resources. The surgical team, medical and non-medical professionals, influence positively or negatively the performance of the learning process through their knowledge, skills and attitude. Hence surgical teams need to be trained and prepared to identify and respond appropriately to any possible complication during the learning process. Patient factors such as complex anatomy and varying case-mix can affect the learning curve. As the surgeons become more experienced, there is a trend to take on more challenging cases which could affect the outcomes in an adverse manner.

Table 1. The hierarchy of influences

Level 1	The specialist community	manuscripts, guidelines
Level 2	The institution	material and human resources
Level 3	The team	knowledge, skills, attitude
Level 4	Case-mix	patient variability
Level 5	Operator characteristics	knowledge, skills, attitude and learning capacity
Level 6	Learning process	learner-centered,

The final level represents the operator characteristics involving the surgeon's attitude, capacity for acquiring new skills and natural ability such as manual dexterity. Previous experience and the type of training the surgeon received are also important. Training on inanimate trainers and animal tissue has been shown to facilitate the process of learning [6].

Other factors could be the presence of structured training schemes, mentoring and a leading authority. Learning curves depend on the frequency of procedures performed in a specified period. Many studies suggest that complication rates are inversely proportional to the volume of surgical workload. However rapidity of learning is not significantly related to the surgeon's age, size of practice or hospital setting.

Evaluation and Analysis of Learning Curves

A reliable and valid method for testing operative skills in surgical training processes is the Objective Structured Assessment of Technical Skill (OSATS) [7]. This model of testing involves direct observation of the surgeon performing a variety of structured operative tasks, during real surgery but also on live animals or bench models. A standard OSATS global rating scale is constructed of 7 categories marked on a Likert scale from 1 to 5, tied with descriptive anchors, giving a possible total of 35 marks.

Respect for tissue scores 1 for frequently used unnecessary force on tissues and or caused damage by inappropriate use of instruments. It is scored 3 if there is careful handling of tissue but occasionally caused inadvertent damage and a score of 5 when the tissues are handled consistently appropriately with minimal damage.

Time and motion scores 1 if there are many unnecessary moves, scores 3 when there is an efficient time and motion with some unnecessary moves and a 5 when there is a clear economy of movement with maximum efficiency.

Instrument handling scores 1 in the presence of repeatedly made tentative or awkward moves with instruments by inappropriate use of instruments. A score of 3 validates a competent use of instruments with an occasional stiff or awkward handling and a score of 5 for fluidity with instruments without any awkward moves.

Knowledge of instruments scores 1 when the wrong instrument is asked of for inappropriate use of an instrument. A score of 3 is reached when most instruments are known and correctly used. A score of 5 represents an obvious familiarity with instruments and their names.

Flow of the operation scores a 1 when the surgeon seems unsure about the next steps. A score of 3 is given if there is some forward planning with reasonable progression of the procedure. An effortless flow on an obviously planned pathway stands for a score of 5.

Use of assistants scores 1 if there is consistently a poor placement or use of assistants. The correct placement and use of assistants most of the time represents a 3 and an always strategically placed and used assistance is a score of 5.

Knowledge of specific procedure scores 1 if specific instructions are needed at most steps. This is upgraded to a 3 if the surgeon knows all important steps of the operation and up to 5 when familiarity with all steps of the operation is demonstrated.

Various statistical methods have been reported to assess the learning curves. Some authors proposed to split data into arbitrary groups and then compared the outcome of interest. The arbitrary division of data in sections may miss the crucial period when 'learning' occurred. More importantly, if learning occurs very early in a sequence of operations it may go undetected especially if the sequences were too long.

Direct observation by a tutor and graphical representation of the learning curve, by use of a cumulative summation (CUSUM) graph may be used to assess individual surgical performance. These qualitative methods, however, have no formal means of indicating when the required level of competence [8] has been reached. Recently a CUSUM test for learning curves (LC-CUSUM) has been proposed; this is a quantitative and individualized statistical tool that may help determine when the learning curve for a surgical procedure is complete [9].

Basic Concept of Adult Learning

To create a more efficient learning process a didactic approach based only on lectures or presentation should be avoided and a more interactive approach between teacher and scholar should be used. Interactive sessions that provide the opportunity for practice are more effective than didactic sessions. Successful adult education should be learner-centered, active rather than passive, relevant to the learner's needs, engaging and reinforcing.

An optimal surgical learning process has two consecutive phases: induced learning and operational learning. In the early English plays, the induction was the preface or the prologue. The word "induction" contains also an element of an active process, driven by influence, persuasion or reasoning. This phase is the process of acquiring a better understanding of cause-effect relationship. It could be called the "know-why". The operational learning, on the other hand, is the process of obtaining validation of action-outcome links. Operational learning is high if a team modifies its actions and observes positive follow up. A high level of operational learning yields "know-how" [10]. The drama of education is that every educational project is considered to add positively to the learning curve. Lapre has clearly identified that this is untrue. Some projects, even with the best intentions, will have no effect, positive effect or sometimes even negative effects on the learning curve. In addition since this information is imbedded in the structure and process of the educational project, the effect can be estimated even before the project is activated.

The objectives of the learning process include gaining knowledge by the digestion of information and its transformation through the process of learning. In order for this transformation to take place effectively, information must be reliable, readily accessible and able to be processed with a maximum of efficiency. Second essential prerequisite are the skills that require the development of psychomotor competencies in process based on regular practice. Third the attitude that refers to how knowledge and skill are combined in the care of patients, including clinical judgment, decision-making, the values of professional behavior and all the components of the competent clinician. The task of integrating knowledge and technical skills with these attitude components is a crucial challenge for surgical training.

To obtain these objectives, the induced learning is again divided in two consecutive phases: the conceptual learning and the virtual learning.

The first step of conceptual learning in surgical training or re-training is the theoretical study of a part or step of the surgical procedure. It is the task of the expert to deconstruct the procedure in "teachable components". Each teachable component needs to be written out and described in detail using all the possible formats of codified knowledge: text, sound, pictures, video… A possible list of the surgical components of OPCAB grafting is presented in Table 2 [11].

The presence of a detailed description of the execution of these elements, the possible problems and difficulties and the adequate solutions for the obstacles permit a structured transfer of a codified knowledge. Table 3 proposes an example of the concept of shunting. Shunting is a two to three seconds maneuver performed under different angles. The different components can change in characteristics through the years and with the accumulated experience, but the repeated update of their descriptions remains fundamental. The testing of this knowledge can be easily performed through automated assessments using learning management systems.

Table 2. Teachable components in OPCAB surgery for the surgeon

Pericardial incision and retraction
Local area stabilization of the anterior wall
Dissection coronary vessel
Shunting
Practice
Anchor stitch placement
Cardiac enucleation and its refinement
Apical suction placement
Local area stabilization of the lateral and inferior wall
Dissection of a vessel in reduced space and with vertical angle of attack
Shunting in reduced space and with vertical angle of attack
Coronary anastomosis on stabilized area but in reduced space and with vertical angle of attack
Jump graft anastomosis (arterial, venous)
Proximal anastomosis (alternative graft, aorta)

Table 3. The concept of coronary shunting

Anastomotic site (general rules)	Reachable by graft As proximal as possible Preferably no distal disease Stabilization possible Place a 4-0 Prolene proximally of the incision site
Anastomotic site (shunting rules)	No proximal disease within 2 cm No proximal side-branching within 2 cm No distal side-branching within 2 cm Preferably a straight vessel
Shunt selection	Appropriate size (leakage, flow, disease) Appropriate brand (tortuosity)
Interface with anesthesia before incision	
Vessel incision	Incise vessel Close the proximal ligature Extend the incision in both directions with Potts or Dietrich scissors
General evaluation	Evaluate that the shunt is indeed in the coronary vessel in both directions by visualizing the epithelial borders Evaluate leakage and if needed change to an appropriate shunt Evaluate distal flow and myocardial contractility Evaluate side branches for flow and myocardial contractility
Interface with anesthesia	That shunt is in place and that continued monitoring is mandatory

SIMULATION

The current method of surgical training is predicated on the apprenticeship model introduced by Halsted at Johns Hopkins over a century ago, after a visit of surgical training units in Germany. Teaching of surgical skills takes place mostly in the operating theatre and on live patients. There are a number of threats and limitations to this style of surgical training with the evolving patterns of the surgical practice. These include working-hour restrictions for medical professionals, an increasing complexity of cases at surgical teaching centers and the ethical concerns for patient's safety. These factors have contributed to fewer opportunities to learn surgical procedures in the operating theatre on live patients. These challenges have stimulated the pursuit of novel techniques for teaching trainees outside the operating theatre. Simulation provides the learner with an opportunity for repetitive and deliberate practice of procedural skills in a low-consequence environment. The utility of simulation in surgical training is gaining widespread recognition; there is increasing literature demonstrating the benefit of deliberate practice of skills in a simulated environment on performance of specific surgical tasks in numerous subspecialties [12,13]. Despite this evidence, the use of simulation in cardiovascular surgery remains relatively limited.

Several simulation models have been proposed recently in training and research. Most of them were high fidelity cadaver or animal models with limited availability, high costs and with zero reusability.

Low fidelity models, based on low fidelity reconstruction of the surgical environment have been applied in several teaching centers. These models are reusable, low cost, safe, portable with a maximal availability and with the possibility to deconstruct the learning process in teachable components [14]. These models are used to practice not only the anastomotic technique but also the insertion of the coronary shunts, the two fundamental elements in off-pump coronary surgery. The low-fidelity model used at the OPCAB training center at the University hospital Leuven is presented in the Figure 1.

This model simulates two major steps in OPCAB surgery: shunt insertion and coronary anastomoses. In addition it allows simulation in different angles with/without a reduction (gradual) of the airspace above the anastomotic zone as in surgical reality.

The OPCAB training with simulation models follows a written down pathway with structured steps that need to be achieved before a next step should be started. The trainee starts working on his lumbar posture and the position of his elbow and forearm. He then learns to support his hand with a soft tissue so that the relation hand-forearm remains relaxed and stable without any pronation, supination, ante-flexion or dorsi-flexion. The Castro-Viejo needle-holder is positioned in the hand so that the first and second fingers remain parallel to the needle-holder. The trainee will now learn to rotate the needle-holder without lifting the hand from the support and without moving the tip of the needle-holder in a three-dimensional space. Next he learns to move the needle-holder backwards and forwards, again without lifting the hand and without moving the axis of the needle-holder. This manoeuver is repeated and practiced over and over again.

In a following phase the needle is held in a half-opened needle-holder. This needle is now moved and rotated by pushing with a closed forceps to obtain every possible angle of the needle versus the needle-holder.

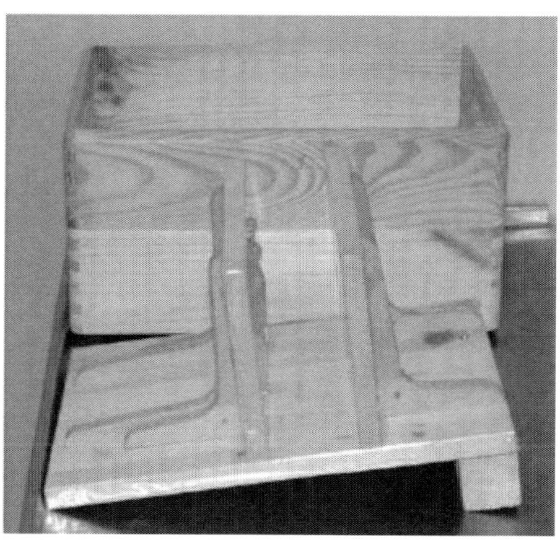

Figure 1. The "Training box" of the OPCAB training center at the University Hospital Leuven.

This maneuver is learned without moving the axis of the needle-holder and without lifting the hand. The hand holding the closed forceps is similarly supported and relaxed. It should also not move from its support.

Once these skills are mastered, the trainee starts with anastomoses, first on a horizontal plane, then on a vertical plane. In this last plane, the angle of vision on the anastomotic site is less than 20°. Gradually the airspace above the anastomotic site is then reduced to 5 cm and later to 2 cm. Shunt insertion (Figure 2) is trained in a similar stepwise fashion. The total number of shunt insertions and anastomoses performed in a simulation environment exceeds 1000 for each process.

The trainer supervises all the phases of the training on the simulator. A strict supervision and control of the use of the forceps and Castro-Viejo needle holder, spacing and needle transfer are mandatory. The K.U.Leuven school uses the FANN OSATS for the simulation training and the PAR matrix [15] for the real procedures.

Several groups have already demonstrated the validity of the simulation laboratory training in coronary anastomosis. Price demonstrated [16] that a period of 2 weeks of deliberate practice on simulators increases the OSATS score and the flow of the procedure, the time and motion of the execution, the use of assistance, the spacing of the sutures and the quality of the anastomosis.

Fann registered a 20% reduction in anastomoses completion times from 351 to 281 seconds, after 1 week of practice in portable task stations to practice end-to-side anastomosis. This improvement was also confirmed in a beating-heart anastomosis model, with a reduction from 426 to 362 seconds.

RESULTS OF TRAINING AND RE-TRAINING IN OPCAB

The unique technical challenges of OPCAB grafting have raised concern that adoption of OPCAB may lead to poorer outcomes during each surgeon's learning curve. Some units have taken a years-long and gradual approach to implementing this new technology by gradually expanding the patient-spectrum and surgeons; other teams have used retraining and guidance by expert centers to accelerate this. Studies have focused on outcome obtained from the re-training process of experienced surgeons and other on the training of surgical residents.

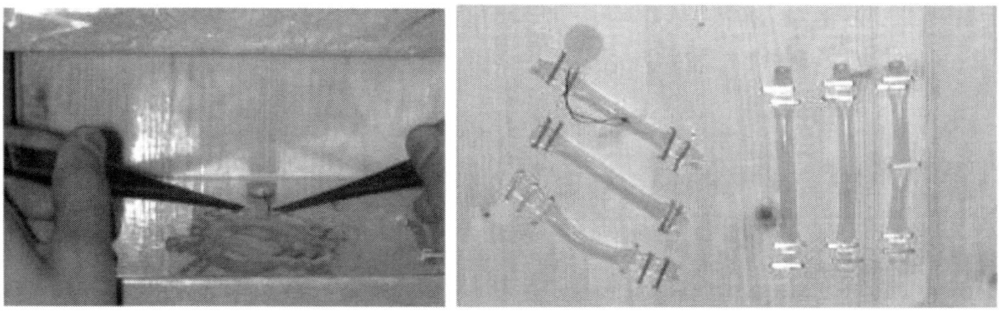

Figure 2. Simulation model for the coronary shunt insertion.

After the re-engineering and re-training process in our unit the propensity towards OPCAB changed abruptly; after October 1999 till January 1st 2003 it was 93.4%, reaching even above 98% in 2000 and 2001. In a consecutive unselected series of 3333 CABG patients operated between January 1997 and January 2003 we studied early morbidity and mortality [17]. Comparing a non risk adjusted dataset of 1593 patients treated on-pump and 1740 treated off-pump we registered a 20% reduction of mortality, 60% reduction of stroke and 20% reduction of dialysis. These differences did not reach a statistical significance, showing the difficulties to demonstrate clinical evidence in favor of one technique with respect to the other. The interactions between risk, number of patients and the risk-reducing effect are still a crucial factor in generating evidence of the superiority of OPCAB, demanding for large dataset and sophisticated statistical instrument.

During the re-engineering process we created CUSUM charts for real-time monitoring of the 30 days mortality, based on a database updated daily. These charts (data not published) indicated the progressive positive OPCAB performance, compared with the EuroSCORE reference (Figure 3). The continuous number of lives saved shows the OPCAB benefit in risk reduction versus the on-pump technique.

Albert [18] assessed the shift to OPCAB using a similar protocol and re-engineering process. The change from conventional CABG to OPCAB was effective in decreasing the incidence and severity of stroke, but this difference lost statistical significance after correction for propensity and event related variation. Again the analysis was not statistically powered to identify a mortality difference for these periods of time and this bias has probably decreased the possibility to detect significant differences.

After the re-engineering process at the University Hospital Leuven, since 2000 we started a Continuing Medical Education of Surgical Technologies program (CMEST). During the last decade more than 450 teams of surgeon and anesthesiologist from 58 countries have visited our center for annual 2 days seminar.

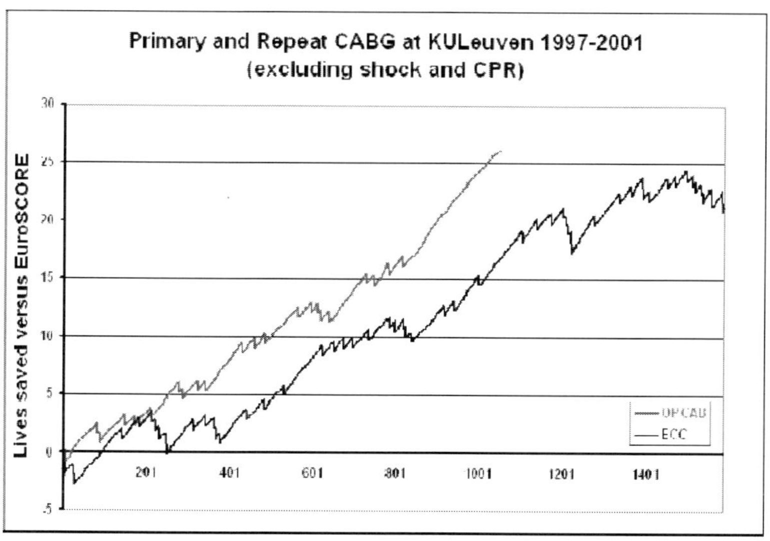

Figure 3. CUSUM chart of primary and repeated CABG (OPCAB and on-pump) between 1997 and 2001 at the University Hospital Leuven.

We evaluate the performance of this re-training program examining the attitude towards OPCAB at the end of the seminar and then three months after the seminar [19]. A second parameter we analyzed was the OPCAB application rate after three months following the seminar. By means of three questionnaires, 50 teams from February through November 2004 were investigated. The OPCAB attitude at exit and at three months was influenced by the training (P <.001, versus at entry); OPCAB was considered beneficial for all patients by 90%, for the low-risk patients only by 2%, and for the high-risk patients only by 6% of the teams, and 2% were uncertain. The OPCAB application rate of the surgeons increased by about 26% (absolute increase) or 110% (relative increase) 3 months after the OPCAB retraining (49% ± 32% versus 23% ± 28% pre-visit; P <.0001). The surgeons were asked to define an OPCAB complexity score, that identifies 10 anatomic and physiologic conditions commonly considered complexity variables for OPCAB. These included redo operation, the presence of left main disease, severe left ventricular hypertrophy, low ejection fraction, intramural or intraseptal coronary vessels, posterolateral wall coronary vessels, sequential arterial grafts, recent infarct (within 7 days), and an unstable ST segment. The total number of positive responses was calculated as "complexity score". The OPCAB complexity score at exit from the seminar was 1.24 ± 1, strongly reduced (P <.001, mean difference –2.4) versus at entry. The OPCAB complexity variables most frequently cited at exit and at three months were intraseptal vessels and intramural vessels. The inferolateral and posterolateral location of coronary anastomoses (10 teams at entry), as well as the sequential arterial grafting (9 teams at entry) and low ejection fraction (16 teams at entry), disappeared from the list at exit and at three months follow up. The multimodal OPCAB re-training resulted in a substantial increase in the application, concomitant with the positive impact on attitude and complexity score.

The group in Bristol was one of the first to publish the results of OPCAB performed by trainees under supervision [20]. Of the 559 operations performed between January 1997 and May 2000, 124 (22%) were carried out by a supervised trainee and 435 by a consultant. In the consultant group more patients had past and recent history of congestive heart failures requiring medical therapy, significantly lower ejection fractions, and higher Parsonnet scores compared with patients operated on by trainees. The average number of grafts and the coronary anatomical distribution was similar in the two groups. Also the rate of stroke, myocardial infarction reoperation for bleeding and respiratory failure did not differ. In both groups there was a significant decrease in the angina class compared to the preoperative status (p = 0.001). No differences were observed in survival or in the incidence of cardiac events in both groups.

The same group demonstrated that the results in term of mortality and morbidity remained unvaried also when the trainees performed the procedure alone without the supervision of the consultant [21].

Caputo in 2004, comparing 474 patients operated by residents and 293 by consultants, reported a similar or better performance of the residents compared with the consultants. Paradoxically the patients operated on by residents tended to be older, more obese, more likely to require urgent operation. In this series also the conversion rate were not significantly different [22].

The effectiveness of OPCAB performed by trainees was also tested in high risk patients [23]. Patients satisfying at least one of the following criteria were classified as high-risk: age older than 75 years, ejection fraction less than 0.30, myocardial infarction in the previous month, current congestive heart failure, previous cerebrovascular accident, creatinine greater than 150 μmol/L, respiratory impairment, peripheral vascular disease, previous cardiac surgery, and left main stem stenosis greater than 50%. Kaplan-Meier cumulative mortality estimates at 24-month follow-up were 10.5% and 6.4% in consultant and trainee groups, respectively (p=0.05), confirming that off-pump coronary artery bypass grafting surgery in high-risk patients can be safely performed by trainees.

Also when the residents performed more technically demanding surgery as minimally invasive access, bilateral mammary artery, "y" graft construction, postoperative outcomes were similar compared to the senior surgeons [23].

Conclusion

The knowledge transfer of OPCAB technology is a complicated and sophisticated process. Only an individualized cognitive approach, based on labor-intensive and interactive discussions, team participation, repeated observations, and hands-on practices, can affect the application of this technology. If this process is conducted by committed and expert training centers the impeding factors can be reduced and a positive effect of the learning process can be achieved.

References

[1] Ebbinghaus, H. Über das Gedächtnis. Untersuchungen zur experimentellen Psychologie. Leipzig: Duncker and Humblot 1885.

[2] Kjerstad, C. The form of the learning curves, *Psychological Monographs: general and applied* 1919;26:1-89

[3] Bills, A. General experimental psychology. *Longmans Psychology Series.* Longmans, Green and Co 1934

[4] Wright, T. Factors affecting the cost of airplanes. *Journal of Aeronautical Sciences* 1936;3:122-128

[5] Ramsay, C., Grant, A., Garthwaite, P., Mon, R. I., Assessment of the learning curve in health technologies, a systematic review. *Int. J. Technol. Assess. Health Care* 2000;16:1095-108

[6] Traxer, O., Gettman, M. T., Napper, C. A., et al. The impact of intense laparoscopic skills training on the operative performance of urology residents. *J. Urol.* 2001;166:1658-61

[7] Martin, J. A., Regehr, G., Reznick, R., et al. Objective structured assessment of technical skill (OSATS) for surgical residents. *Br. J. Surg.* 1997;84:273-8.

[8] De Leval, M. R., Francois, K., Bull, C., Brawn, W., Spiegelhalter, D. Analysis of a cluster of surgical failures. Application to a series of neonatal arterial switch operations. *J. Thorac. Cardiovasc. Surg.* 1994;107:914-23.

[9] Biau, D. J., Williams, S. M., Schlup, M. M., Nizard, R. S., Porcher, R. Quantitative and individualized assessment of the learning curve using LC-CUSUM. *Br. J. Surg.* 2008;95:925-9.

[10] Lapre, M. A., Van Wassenhove, L. N. Managing learning curves in factories by creating and transferring knowledge. *California Management Review* 2003;46:53-71.

[11] Davis, D., O'Brien, M. A., Freemantle, N., Wolf, F. M., Mazmanian, P., Taylor-Vaisey, A. Impact of formal continuing medical education: do conferences, workshops, rounds, and other traditional continuing education activities change physician behavior or health care outcomes? *JAMA* 1999;282:867-74.

[12] Pandey, V. A., Black, S. A., Lazaris, A. M., et al. Do workshops improve the technical skill of vascular surgical trainees? *Eur. J. Vasc. Endovasc. Surg*. 2005;30:441-7.

[13] Grober, E. D., Hamstra, S. J., Wanzel, K. R., et al. The educational impact of bench model fidelity on the acquisition of technical skill: the use of clinically relevant outcome measures. *Ann. Surg*. 2004;240:374-81.

[14] Fann, J. I., Caffarelli, A. D., Georgette, G., Howard, S. K., Gaba, D. M., Youngblood, P., Mitchell, R. S., Burdon, T. A. Improvement in coronary anastomosis with cardiac surgery simulation. *J. Thorac. Cardiovasc. Surg*. 2008;136:1486-91.

[15] Papaspyros, S. C., Javangula, K. C., O'Regan, D. J. Surgical training in the 48-h week: a novel simulation and educational tool. From amateur golfer to professional pilot. *Eur. J. Cardiothorac. Surg*. 2009;36:511-5.

[16] Price, J., Naik, V., Boodhwani, M., Brandys, T., Hendry, P., Lam, B.-K. A randomized evaluation of simulation training on performance of vascular anastomosis on a high-fidelity in vivo model: The role of deliberate practice. *J. Thorac. Cardiovasc. Surg*. 2011;142:496-503.

[17] Sergeant, P., Wouters, P., Meyns, B., et al. OPCAB versus early mortality and morbidity: an issue between clinical relevance and statistical significance. *Eur. J. Cardiothorac. Surg*. 2004;25:779-85.

[18] Albert, A., Sergeant, P., Florath, I., Ismael, M., Rosendahl, U., Ennker, J. Process review of a departmental change from conventional coronary artery bypass grafting to totally arterial coronary artery bypass and its effects on the incidence and severity of postoperative stroke. *Heart Surg. Forum*. 2011;14: E73-80.

[19] Albert, A., Peck, E. A., et al. Performance analysis of interactive multimodal CME retraining on attitude toward and application of OPCAB. *J. Thorac. Cardiovasc. Surg*. 2006;131:154-162.

[20] Caputo, M., Chamberlain, M. H., Ozalp, F., Underwood, M. J., Ciulli, F., Angelini, G. D. *Ann. Thorac. Surg*. 2001;71:1215-9.

[21] Caputo, M., Bryan, A. J., Capoun, R., et al. The evolution of training in off-pump coronary surgery in a single institution. *Ann. Thorac. Surg*. 2002;74:S1403-7.

[22] Caputo, M., Reeves, B. C., Rogers, C. A., Ascione, R., Angelini, G. D. Monitoring the performance of residents during training in off-pump coronary surgery. *J. Thorac. Cardiovasc. Surg*. 2004;128:907-15.

[23] Ascione, R., Reeves, B. C., Pano, M., Angelini, G. D. Trainees operating on high-risk patients without cardiopulmonary bypass: a high-risk strategy? *Ann. Thorac. Surg*. 2004;78:26-33.

In: Off-Pump Coronary Artery Bypass Grafting
Editors: S.G. Raja and M. Amrani
ISBN 978-1-62081-575-5

Chapter 19

HYPERCOAGULABLE STATE AFTER OFF-PUMP CORONARY ARTERY BYPASS GRAFTING

***Shahzad G. Raja*[1] *and Robert S. Poston*[2]**
[1]Cardiac Surgeon, Harefield Hospital, London, UK
[2]Chief Division of Cardiothoracic Surgery,
Jack G. Copeland Endowed Chair of Cardiovascular Surgery,
Michael Drummond Distinguished Professor of Cardiovascular and Thoracic Surgery,
University of Arizona, Tucson, AZ, US

ABSTRACT

During the past decade, there has been a dramatic resurgence in the adoption of off-pump technology in coronary artery bypass surgery. This has inspired remarkable advances in the techniques of localized tissue stabilization and a greater understanding of the physiology of beating heart mobilization and exposure. An avalanche of reports in the literature has demonstrated the early safety and efficacy of the procedure. However, despite abundant evidence validating safety and efficacy of off-pump coronary artery bypass surgery considerable controversy still persists regarding the long-term outcomes of this approach to myocardial revascularization. One area of concern, and even greater uncertainty, surrounds the issue of the existence of a hypercoagulable state after off-pump coronary artery bypass surgery. This chapter provides an overview of the impact of off-pump coronary artery bypass surgery on coagulation, fibrinolysis and platelet activation, discusses the issue of hypercoagulability with emphasis on the mechanisms responsible for this actual or potential hypercoagulability and explores the implications of this issue for clinical practice.

INTRODUCTION

In an attempt to prevent cardiopulmonary bypass (CPB)-related morbidity and end-organ dysfunction during surgical myocardial revascularization, off-pump coronary artery bypass (OPCAB), a revascularization technique that does not require CPB, has seen resurgence in the last decade or so. OPCAB, first introduced in the late 1960s [1], has recently become more popular. Proponents of OPCAB argue that all surgical myocardial revascularizations should be performed without the use of CPB. However, skepticism regarding the technical difficulty of OPCAB and concerns that incompleteness of revascularization with this strategy compromises patient outcomes has prevented OPCAB from being universally adopted [2]. As a result, numerous studies have been performed in an effort to address these issues.

Evidence in the form of randomized controlled trials (RCTs) [3-6], meta-analyses [7-12], systematic reviews [13-15], and non-randomized observational studies [16,17] shows that compared to conventional surgical myocardial revascularization on CPB, OPCAB is associated with similar completeness of revascularization, similar early outcomes, shorter length of hospital stay, reduced transfusion requirements, reduced pulmonary morbidity, and fewer postoperative neurologic events.

Despite abundant evidence validating safety and efficacy of OPCAB, one area of concern, and even greater uncertainty, surrounds the issue of the existence of a hypercoagulable state after OPCAB that potentially can endanger the patency of coronary anastomoses [18]. This chapter discusses in detail the controversial issue of presence of hypercoagulable state after OPCAB and its clinical implications.

Current Evidence Regarding Hemostasis Preserving Effect of OPCAB

A systematic search for current best evidence on the topic retrieved eleven manuscripts comparing the impact of on-pump and off-pump coronary artery bypass grafting on preservation of hemostasis [19-29] (Figure 1). All of these were RCTs (Table 1). Majority of the studies [19,21-24,27-29] showed that on-pump CABG caused earlier and more significant generation of thrombin, however OPCAB caused a late and sustained generation of thrombin. On-pump CABG caused intraoperative activation of fibrinolysis and fibrin degradation, however, at 24h these parameters were equally elevated in both groups. More importantly, early postoperative decrease in platelet count and increase in platelet activation occurs to a much lesser extent and does not alter bleeding time or adenosine diphosphate-induced platelet aggregation in patients undergoing OPCAB. This lack of significant effects on platelets might in part account for the potential decreased risk in bleeding and for the preserved hemostasis seen in patients undergoing OPCAB compared with those undergoing on-pump CABG.

Interestingly, the RCT by Paulitsch et al. [20] contrary to other RCTs concluded that on-pump CABG was associated with biochemical evidence of a prothrombotic state early after surgery but no greater incidence of thrombotic events was observed. They assigned patients prospectively and randomly to either on-pump ($n = 41$) or off-pump ($n = 51$). The concentrations of C-reactive protein, fibrinogen, D-dimer, and plasminogen activator inhibitor type-1 in blood were quantified before and after (1 and 24 h) surgery. Clinical events were assessed during initial hospitalization and at the end of 1 year. The results of this RCT showed that the concentrations of plasminogen activator inhibitor type-1 and D-dimer were greater compared with preoperative values 1 and 24 h after surgery in both groups, but their concentrations increased to a greater extent 24 h after surgery in the on-pump group ($P<0.01$). The concentration of C-reactive protein did not change appreciably immediately after surgery in either group but increased in a parallel manner 24 h after either on-pump or off-pump surgery ($P<0.01$). Bypass surgery in the on-pump group was associated with greater blood loss during surgery and more bleeding after surgery ($P<=0.01$). The incidence of all other complications was similar in the two groups. According to the authors the prothrombotic state might be a consequence of extracorporeal bypass, compensation in response to more bleeding, or both in patients undergoing on-pump surgery.

It is important to stress that all of the RCTs comparing impact of OPCAB and on-pump CABG on activation of coagulation system have several limitations. The number of patients is rather small, so these should be considered more as pilot investigations to direct the most appropriate analyses of coagulation variables in a larger cohort. Because the small sample size precludes excluding Type II error, small differences between groups at certain time points could have been missed.

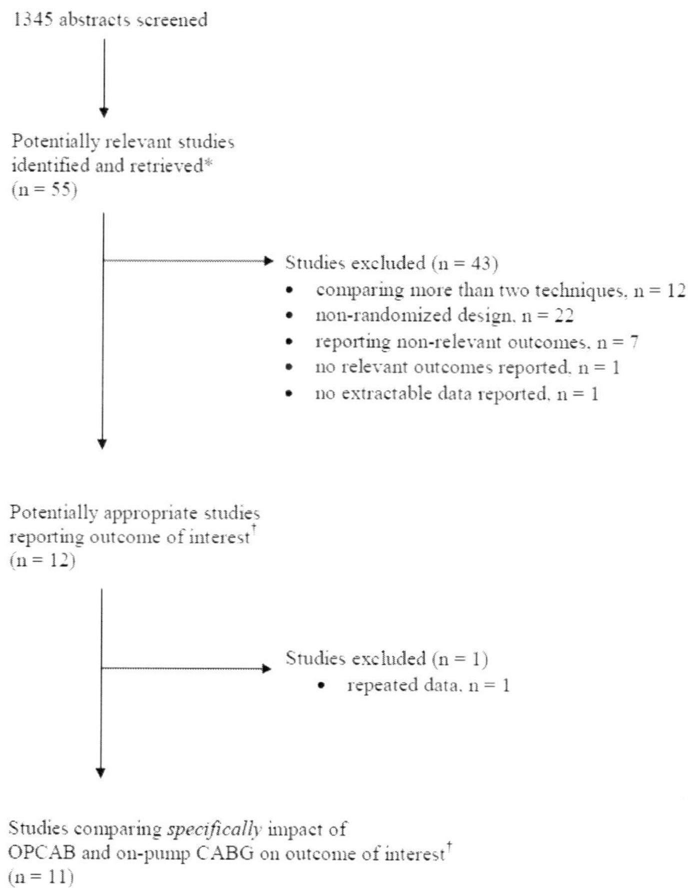

*Randomized controlled trials.
CABG = coronary artery bypass grafting; OPCAB = off-pump coronary artery bypass.
†Coagulation, hemostasis, fibrinolysis or platelet activation.

Figure 1. Identification of eligible studies.

In addition, the number of sampling periods is limited, so only data from these predefined sampling periods can be supplied; therefore, hemostatic abnormalities at other time points after CABG could have been missed. Second, a number of additional factors associated with the on-pump procedure that could have influenced the results varied between the RCTs. These include 1) use of dexamethasone (to mitigate the systemic inflammatory response), 2) use of moderate hypothermia, 3) use of cardioplegia to arrest the heart, and 4) use of different anticoagulation strategies (target activated coagulation time [ACT] >450 vs 250 seconds). Furthermore, several trials used a fixed protamine dosage for heparin reversal. Because ACT may be influenced by other factors, such as hypothermia and hemodilution, it may not accurately reflect the extent of anticoagulation by heparin [30]. This could have led to relative protamine overdose and therefore might have influenced the results in the immediate postoperative period [30].

MECHANISMS OF HYPERCOAGULABILITY AFTER OPCAB

Thrombocytopenia has been well documented in patients undergoing on-pump surgery and has been attributed to many factors, including hemodilution, mechanical disruption, adhesion to the extracorporeal circuit, and sequestration in organs [31]. Additionally, platelet dysfunction has also been shown to occur during on-pump surgery, resulting both in the prolongation of the bleeding time and the decrease in ADP-induced platelet aggregation. Similarly, enhanced platelet activation after use of CPB is a recognized phenomenon [32]. Although there is a lack of consensus as to the pathophysiology of platelet activation, many potential explanations have been entertained. Notable among these are exposure to synthetic material of the extracorporeal circuits, generation of thrombin, and use of heparin and protamine [33-35]. These decreases in platelet counts and abnormalities of platelet function and activity have been implicated by many in the bleeding complications in the postoperative period [36,37]. The fact that these changes are less pronounced in the OPCAB patients compared with on-pump patients could partly explain the relatively "preserved hemostasis" in the former group compared with the latter cohort.

Another plausible mechanism by which OPCAB may induce hypercoagulability is via the obligatory periods of regional warm ischemia that accompany the distal anastomoses. Animal models have demonstrated an induction of thrombin production during periods of warm ischemia as little as 15 minutes [38,39]. Kon et al. in their pilot study, using transcardiac assays, illustrated that regional coagulation was enhanced after off- compared with on-pump CABG [40].

It is also important to highlight that there are temporal differences in the activation of coagulation as seen after on-pump CABG and OPCAB. In fact two discrete phases can be distinguished: an early phase, occurring only after on-pump CABG, characterized by a sharp activation of coagulation and fibrinolysis, which may be ascribable to the use of extracorporeal circulation; and a later phase, occurring in patients undergoing either on-pump CABG or OPCAB, probably consequent to an inflammatory reaction induced by general surgical trauma [26].

Table 1. Impact of off-pump coronary artery bypass surgery on coagulation, fibrinolysis and platelet activation

Author Year	Study type Level of Evidence	No of patients OPCAB	 CABG	Outcomes	Key result	Hypercoagulable state OPCAB	 CABG	Ref.
Vallely et al. 2009	RCT (Level 1b)	10	10	Tissue factor pathway-factor VIIa, von Willebrand Factor antigen, prothrombin fragments FI+II, D-Dimer, platelet counts and soluble P-selectin quantified upto 24 hrs post-operatively	Late thrombin generation, reduced fibrinolysis and intact functioning platelets after OPCAB	Yes	No	[19]
Paulitsch et al. 2009	RCT (level 1b)	51	41	CRP, fibrinogen, D-Dimer and plasminogen activator inhibitor type-1 quantified before (1 hr) and after (24 hr) surgery Clinical events assessed during initial hospitalization and after 1 yr	Significantly greater increase in plasminogen activator inhibitor type-1and D-dimer concentrations after CABG ($P < 0.01$) No greater incidence of thrombotic events	No	Yes	[20]
Bednar et al. 2008	RCT (level 1b)	40	40	Platelet activity assessed by P selectin expression Aspirin efficacy assessed by AA-induced platelet aggregation before operation, immediately after surgery, on days 1, 2, 5 and 30	Markedly increased P-selectin expression in OPCAB group on day 2and day 5 Similar P-selectin expression at day 30 AA-induced platelet aggregation increased in OPCAB group on day 2	Yes	No	[21]
Jares et al. 2007	RCT (level 1b)	10	10	roTEG results obtained pre-op, at15 min after sternotomy, completion of anastomoses and at the end of surgey D-dimer levels before operation, at the end of surgeryand 24 hrs later	Slightly greater activation of fibrinolysis after CABG	Yes	No	[22]

Table 1. (Continued)

Author	Study type	No of patients		Outcomes	Key result	Hypercoagulable state		Ref.
Year	Level of Evidence	OPCAB	CABG			OPCAB	CABG	
Ballotta et al. 2007	RCT (level 1b)	30	30	Platelet count and function assessed2 hr before and after surgery	Significant decrease in platelet count and increase in platelet activation after CABG	Yes	No	[23]
Paparella et al. 2006	RCT (level 1b)	16	16	Activation of coagulation and fibrinolysis and platelet function assessed at 7 times up to day 6 post-operatively	Normally functioning plateletsand weak activation of fibrinolytic sytem	Yes	No	[24]
Parolari et al. 2005	RCT (level 1b)	15	15	Plasma, monocyte-bound and platelet-bound tissue factor expression Platelet and soluble P-selectin expression assessed before surgery, after protamine administration and 4, 8 and 30 days after surgery	Similar tissue factor and P-selectin expression after CABG and OPCAB	Yes	Yes	[25]
Parolari et al. 2005	RCT (level 1b)	17	18	Prothrombin fragment F1.2, thrombin-antitrombin complex, D-dimer, vWF and VCAM1 levels measured before surgeryand 1 month after surgery	Similar rise in markers of activation of coagulation, fibrinolysis and endothelium after CABG and OPCAB	Yes	Yes	[26]
Vedin et el. 2005	RCT (level 1b)	17	14	Fibrin D-dimer, prothrombin fragment 1.2, α-2macroglobulin, protein C1 esterase inhibitor, fibronectin and vWF levels assessed up to 24 hrs after surgery	Less activation of fibrinolysisand coagulation after OPCAB	Yes	No	[27]

Author Year	Study type Level of Evidence	No of patients OPCAB	CABG	Outcomes	Key result	Hypercoagulable state OPCAB	CABG	Ref.
Lo et al. 2004	RCT (level 1b)	20	20	Platelet count, fibrin D-dimer, prothrombin fragment 1.2, soluble fibrin, P-selectin and vWF levels measured up to day 4 after surgery	OPCAB group had delayed activation of hemostasis and it became equivalent to CABG group in the later post-operative period (20-96 hrs)	Yes	No	[28]
Møller et al. 2003	RCT (level 1b)	15	15	Platelet function assessed pre-op, immediate post-op, 4 hr post-op and1 day postop	Significant increase in PAF-induced platelet aggregation after OPCAB compared to CABG	Yes	No	[29]

AA = arachidonic acid; CABG = on-pump coronary artery bypass grafting; CRP = C-reactive protein; OPCAB = off-pump coronary artery bypass; PAF = platelet activating factor; RCT = Randomized controlled trial; roTEG = rotation thromboelastography; VCAM = vascular cell adhesion molecule; vWF = von Willebrand factor.

Clinical Implications

Traditional on-pump CABG has established a low incidence of postoperative thrombotic events [41] that is believed to be mediated in part by the anticoagulating effect of CPB [42]. By circumventing CPB, OPCAB is widely believed to be associated with a "hypercoagulable state" akin to that described after general surgical procedures [43]. Current best available evidence from RCTs confirms that there is a tendency towards decreased activation of both coagulation and fibrinolysis with less pronounced changes in platelet counts and function after OPCAB resulting in a procoagulant state.

It important to mention that there is no consensus amongst various researchers regarding a definition for this "hypercoagulable state". Whether activation of enzymatic component of the coagulation cascade or platelet hyperactivity is synonymous with postoperative "hypercoagulable state" remains unclear at present. One could argue that perhaps a more suitable definition for this hypercoagulability could be based on an endpoint of early failure of the coronary artery bypass graft. However, as graft patency is dependent upon multiple factors a better definition for "hypercoagulability" could perhaps be achieved by performing simple functional tests such as thromboelastography (TEG) or aggregometry which are cost-effective and can be easily performed and interpreted.

Interestingly, despite the preservation of hemostasis and procoagulant state after OPCAB correlation between this procoagulant and clinical outcome (namely graft patency) is still a matter of debate. Vein graft failure remains a major problem after CABG. Occlusion in the first weeks is secondary to thrombosis, whereas intimal hyperplasia and eventually atherosclerotic changes with superimposed thrombus formation underlie subsequent closure [24]. There are several possible explanations for the poorer graft performance in patients operated on by the off-pump technique: the poorer coronary vessel exposure, heart movement, poor coronary visualization provoked by bleeding, all render the distal anastomosis more difficult to perform and sometimes less accurate than those made with the heart arrested. The tools used during the anastomoses (intracoronary shunts, coronary occluding stitch, carbon dioxide blower) to improve visualization may all potentially damage the coronary and graft endothelium [44].

To date, none of the RCTs has shown a correlation between procaoagulant state and early graft occlusion. This could be attributed to variable sampling periods in these RCTs with none of the trials powered or designed to detect impact of procoagulant state on thrombotic events.

Another important issue that stems from the presence of procoagulant state after OPCAB and merits further research is the perioperative anticoagulation policy for patients undergoing OPCAB. It is important to highlight that the postoperative anticoagulation treatment may differ quite significantly between off- and on-pump patients. It is uncertain at present whether for OPCAB patients the perioperative anticoagulation should be more aggressive than that for patients undergoing conventional on-pump CABG. Furthermore, the suitable dose of heparin administered intraoperatively and the need to antagonize the heparin with protamine at the end of the procedure are potential avenues for further research.

There is evidence to suggest that there is a significant increase in platelet resistance to aspirin effect in off-pump patients with early graft thrombosis [45]. The presence of hypercoagulability after OPCAB along with aspirin resistance in the early postoperative period is extremely risky for early graft failure because of thrombosis. There arises a question whether modification or intensification of the dose regimen of aspirin or different anti-platelet strategies after off-pump and on-pump bypass surgery could lead to a more effective inhibition of platelet aggregation with a minimum influence on postoperative bleeding and thus possibly improved clinical outcomes.

Antiplatelet therapy has been shown to improve vein graft patency [46]. Study by Chesebro et al. [47] demonstrated that the combination of dipyridamol and aspirin was effective. More agressive antiplatelet therapy, including clopidogrel, could potentially increase graft patency similar to the effect on intracoronary stents. The American College of Chest Physicians (ACCP) seventh conference on antithrombotic and thrombolytic therapy published their guidelines in 2004 [48]. For patients who undergo CABG for non-ST segment elevation acute coronary syndrome (ACS), they recommend that clopidogrel should be started in addition to aspirin post-surgery and continued for 9–12 months. This recommendation is based on the Clopidogrel versus Aspirin in Patients at Risk of Ischemic Events (CAPRIE) study [49] and the Clopidogrel in Unstable angina to prevent Recurrent Events (CURE) study [50].

The CAPRIE study reported an 8.7% relative risk reduction in the primary composite endpoint (first occurrence of ischaemic stroke, myocardial infarction or vascular death) in favour of clopidogrel (75 mg/day) over aspirin (325 mg/day) in a multicentre RCT of 19,185 patients with a history of recent ischaemic stroke, recent myocardial infarction or symptomatic peripheral arterial disease [49]. A sub-analysis of the CAPRIE database showed that in 1480 patients with a previous history of cardiac surgery, clopidogrel was associated with a relative risk reduction of 39% for vascular death, 38% for myocardial infarction, 25% for all-cause rehospitalization, and 27% for rehospitalization for ischemia or bleeding. A major drawback of this study is the lack of information about the type of cardiac surgery previously performed in these patients.

The CURE trial randomized patients with acute coronary syndromes (n = 12,562) to treatment with clopidogrel (300 mg then 75 mg/day) or placebo in addition to aspirin (75–325 mg/day). The antiplatelet combination resulted in a 20% risk reduction relative to aspirin alone (9.3% vs. 11.4%, $p < 0.001$) in the primary endpoint of cardiovascular death, myocardial infarction or stroke over a mean nine-month treatment period [50]. The antiplatelet combination produced a 19.0% reduction relative to aspirin alone in the risk of cardiovascular death, myocardial infarction or stroke among those patients who underwent CABG surgery during the initial hospitalisation and an 11.0% relative risk reduction among patients who underwent CABG surgery at any time during the treatment period. The clinical benefits of aspirin plus clopidogrel were mainly evident during the preoperative period with 18% relative risk reductions in the primary endpoint seen before CABG surgery compared to 3% relative risk reduction following CABG surgery relative to aspirin alone [51]. The main pitfall of the study is that patients who did not take the drug after surgery were still included in the clopidogrel group and the effect of clopidogrel was not adjusted for other risk factors.

The Clopidogrel for the Reduction of Events During Observation (CREDO) trial evaluated the short-term benefits of combined aspirin and clopidogrel pre-treatment and the long-term benefits of sustained therapy in the setting of percutaneous coronary intervention (PCI) in an RCT of 2116 patients. After one year of treatment, patients receiving clopidogrel (75 mg/day) plus aspirin (81–325 mg/day) had a significant 26.9% relative risk reduction in the combined endpoint of death, myocardial infarction or stroke [52]. A subgroup analysis of patients who underwent CABG without PCI had a modest reduction of 1-year events (risk reduction rate = 16.7%) with clopidogrel [53]. But this was a post hoc analysis and the number of patients in this group was small.

With regard to the other high risk group of patients, namely patients post PCI having CABG, at present there are no studies that report the outcome of stent patency post-CABG. The ACCP guidelines [54] recommend clopidogrel in addition to aspirin for all patients post PCI for 9–12 months. A small study by Kaluza et al. [55] demonstrated that there was an instent thrombosis rate of around 20% with a similar mortality in patients having surgery of any type shortly post PCI. Therefore, if the stent is not covered by a graft intraoperatively then it would seem reasonable to follow the ACCP guideline with 9–12 months of clopidogrel. However, if the stent is covered by a graft more distally, there is no evidence to support continuation of clopidogrel.

Gao et al. [56] in their study, of one-hundred and ninety-seven selected patients undergoing CABG, assigned the patients to two groups according to antiplatelet drug: the clopidogrel group of 102 patients who received clopidogrel (75 mg) daily; and the combination group of 95 patients who received clopidogrel (75 mg) plus aspirin (100 mg) daily. Multislice computed tomography angiography was performed to evaluate graft patency at 1 month and 12 months after CABG. At 1 month and 12 months after CABG graft patency rates of clopidogrel group were, respectively, 99.0% and 96.9% for the left internal mammary artery (LIMA) and 98.1% and 93.5% for the saphenous vein grafts; those of the combination group were, respectively, 98.9% and 97.8% for LIMA, and 98.2% and 96.3% for saphenous vein grafts. There were no significant differences in graft patency between the two groups ($p > 0.05$). On the other hand, an RCT [57] to evaluate the effect of aspirin plus clopidogrel versus aspirin alone on SVG occlusion at 3 months after CABG showed that SVG patency was 91.6% (219 of 239) in the dual antiplatelet therapy group versus 85.7% (198 of 231) in the aspirin alone group ($p = 0.043$). In multivariate analysis, combined antiplatelet therapy independently increased venous graft patency ($p = 0.045$). Multislice computed tomography angiography was used to evaluate graft patency in this RCT. Similar conclusions were reached by Sun et al. [58] in their RCT which showed a high rate of graft occlusion after CABG surgery and suggested that the addition of clopidogrel to aspirin is feasible and safe.

Interestingly, the CASCADE (Clopidogrel After Surgery for Coronary Artery Disease) trial [59] undertaken to evaluate whether the addition of clopidogrel to aspirin inhibits saphenous vein graft (SVG) disease after CABG, as assessed at 1 year by intravascular ultrasound, concluded that compared with aspirin monotherapy, the combination of aspirin plus clopidogrel did not significantly reduce the process of SVG intimal hyperplasia 1 year after CABG.

The published evidence for the use of dual antiplatelet therapy after OPCAB is extremely scant at present unlike that for on-pump CABG. Nielsen et al. [60] randomly assigned twenty nine patients to receive aspirin alone or clopidogrel and aspirin until 30 days after OPCAB. The follow-up time was 2 months including standard blood samples and TEG with a specific platelet inhibition assay. In both groups a significant increase in TEG maximum amplitude was found 5 days after surgery. Platelet inhibition showed great variations but was significantly increased in the clopidogrel group (34.1%) vs. control group (11.0%) after 1 month. This study showed that hypercoagulability was seen 5 days after OPCAB and could not be demonstrated after 1 month. An observational study by Gurbuz et al. [61] showed that clopidogrel therapy with aspirin was independently associated with decreased symptom recurrence and adverse cardiac events following OPCAB. However, extending clopidogrel use beyond 30 days did not have a significant effect on defined end points. A small recently published RCT [62] recruiting twenty patients undergoing OPCAB concluded that early administration of a combined regimen of clopidogrel and aspirin after OPCAB grafting is not associated with increased postoperative bleeding or other major complications. Despite the small number of patients in this study and small number of examined grafts, the results of this RCT suggest that the addition of clopidogrel may increase graft patency after OPCAB grafting.

Hence, additional studies are needed to address the need for dual anti-platelet therapy after OPCAB particularly when it is known that clopidogrel, unlike aspirin, inhibits not only platelet aggregation but also P-selectin expression [21].

Conclusion

Cardiopulmonary bypass induces clotting disorders and platelet dysfunction. However, such an effect on hemostasis, which increases postoperative bleeding and is usually considered as adverse, also has a desirable effect in protecting anastomosis patency. An impaired hemostasis is thought to prevent thrombosis of the coronary grafts, presumably until a full postoperative regimen of antiplatelet therapy is established. Avoidance of CPB preserves hemostasis which may result in a hypercoagulable state after OPCAB surgery. At present however, it is not clear whether this hypercoagulable state translates into increased graft occlusion or adverse outcomes after OPCAB. It is expected that future laboratory and clinical research will provide greater insight into the mechanisms of this hypercoagulable state after OPCAB and its impact on clinical outcomes of relevance (graft patency and thrombotic events). Furthermore, any future research in this area will hopefully provide important information regarding the routine adoption of dual anti-platelet therapy and appropriate perioperative anticoagulation protocols to allay the anxiety attributed to presence of hypercoagulable state after OPCAB.

References

[1] Puskas JD, Wright CE, Ronson RS, Brown WM 3rd, Gott JP, Guyton RA. Off-pump multivessel coronary bypass via sternotomy is safe and effective. *Ann Thorac Surg* 1998;66:1068-72.

[2] Raja SG. Safety of off-pump coronary artery surgery: no more skepticism please! *Eur J Cardiothorac Surg* 2004;26:1229.

[3] Angelini GD, Taylor FC, Reeves BC, Ascione R. Early and midterm outcome after off-pump and on-pump surgery in Beating Heart Against Cardioplegic Arrest Studies (BHACAS 1 and 2): a pooled analysis of two randomised controlled trials. *Lancet* 2002;359:1194-1199.

[4] Nathoe H M, Van Dijk D, Jansen EW, et al; Octopus Study Group. A comparison of on-pump and off-pump coronary bypass surgery in low-risk patients. *N Engl J Med* 2003; 348,394-402.

[5] Puskas JD, Williams WH, Duke PG, et al. Off-pump coronary artery bypass grafting provides complete revascularization with reduced myocardial injury, transfusion requirements, and length of stay: a prospective randomized comparison of two hundred unselected patients undergoing off-pump versus conventional coronary artery bypass grafting. *J Thorac Cardiovasc Surg* 2003;125:797-808.

[6] Al-Ruzzeh S, George S., Bustami M, et al. Effect of off-pump coronary artery bypass surgery on clinical, angiographic, neurocognitive, and quality of life outcomes: randomised controlled trial. *BMJ* 2006;332:1365.

[7] Sedrakyan A, Wu AW, Parashar A, Bass EB, Treasure T. Off-pump surgery is associated with reduced occurrence of stroke and other morbidity as compared with traditional coronary artery bypass grafting: a meta-analysis of systematically reviewed trials. *Stroke* 2006;37:2759-69.

[8] Møller CH, Penninga L, Wetterslev J, Steinbrüchel DA, Gluud C. Clinical outcomes in randomized trials of off- vs. on-pump coronary artery bypass surgery: systematic review with meta-analyses and trial sequential analyses. *Eur Heart J* 2008;29:2601-16.

[9] Cheng DC, Bainbridge D, Martin JE, Novick RJ; Evidence-Based Perioperative Clinical Outcomes Research Group. *Anesthesiology* 2005;102:188-203.

[10] Reston JT, Tregear SJ, Turkelson CM. Meta-analysis of short-term and mid-term outcomes following off-pump coronary artery bypass grafting. *Ann Thorac Surg* 2003;76:1510-5.

[11] Parolari A, Alamanni F, Cannata A, et al. Off-pump versus on-pump coronary artery bypass: meta-analysis of currently available randomized trials. *Ann Thorac Surg* 2003;76:37-40.

[12] Kuss O, Von Salviati B, Börgermann J. Off-pump versus on-pump coronary artery bypass grafting: a systematic review and meta-analysis of propensity score analyses. *J Thorac Cardiovasc Surg* 2010;140:829-35.

[13] Raja SG, Berg GA. Impact of off-pump coronary artery bypass surgery on systemic inflammation: current best available evidence. *J Card Surg* 2007;22:445-55.

[14] Raja SG, Dreyfus GD. Impact of off-pump coronary artery bypass surgery on post-operative pulmonary dysfunction: current best available evidence. *Ann Card Anaesth* 2006;9:17-24.

[15] Raja SG, Dreyfus GD. Impact of off-pump coronary artery bypass surgery on graft patency: current best available evidence. *J Card Surg* 2007;22:165-9.

[16] Biancari F, Mahar MA, Mosorin M, et al. Immediate and intermediate outcome after off-pump and on-pump coronary artery bypass surgery in patients with unstable angina pectoris. *Ann Thorac Surg* 2008;86:1147-52.

[17] Ferreira-González IJ, Ribera A, Cascant P, Permanyer-Miralda G; ARCA study group. Outcomes in off-pump vs. on-pump coronary artery bypass grafting stratified by pre-operative risk profile: an assessment using propensity score. *Eur Heart J* 2006;27:2473-80.

[18] Mariani MA, Gu YJ, Boonstra PW, Grandjean JG, Van Oeveren W, Ebels T. Procoagulant activity after off-pump coronary operation: is the current anticoagulation adequate? *Ann Thorac Surg* 1999;67:1370-5.

[19] Vallely MP, Bannon PG, Bayfield MS, Hughes CF, Kritharides L. Quantitative and temporal differences in coagulation, fibrinolysis and platelet activation after on-pump and off-pump coronary artery bypass surgery. *Heart Lung Circ* 2009;18:123-30.

[20] Paulitsch FS, Schneider D, Sobel BE, et al. Hemostatic changes and clinical sequelae after on-pump compared with off-pump coronary artery bypass surgery: a prospective randomized study. *Coron Artery Dis* 2009;20:100-5.

[21] Bednar F, Osmancik P, Vanek T, et al. Platelet activity and aspirin efficacy after off-pump compared with on-pump coronary artery bypass surgery: results from the prospective randomized trial PRAGUE 11-Coronary Artery Bypass and REactivity of Thrombocytes (CABARET). *J Thorac Cardiovasc Surg* 2008;136:1054-60.

[22] Jares M, Vanek T, Bednar F, Maly M, Snircova J, Straka Z. Off-pump versus on-pump coronary artery surgery. *Int Heart J* 2007;48:57-67.

[23] Ballotta A, Saleh HZ, El Baghdady HW, et al. Comparison of early platelet activation in patients undergoing on-pump versus off-pump coronary artery bypass surgery. *J Thorac Cardiovasc Surg* 2007;134:132-8.

[24] Paparella D, Galeone A, Venneri MT, et al. Activation of the coagulation system during coronary artery bypass grafting: comparison between on-pump and off-pump techniques. *J Thorac Cardiovasc Surg* 2006;131:290-7.

[25] Parolari A, Mussoni L, Frigerio M, et al. The role of tissue factor and P-selectin in the procoagulant response that occurs in the first month after on-pump and off-pump coronary artery bypass grafting. *J Thorac Cardiovasc Surg* 2005;130:1561-6.

[26] Parolari A, Mussoni L, Frigerio M, et al. Increased prothrombotic state lasting as long as one month after on-pump and off-pump coronary surgery. *J Thorac Cardiovasc Surg* 2005;130:303-8.

[27] Vedin J, Antovic A, Ericsson A, Vaage J. Hemostasis in off-pump compared to on-pump coronary artery bypass grafting: a prospective, randomized study. *Ann Thorac Surg* 2005;80:586-93.

[28] Lo B, Fijnheer R, Castigliego D, Borst C, Kalkman CJ, Nierich AP. Activation of hemostasis after coronary artery bypass grafting with or without cardiopulmonary bypass. *Anesth Analg* 2004; 99:634-40.

[29] Møller CH, Steinbrüchel DA. Platelet function after coronary artery bypass grafting: is there a procoagulant activity after off-pump compared with on-pump surgery? *Scand Cardiovasc J* 2003;37:149-53.

[30] Despotis GJ, Joist JH. Anticoagulation and anticoagulation reversal with cardiac surgery involving cardiopulmonary bypass: an update. *J Cardiothorac Vasc Anesth* 1999;13(4 Suppl. 1):18-29.

[31] Muriithi EW, Belcher PR, Day SP, Menys VC, Wheatley DJ. Heparin-induced platelet dysfunction and cardiopulmonary bypass. *Ann Thorac Surg* 2000;69:1827-1832.

[32] Muriithi EW, Belcher PR, Rao JN, Chaudhry MA, Nicol D, Wheatley D. J. The effects of heparin and extracorporeal circulation on platelet counts and platelet microaggregation during cardiopulmonary bypass. *J Thorac Cardiovasc Surg* 2000;120:538-543.

[33] Khuri SF, Valeri CR, Loscalzo J, et al. Heparin causes platelet dysfunction and induces fibrinolysis before cardiopulmonary bypass. *Ann Thorac Surg* 1995;60:1008-1014.

[34] Li N, Astudillo R, Ivert T, Hjemdahl P. Biphasic pro-thrombotic and inflammatory responses after coronary artery bypass surgery. *J Thromb Haemost* 2003;1:470-476.

[35] Tzima E, Walker JH. Platelet Annexin V: the ins and outs. *Platelets* 2000;11:245-251.

[36] Ascione R, Williams S, Lloyd CT, Sundaramoorthi T, Pitsis AA, Angelini GD. Reduced postoperative blood loss and transfusion requirement after beating-heart

coronary operations: a prospective randomized study. *J Thorac Cardiovasc Surg* 2001;121:689-96.

[37] Frankel TL, Stamou SC, Lowery RC, et al. Risk factors for hemorrhage-related reexploration and blood transfusion after conventional versus coronary revascularization without cardiopulmonary bypass. *Eur J Cardiothorac Surg* 2005;27:494-500.

[38] Chong AJ, Pohlman TH, Hampton CR, et al. Tissue factor and thrombin mediate myocardial ischemia-reperfusion injury. *Ann Thorac Surg 2003;*75:S649–55.

[39] Kloner RA, Jennings RB. Consequences of brief ischemia: stunning, preconditioning, and their clinical implications: part 2. *Circulation 2001;*104:3158–67.

[40] Kon ZN, Kwon MH, Collins MJ, et al. Off-Pump coronary artery bypass leads to a regional hypercoagulable state not detectable using systemic markers. *Innovations* (Phila)2006;1:232-238.

[41] Goldman S, Zadina K, Moritz T, et al. Long-term patency of saphenous vein and left internal mammary artery grafts after coronary artery bypass surgery: results from a Department of Veterans Affairs Cooperative Study. *J Am Coll Cardiol 2004;*44:2149-56.

[42] MacGillivray TE, Vlahakes GJ. Patency and the pump–the risks and benefits of off-pump CABG. *N Engl J Med 2004;*350:3-4.

[43] White RH, Henderson MC. Risk factors for venous thromboembolism after total hip and knee replacement surgery. *Curr Opin Pulm Med 2002;*8:365-71.

[44] Okazaki Y, Takarabe K, Murayama J, et al. Coronary endothelial damage during off-pump CABG related to coronary-clamping and gas insufflation. *Eur J Cardiothorac Surg* 2001;19:834-839.

[45] Poston R, Gu J, Manchio J, et al. Platelet function tests predict bleeding and thrombotic events after off-pump coronary bypass grafting. *Eur J Cardiothorac Surg* 2005;27:584-91.

[46] Goldman S, Copeland J, Moritz T, et al. Improvement in early saphenous vein graft patency after coronary artery bypass surgery with antiplatelet therapy: results of a Veterans Administration Cooperative Study. *Circulation* 1988;77:1324-1332.

[47] Chesebro JH, Fuster V, Pugo FJ. Aspirin and mortality from coronary bypass surgery. *N Engl J Med* 2003;348:1057-1059.

[48] Stein PD, Schunemann HJ, Dalen JE, Gutterman D. Antithrombotic therapy in patients with saphenous vein and internal mammary artery bypass grafts: the seventh ACCP conference on antithrombotic and thrombolytic therapy. *Chest* 2004;126:600S-608S.

[49] Bhatt DL, Chew DP, Hirsch AT, Ringleb PA, Hacke W, Topol EJ. Superiority of clopidogrel versus aspirin in patients with prior cardiac surgery. *Circulation* 2001;103:363-368.

[50] Yusuf S, Zhao F, Mehta SR, Chrolavicius S, Tognoni G, Fox KK. Effects of clopidogrel in addition to aspirin in patients with acute coronary syndromes without ST-segment elevation. *N Engl J Med* 2001;345:494-502.

[51] Fox KA, Mehta SR, Peters R, et al. Benefits and risks of the combination of clopidogrel and aspirin in patients undergoing surgical revascularisation for non-ST-elevation acute coronary syndrome: the Clopidogrel in Unstable angina to prevent Recurrent ischemic Events (CURE) Trial. *Circulation* 2004;110:1202-1208.

[52] Steinhubl SR, Berger PB, Mann JT 3rd, Fry ET, De Lago A, Wilmer C, Topol EJ. Early and sustained dual oral antiplatelet therapy following percutaneous coronary intervention: a randomised controlled trial. *J Am Med Assoc* 2002;288:2411-2420.

[53] Topol EJ, Steinhubl SR, Brennan D, Berger PB, Moliterno DJ. CREDO Investigators. Comparison of long-term usefulness of clopidogrel therapy after the first percutaneous coronary intervention or coronary artery bypass grafting versus that after the second or repeat intervention. *Am J Cardiol* 2004;94:623-625.

[54] Popma JJ, Berger P, Ohman E M, Harrington RA, Grines C, Weitz JI. Antithrombotic therapy during percutaneous coronary intervention: Seventh ACCP conference on antithrombotic and thrombolytic therapy. *Chest* 2004;126:576-599.

[55] Kaluza GL, Joseph J, Lee JR, Raizner ME, Raizner AE. Catastrophic outcomes of noncardiac surgery soon after coronary stenting. *J Am Coll Cardiol* 2000;35:1288-1294.

[56] Gao C, Ren C, Li D, Li L. Clopidogrel and aspirin versus clopidogrel alone on graft patency after coronary artery bypass grafting. *Ann Thorac Surg* 2009;88:59-62.

[57] Gao G, Zheng Z, Pi Y, Lu B, Lu J, Hu S. Aspirin plus clopidogrel therapy increases early venous graft patency after coronary artery bypass surgery a single-center, randomized, controlled trial. *J Am Coll Cardiol* 2010;56:1639-43.

[58] Sun JC, Teoh KH, Lamy A, et al. Randomized trial of aspirin and clopidogrel versus aspirin alone for the prevention of coronary artery bypass graft occlusion: the Preoperative Aspirin and Postoperative Antiplatelets in Coronary Artery Bypass Grafting study. *Am Heart J* 2010;160:1178-84.

[59] Kulik A, Le May MR, Voisine P, et al. Aspirin plus clopidogrel versus aspirin alone after coronary artery bypass grafting: the clopidogrel after surgery for coronary artery disease (CASCADE) Trial. *Circulation* 2010;122:2680-7.

[60] Nielsen AB, Bochsen L, Steinbrüchel DA. Hypercoagulability and platelet inhibition after OPCAB. Randomized intervention with clopidogrel. *Scand Cardiovasc J* 2007;41:325-30.

[61] Gurbuz AT, Zia AA, Vuran AC, Cui H, Aytac A. Postoperative clopidogrel improves mid-term outcome after off-pump coronary artery bypass graft surgery: a prospective study. *Eur J Cardiothorac Surg* 2006;29:190-195.

[62] Mujanovic E, Nurkic M, Caluk J, Terzic I, Kabil E, Bergsland J. The effect of combined clopidogrel and aspirin therapy after off-pump coronary surgery: a pilot study. *Innovations* 2009;4:265-268.

In: Off-Pump Coronary Artery Bypass Grafting
Editors: S.G. Raja and M. Amrani

ISBN 978-1-62081-575-5

Chapter 20

CONVERSION TO CARDIOPULMONARY BYPASS IN OFF-PUMP CORONARY ARTERY BYPASS GRAFTING

Antonios Kourliouros,[1] Dayal Mukherjee[2] and Thanos Athanasiou[3]

[1]Specialist Registrar, Department of Cardiac Surgery, St Thomas' Hospital, London, UK
[2]Research Fellow in Cardiac Surgery, Imperial College of Medicine, London, UK
[3]Professor of Cardiovascular Sciences and Cardiac Surgery, Imperial College Healthcare Trust, Hammersmith Hospital, London, UK

ABSTRACT

Conversion is the process of institution of cardiopulmonary bypass as a preemptive or, more frequently, emergency measure to manage intraoperative complications arising during off-pump coronary artery bypass surgery. The incidence of conversion appears to be around 8% and in most cases is the result of hemodynamic compromise or anatomical considerations hindering the safe conduct of off-pump surgery. Although clinical outcomes following conversion have not been systematically analyzed until recently, it has been shown that it can lead to 6-fold increase in mortality, as well as a considerable increase in stroke, myocardial infarction, renal and respiratory failure and infection. This chapter provides an overview of the definitions, frequency and risk factors for conversion, examines its effect on postoperative outcomes, focuses on the implications of conversion in clinical practice and recommends strategies to prevent its occurrence.

INTRODUCTION

The enthusiastic resurgence of coronary artery bypass surgery (CABG) without the use of cardiopulmonary bypass (CPB) was followed by skepticism and, recently, by a more balanced and targeted approach based on coronary disease characteristics, patient co-morbidity and, ultimately, surgeon's experience and competency in off-pump revascularization techniques. In an era where postoperative outcomes following coronary surgery are closely monitored and mortality rarely exceeds 1-2%, most advancements in CABG, including off-pump revascularization, mainly aim at the amelioration of morbidity as well as enhanced recovery. Off-pump coronary artery bypass (OPCAB) appears to be non-inferior, at least, to conventional on-pump CABG in achieving these goals. However, OPCAB requires appropriate preoperative planning, prompt management of intraoperative hemodynamic changes and a different revascularization strategy in order to avoid the utilization of CPB with its known adverse consequences on patient physiology and outcomes. But what happens when there is a need for institution of CPB in a case that was planned and initiated as off-pump? This process, known as conversion, is a relatively unexplored phenomenon and its incidence and causation, as well its impact on patient morbidity and mortality have not been systematically analyzed until recently. This chapter aims to highlight the importance of conversion as a contributing factor to morbidity and mortality and discusses available measures to prevent its occurrence.

DEFINITIONS AND INCIDENCE OF CONVERSION

Conversion is the utilization of CPB during a CABG procedure that was planned to be performed off-pump. The overall rate of conversion across more than 20,000 OPCAB cases was found to be 8.4% [1]. However, it appears that there is great variability among studies demonstrating that in high-volume centers with relevant expertise in OPCAB the incidence of conversion is remarkably less [2].

Conversion may be urgent or non-urgent, and as no unified definitions existed in the literature we have previously categorized conversion as being either 'emergency' or 'elective' and defined them as follows:

- Emergency conversion – an urgent institution of CPB (with or without cardioplegia) to manage clinical instability, usually after commencement of coronary anastomoses.
- Elective conversion – conversion occurring as a planned measure to prevent clinical instability, usually prior to the commencement of coronary anastomoses.
- Overall conversion – all conversions, whether emergency or elective.

Although a large number of studies did not specify the status of 'urgency' of conversion in their reports, it appears that in most cases establishment of CPB was a 'hurried' process and the ratio of emergency to elective conversions appears to be approximately 4:1 [1].

The clinical reasons for intraoperative conversion are several, however, the predominant cause was found to be hemodynamic compromise, which accounted for two-thirds of all cases (Figure 1).

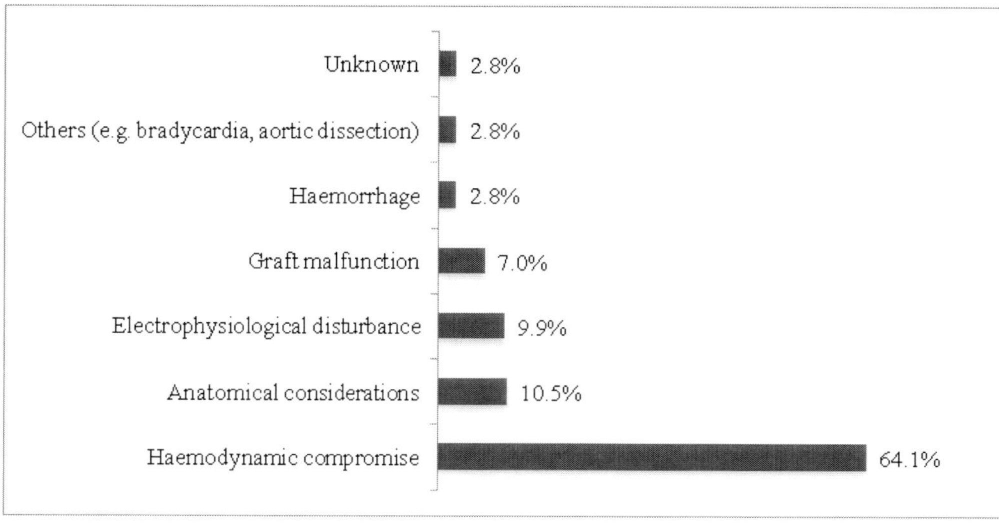

Figure 1. Causes of overall conversion.

Anatomical considerations (such as poor coronary targets, deeply intramyocardial coronary vessels, adhesions, excessive epicardial fat, and cardiac enlargement), a visual evaluation of which could lead the surgeon to convert electively due to unfeasibility of a beating heart procedure, were the second commonest cause of conversions. With regards to the operative timing of conversions, it appears that almost three-quarters of all conversions occurred during either left anterior descending (LAD) or circumflex anastomosis in keeping with the hemodynamic importance of their respective coronary territories [1].

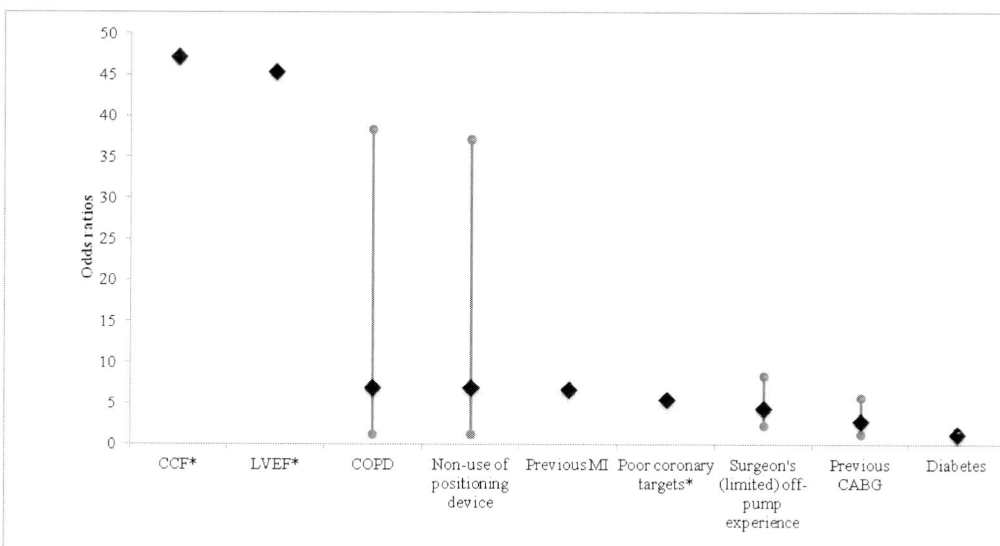

Figure 2. Predictors of conversion.

PREDICTORS OF CONVERSION

Regression analysis was used by several studies to identify factors that are predictive of conversion. The most notable of these factors include pre-existing cardiac dysfunction [3,4] or failure [4,5] chronic obstructive pulmonary disease [6,7], non-use of a cardiac positioning device [6,8], previous myocardial infarction (MI) [4,9], poor coronary targets [4,10], surgeon's off-pump experience [3,5], previous CABG [5,9] and diabetes [9,10]. Figure 2 demonstrates the predictors of conversion, which have each been identified in two or more unrelated studies.

IMPACT OF CONVERSION ON POSTOPERATIVE OUTCOMES

Effect of Conversion on Mortality

The outcomes of elective conversions have not been reported extensively, but the 3 studies [5,11,12] which have done so report outcomes similar to successful, non-converted OPCAB (or risk-matched on-pump) cases. Emergency conversion however has consistently been associated with poorer outcomes, with the rate of in-hospital mortality ranging from 5.4% to 32.1%, whereas the highest mortality rate encountered in the non-converted cohorts was 3.6%. The analysis by Edgerton and colleagues [5] warrants special mention, as probably the most comprehensive study into conversion mortality prior to our recently published meta-analysis [13]. Emergency conversions were found to carry a 5-fold higher mortality than elective conversions and conversions occurring after commencement of any coronary anastomosis carried a 12-fold higher mortality rate than those occurring prior to arteriotomy.

Using random effects modeling of assimilated data for 18,870 OPCAB cases (between 1998 and 2008) we found that conversion in general produced an odds ratio for mortality of 6.18, when compared to non-converted cases [13]. For emergency conversion specifically, this odds ratio was 6.99. This suggests an approximate 6-fold rise in the risk of mortality with any conversion, and a nearly 7-fold rise in mortality risk with emergency conversion.

Effect of Conversion on Morbidity

It is evident that intraoperative hemodynamic compromise, which constitutes the main driver of conversion, could result in end-organ ischemia and cause significant morbidity. Although many studies have previously reported adverse outcomes associated with conversion, this association had not been systematically approached and quantified. By incorporating data from 15 independent studies comprising 25,409 OPCAB cases we recently assessed the extent to which conversion raised the occurrence of organ damage and other morbidity [14]. Stroke, MI, bleeding requiring reoperation, renal failure requiring dialysis, deep sternal wound infection, red cell transfusions, respiratory complications, gastrointestinal complications, as well as intraoperative or postoperative requirement for an intra-aortic balloon pump (IABP), were all complications that were significantly more common after conversion to CPB (Figure 3).

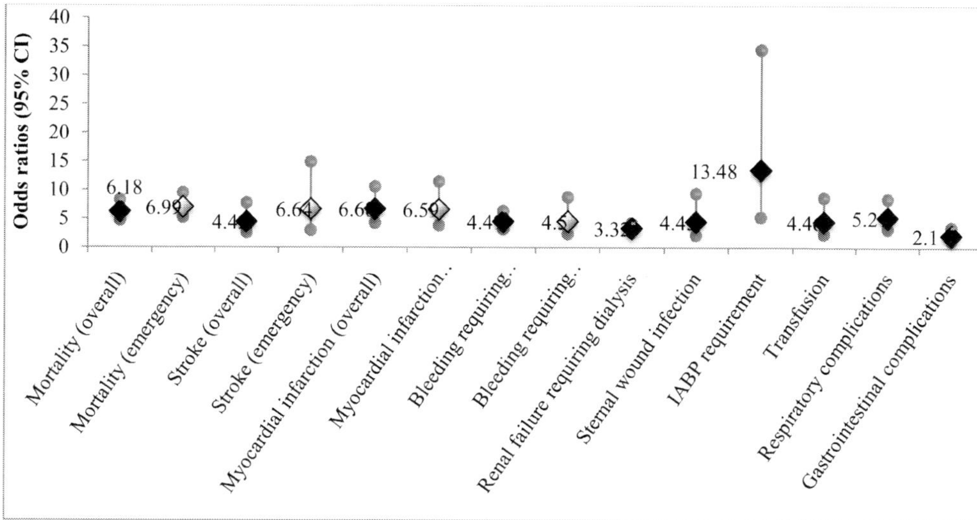

Figure 3. Effect of conversion on mortality and morbidity.

Economic Impact of Conversion

Within the debate of off-pump and on-pump revascularization, two important studies [15,16] have shown favourably lower economic costs for OPCAB and this cost benefit maintained at 1 year [16]. A unique decision model based analysis by Shiga and colleagues [17] suggests that the mean lifetime cost (per patient) of an OPCAB procedure is $91,282, which is marginally lower than for an on-pump procedure ($91,685).

However, if conversion were to occur, the cost of the off-pump operation would rise by almost 14% to $103,909. Therefore conversion may have a significant impact on the cost-benefit analysis of off- versus on-pump surgery and this remains to be further elucidated.

Possible Pathogenetic Explanations

The occurrence of conversion, especially as an emergency measure, has a negative impact on postoperative outcomes, as shown earlier, increasing the odds of stroke, MI and IABP use, bleeding requiring reoperation, kidney injury and respiratory failure as well as overall mortality.

It is evident that the risk factors predisposing to conversion are also strong predictors of adverse outcomes in conventional coronary surgery with the use of CPB [18]. The causal and direct relationship between conversion and increased morbidity cannot be supported with the available clinical data while such an often frequent bailout measure cannot be standardised for a targeted cause-effect study. Nevertheless, there are certain inherent characteristics of conversion that can give rise to pathophysiological sequelae and influence postoperative outcomes:

- Manipulation of the aorta and embolic phenomena: Aortic handling increases the risk of dislodgement of atheromatous debris, which can pass through the carotid arteries into the cerebral circulation blocking supply arteries and causing ischemic stroke. Off-pump surgery without conversion involves relatively little handling or manipulation of the aorta except during the utilization of the side-biting clamp. However, in emergency conversion two elements change this practice: the need for CPB involving aortic cannulation and cross-clamping, and haste. Arguably the risk of dislodging emboli during aortic cannulation or cross-clamping is greater under conditions of haste. Particularly in patients where severe atheromatous disease of the aorta was the criterion for an off-pump strategy, conversion and aortic manipulation may not be tolerated.
- Intraoperative hypoperfusion and ischemic damage: Verticalization of the heart during posterolateral anastomoses, especially in patients with poor left ventricular function, could cause transient but sometimes intractable hemodynamic compromise necessitating emergency conversion. Sustained episodes of ventricular tachycardia or fibrillation of the ischemic and often hypertrophied heart can also lead to hemodynamic compromise. This period of hypoperfusion may have a detrimental effect to the nephrons, leading to acute kidney injury, but it also contributes to the development of cerebrovascular or transient ischemic attacks. Although it appears that the leading cause of brain injury is dislodgement of aortic atheromatous debris, this process is more pronounced in situations of cerebral hypoperfusion. Lower mean arterial pressures during cardiac surgery give the potential for 'watershed' ischemia or infarction, not only to the brain but to other end-organs too. In a study by Tufo and colleagues [19] signs of neurological deficit were found in 27% of patients maintained at a mean arterial pressure of 60mmHg, but in as much as 78% of those maintained at 40mmHg. The majority of microemboli may be migratory and therefore be 'washed out' without any residual harm, but at lower blood pressures this process may be compromised [20]. The concept of 'watershed' cerebral ischemia may be particularly relevant for patients with pre-existing carotid or cerebrovascular disease, as well as those who are elderly or hypertensive.
- Suboptimal coronary anastomosis: We have previously demonstrated the effect of conversion on the incidence of MI, IABP requirement, and postoperative bleeding. However, for all these outcomes a fundamental link may be present; a suboptimal coronary anastomosis requiring revision. This revision may be necessitated immediately or may not be realized until later, occasionally leading to reoperation. If immediate revision is needed, the operation and CPB time are prolonged with a consequent increase in surgical or coagulopathic bleeding. Achievement of satisfactory coronary anastomoses is a greater challenge to the surgeon when the operation is off-pump and the heart is beating, where coronaries may be friable upon manipulation and the visibility is poor due to a bloody surgical field. The haste of an emergency conversion may unsettle a surgeon and affect his/her physical and psychological control over the situation.

Ischemic damage during conversion to other end organs, such as kidney, bowel, and lung, may be caused by the same mechanisms that potentiate stroke namely the combination of micro-embolism and hypoperfusion. When emergency conversion is coupled with the pulmonary edema resulting from intraoperative hemodynamic compromise and the distension of an ischemic heart, a catastrophic cascade of clinical events may ensue involving systemic inflammatory response syndrome with peripheral vasodilatation, hypotension, leading to further pronounced hypoperfusion. To propose specific pathogenetic mechanisms linking conversion to mortality is probably impossible. However, this may not be necessary as mortality is in general the product of the entire clinical situation, and many permutations of the clinical consequences of conversion discussed above could be seen to promote mortality.

Implications of Conversion Outcomes for Clinical Practice

There is certainly the evocation that conversion as a concept has been neglected and under-reported in the majority of literature comparing OPCAB and on-pump CABG, and that the significant proportion of patients who undergo conversion may be entering a territory of unknown risk. If it is then accepted that conversion is a significant complication of coronary surgery, and that the conversion-related mortality risk is substantially higher, the important matters relating to the consent process and training of off-pump surgeons will have to be addressed.

The consent process is one where the surgeon requests the explicit, unwavering, and unrestricted trust of the patient on the basis of the information of the potential benefits and risks involved in an operation. Consent is very important in cardiac surgery, as it takes into account the small but significant risk of death. Putting in context our recent meta-analytic findings [13] there is a 7-fold increase in operative mortality associated with emergency conversion transforming the mortality risk from a '1 in 100' to a '1 in 14'. It is reasonable to question, therefore, if it is possible to obtain true informed consent from the patient without incorporating and explaining the risks of conversion and conversion-related mortality. While straightforward pathology and lack of comorbidities may arguably not pose a great risk for conversion, in cases where patients present with risk factors predictive of conversion (as in Figure 2), the consideration of conversion risk in the consent process becomes all the more relevant. An empirical solution to this ethical question surrounding consent would be to include a metric accounting for conversion risk in future revisions of commonly used risk stratification models.

A surgeon's degree of inexperience in off-pump surgery is an identified and relatively well investigated predictor of conversion [3,5]. Although overall mortality rates may not differ between trainees and established off-pump surgeons (albeit in the setting of non-randomized and possibly selection-bias prone studies [21]), in those with an experience of less than 25 previous OPCAB cases, the risk of conversion may be 4.5 times higher compared to surgeons with an experience exceeding 100 cases [5]. Mentoring of novices by established OPCAB surgeons throughout the learning curve is of paramount importance in managing the increased risk to the patient. 'Off-pump mentorship' in this way is preferable to an en masse uptake of off-pump surgery at an institution composed only of skilled on-pump surgeons [2]. It is valid to consider that established on-pump surgeons may have a higher predilection to convert an off-pump procedure back to CPB, which is their familiar territory, and, furthermore, they may well take on off-pump cases at a lower rate than required to traverse the learning curve.

Prevention Strategies for Conversion

Having previously identified the commonest reported causes of conversion (Figure 1) as well as those variables that could predict conversion (Figure 2) we approach the challenge of prevention in a conceptual but practical model addressing individually the cause-based factors and the predictor-based ones (Table 1).

Table 1. Prevention strategies for conversion

		Preventive measures
Cause – based strategies	Hemodynamic compromise and unfavourable anatomy	Comprehensive preoperative imaging of coronary tree and LV function
		Post-sternotomy inspection of coronary anatomy – elective conversion if unfavorable
		Pre-arteriotomy positioning to test for hemodynamic instability
		Trendelendburg position with rightward tilt
		Minimization of ventricular compression with "Lima stitch" or positioning devices
		Optimal sequence of anastomosis (grafting LAD or dominant vessels first, creating proximal anastomoses before distals, grafting culprit vessel causing papillary dysfunction and MR first etc)
		Transesophageal echocardiography to assess thoracic aortic blood flow
		"CPB – readiness" including perfusionist stand by, ready CPB pump, pre-placement of aortic purse-strings
Predictor – based strategies	Surgeon - specific	Traverse off-pump learning curve through structured training
		Mentorship and communication
		Prevention and appropriate management of emergency conversion
	Patient – specific	Patient selection
		Risk – benefit approach to off-pump surgery
	Technology - specific	Cardiac positioning devices (apical suction)
		Epicardial stabilizer
		Intraluminal shunts
		Circulatory support devices (e.g. IABP, VAD)
		Transesophageal echochardiography

CPB = cardiopulmonary bypass; IABP = intra-aortic balloon pump; LV = left ventricle; VAD = ventricular assist device.

Since certain strategies apply to the optimal conduct of off-pump surgery in general (such as use of adjuncts) in addition to their potential role in conversion prevention, we will only provide a concise description and not expand to areas that are covered elsewhere in this book.

Cause-Based Strategies

Unfavorable anatomy is usually associated with elective conversion, as the surgeon inspects the heart and coronary vessels intraoperatively before commencing any anastomoses, and makes the decision that off-pump surgery is too risky. Any comprehensive strategy for prevention of emergency conversion must include adequate preoperative imaging, a post-sternotomy inspection of coronary and cardiac anatomy, and pre-arteriotomy positional manipulation of the heart to test for hemodynamic instability. According to Vassiliades and colleagues [22], patients who suffered intraoperative hemodynamic collapse were much more likely to have cardiomegaly than the general OPCAB population.

Important considerations in the prevention of hemodynamic compromise are patient position, heart size, sequence of anastomoses, and existence of concomitant mitral regurgitation. The 'OPCAB position' is the Trendelenburg position but with a rightward tilt. This position increases preload and therefore cardiac output, and improves hemodynamic stability during manipulation of the heart. The rightward tilt facilitates exposure of posterolateral and inferior vessels [23].

Hypertrophied hearts are not only difficult to verticalize and position optimally for posterolateral coronary targets; manipulation and right ventricular compression causes a transient compromise in preload which, in a hypertrophied heart with pre-existent left ventricular diastolic dysfunction, may not be well tolerated. Clearly, if manipulation is likely to cause a hemodynamic problem, OPCAB may not be suitable. A traditional and safe means of cardiac displacement during OPCAB is the use of pericardial sutures placed in the configuration of the 'Lima stitch', which can displace the heart without compression [24]. Newer, highly successful alternatives are cardiac positioning devices, which are discussed later.

In deciding the ideal sequence of anastomoses the surgeon needs to ascertain the approach that will minimize transient regional myocardial ischemia. General approaches include performing all proximal anastomoses first, grafting the LAD or dominant artery first, and grafting collateralized arteries before those from which the collaterals arise. The latter rule can be particularly useful in deciding the optimum grafting sequence, especially when surgical instinct may be to graft the LAD first. For example, if the posterior descending artery (PDA) is completely stenosed, it may depend on collaterals from LAD, in which case grafting the LAD first would impose transient ischemia not only on the anterior ventricular wall but also the posteroinferior wall. This may not be tolerated in an already infracted or failing heart.

Mitral regurgitation (MR) can pose a difficult problem during displacement or verticalization of the heart, when access to posterolateral coronary targets is required. Regurgitation will be more marked during verticalization, such that pre-existent MR that was mild to moderate becomes severe, and the consequence is raised pulmonary arterial pressures, massive pulmonary edema and cardiorespiratory compromise [23]. In mild MR caused by an evolving or recent MI, a potential strategy may be to revascularize the culprit vessel causing papillary muscle dysfunction first [6]. In most cases, however, the MR will be well-established, therefore co-existence of MR with the need for revascularization of a posterolateral target should preclude an off-pump operation.

Hemodynamic compromise, however transient, is capable of causing significant end-organ hypoperfusion. Thoracic aortic blood flow is a proxy measure of perfusion during

OPCAB, and we recommend the use of transesophageal Doppler echocardiography as a tool for its real-time measurement [25].

We also recommend the routine adoption of one or more 'CPB-readiness' measures, which allow the institution of CPB with relative speed and ease, and include the following: a perfusionist on standby in the operating theatre, a primed or unprimed ('dry-ready') CPB pump, and pre-inserted purse-string sutures. Other safety measures include cardiac positioning devices and intraluminal coronary shunts (discussed later). It has been previously shown that conversion mortality tended to decrease as the number of OPCAB safety measures used increased [1].

Predictor-Based Strategies

Predictors of conversion can be divided according to those that are surgeon-specific, patient-specific, and device- or technology-specific.

Surgeon-Specific

As mentioned earlier in the chapter, surgeons early in their OPCAB learning curve present a higher risk of conversion. This has been demonstrated in two ways; regression analysis has isolated surgical inexperience as a predictor of conversion and the annual rate of conversion has been seen to consistently fall with increasing OPCAB experience over time [2, 3, 5, 8, 11]. The implications on surgical training in OPCAB have also been discussed earlier. In general, it is important not only to traverse the off-pump learning curve as a trainee, but also to become competent in the prevention and management of emergency conversion, for which communication and early decision-making as leaders of a multidisciplinary OPCAB team are key skills.

Patient-Specific

A 'conversion paradox' is apparent; whereas OPCAB is generally indicated for high-risk patients with comorbidities (such as poor cardiac function, left main stem disease, even in those with previous CABG), it is these comorbidities that in turn appear to raise the risk of conversion. Once again, it is the responsibility of accomplished cardiac surgeon to tailor the surgical strategy according to the patient needs and offer OPCAB to those who would benefit the most from it without compromising safety and optimal outcomes.

Technology-Specific

We have already commented earlier on the use of transesophageal echocardiography as a proxy measure of end organ perfusion. In addition, several technologies are widely accepted and used in cardiac surgery, mainly for myocardial protection and hemodynamic support.

Cardiac positioning devices have been developed to overcome the problem of hemodynamic upset during cardiac manipulation. These are generally suction-based devices, which pull at the cardiac apex in its long axis, thereby allowing sufficient grip for manipulation, but without ventricular compression and therefore avoiding deformational dysfunction of the cardiac chambers. Positioning devices usually come with an epicardial stabilizer, which enables relative stabilization of the coronary target against a beating myocardium, facilitating the formation of competent anastomoses. Positioning device systems have been found to both improve hemodynamic control [26] and reduce the incidence of conversion [8].

Intraluminal coronary shunts are useful tools in myocardial protection during off-pump surgery. While many studies [27-29] have demonstrated benefit from the use of shunts, in terms of a reduction in regional ischemia and perhaps improved patency, some reports exist of coronary shunts having a denuding effect on the vascular endothelium [30]. If significant, such damage could itself initiate the vicious cascade of plaque rupture, intimal hyperplasia, and ultimately coronary thrombosis. A formal large-scale randomized assessment of coronary shunts, and their effect on conversion rates, remains to be performed. However, given their clear potential in reducing ischemia during grafting, which is a significant cause of hemodynamic instability, it may be postulated that coronary shunts prevent such instability and therefore are likely to reduce the need for conversion.

Devices used for mechanical circulatory support including IABPs and ventricular assist devices (VADs) have been successfully used during off-pump revascularization in patients who were in near-total cardiogenic shock [31,32].

Conclusions

Conversion has been an underestimated and under-reported occurrence in OPCAB. All available evidence to date suggests that emergency conversion can lead to significantly worse outcomes both in terms of morbidity and mortality. As such it may be described as the Trojan horse in off-pump revascularization. This has implications for surgical training, but more importantly for patient safety and equity of the consent process. We have highlighted the effects and implications of conversion, and proposed a general framework through which conversion and its sequelae may be comprehensively prevented.

References

[1] Mukherjee, D., Ahmed, K., Baig, K., Patel, V. M., Darzi, A., Athanasiou, T. Conversion and safety in off-pump coronary artery bypass: a system failure that needs re-emphasis. *Ann. Thorac. Surg.* 2011;91:630-639.

[2] Reeves, B. C., Ascione, R., Caputo, M., Angelini, G. D. Morbidity and mortality following acute conversion from off-pump to on-pump coronary surgery. *Eur. J. Cardiothorac. Surg.* 2006;29:941-947.

[3] Hovakimyan, A., Manukyan, V., Ghazaryan, S., et al. Predictors of emergency conversion to on-pump during off-pump coronary surgery. *Asian Cardiovasc. Thorac. Ann.* 2008;16:226-230.

[4] Mishra, M., Shrivastava, S., Dhar, A., et al. A prospective evaluation of hemodynamic instability during off-pump coronary artery bypass surgery. *J. Cardiothorac. Vasc. Anesth.* 2003;17:452-458.

[5] Edgerton, J. R., Dewey, T. M., Magee, M. J., et al. Conversion in off-pump coronary artery bypass grafting: an analysis of predictors and outcomes. *Ann. Thorac. Surg.* 2003;76:1138-1142.

[6] Tabata, M., Takanashi, S., Horai, T., Fukui, T., Hosoda, Y. Emergency conversion in off-pump coronary artery bypass grafting. *Interact. Cardiovasc. Thorac. Surg.* 2006;5:555-559.

[7] Landoni, G., Pappalardo, F., Crescenzi, G., et al. The outcome of patients requiring emergency conversion from off-pump to on-pump coronary artery bypass grafting. *Eur. J. Anaesthesiol.* 2007;24:317-322.

[8] Patel, N. C., Patel, N. U., Loulmet, D. F., McCabe, J. C., Subramanian, V. A. Emergency conversion to cardiopulmonary bypass during attempted off-pump revascularization results in increased morbidity and mortality. *J. Thorac. Cardiovasc. Surg.* 2004;128:655-661.

[9] Jin, R., Hiratzka, L. F., Grunkemeier, G. L., Krause, A., Page, U. S., 3rd. Aborted off-pump coronary artery bypass patients have much worse outcomes than on-pump or successful off-pump patients. *Circulation* 2005;112:I332-337.

[10] Lund, O., Christensen, J., Holme, S., et al. On-pump versus off-pump coronary artery bypass: independent risk factors and off-pump graft patency. *Eur. J. Cardiothorac. Surg.* 2001;20:901-907.

[11] Soltoski, P., Salerno, T., Levinsky, L., et al. Conversion to cardiopulmonary bypass in off-pump coronary artery bypass grafting: its effect on outcome. *J. Card. Surg.* 1998;13:328-334.

[12] Novick, R. J., Fox, S. A., Stitt, L. W., et al. Effect of off-pump coronary artery bypass grafting on risk-adjusted and cumulative sum failure outcomes after coronary artery surgery. *J. Card. Surg.* 2002;17:520-528.

[13] Mukherjee, D., Ashrafian, H., Kourliouros, A., Ahmed, K., Darzi, A., Athanasiou, T. Intra-operative conversion is a cause of masked mortality in off-pump coronary artery bypass: a meta-analysis. *Eur. J. Cardiothorac.* 2012;41:291-299.

[14] Mukherjee, D., Rao, C., Ibrahim, M., et al. Meta-analysis of organ damage after conversion from off-pump coronary artery bypass procedures. *Ann. Thorac. Surg.* 2011;92:755-761.

[15] Ascione, R., Lloyd, C. T., Underwood, M. J., Lotto, A. A., Pitsis, A. A., Angelini, G. D. Economic outcome of off-pump coronary artery bypass surgery: a prospective randomized study. *Ann. Thorac. Surg.* 1999;68:2237-2242.

[16] Puskas, J. D., Williams, W. H., Mahoney, E. M., et al. Off-pump vs conventional coronary artery bypass grafting: early and 1-year graft patency, cost, and quality-of-life outcomes: a randomized trial. *JAMA* 2004;291:1841-1849.

[17] Shiga, T., Apfel, C. C., Wajima, Z., Ohe, Y. Influence of intraoperative conversion from off-pump to on-pump coronary artery bypass grafting on costs and quality of life: a cost-effectiveness analysis. *J. Cardiothorac Vasc. Anesth.* 2007;21:793-799.

[18] Biancari, F., Kangasniemi, O. P., Luukkonen, J., et al. EuroSCORE predicts immediate and late outcome after coronary artery bypass surgery. *Ann. Thorac. Surg.* 2006;82:57-61.

[19] Tufo, H. M., Ostfeld, A. M., Shekelle, R. Central nervous system dysfunction following open-heart surgery. *JAMA* 1970;212:1333-1340.

[20] Caplan, L. R., Hennerici, M. Impaired clearance of emboli (washout) is an important link between hypoperfusion, embolism, and ischemic stroke. *Arch. Neurol.* 1998;55:1475-1482.
[21] Karagounis, A., Asimakopoulos, G., Niranjan, G., Valencia, O., Chandrasekaran, V. Complex off-pump coronary artery bypass surgery can be safely taught to cardiothoracic trainees. *Interact. Cardiovasc. Thorac. Surg.* 2006;5:222-226.
[22] Vassiliades, T. A., Jr., Nielsen, J. L., Lonquist, J. L. Hemodynamic collapse during off-pump coronary artery bypass grafting. *Ann. Thorac. Surg.* 2002;73:1874-1879.
[23] Halkos, M. E., Puskas, J. D. Teaching off-pump coronary artery bypass surgery. *Semin. Thorac. Cardiovasc. Surg.* 2009;21:224-228.
[24] Lima, R. Surgical techniques of coronary artery exposure. In: Salerno, T., Ricci, M., Karamanoukian, H., D'Ancona, G., Bergsland, J., editors. *Beating Heart Coronary Surgery.* New York: Futura Publishing Company, 2001:23-34.
[25] Decoene, C., Modine, T., Al-Ruzzeh, S., et al. Analysis of thoracic aortic blood flow during off-pump coronary artery bypass surgery. *Eur. J. Cardiothorac. Surg.* 2004;25:26-34.
[26] Sepic, J., Wee, J. O., Soltesz, E. G., et al. Cardiac positioning using an apical suction device maintains beating heart hemodynamics. *Heart Surg. Forum.* 2002;5:279-284.
[27] Bergsland, J., Lingaas, P. S., Skulstad, H., et al. Intracoronary shunt prevents ischemia in off-pump coronary artery bypass surgery. *Ann. Thorac. Surg.* 2009;87:54-60.
[28] Gurbuz, A., Emrecan, B., Yilik, L., et al. Intracoronary shunt reduces postoperative troponin leaks: a prospective randomized study. *Eur. J. Cardiothorac. Surg.* 2006;29:186-189.
[29] Menon, A. K., Albes, J. M., Oberhoff, M., Karsch, K. R., Ziemer, G. Occlusion versus shunting during MIDCAB: effects on left ventricular function and quality of anastomosis. *Ann. Thorac. Surg.* 2002;73:1418-1423.
[30] Hangler, H., Mueller, L., Ruttmann, E., Antretter, H., Pfaller, K. Shunt or snare: coronary endothelial damage due to hemostatic devices for beating heart coronary surgery. *Ann. Thorac. Surg.* 2008;86:1873-1877.
[31] Gregoric, I. D., Poglajen, G., Span, M., Frazier, O. H., Loyalka, P., Kar, B. Percutaneous ventricular assist device support during off-pump surgical coronary revascularization. *Ann. Thorac. Surg.* 2008;86:637-639.
[32] Strecker, T., Fischlein, T., Pfeiffer, S. Impella Recover 100: successful perioperative support for off pump coronary artery bypass grafting surgery in a patient with end-stage ischemic cardiomyopathy. *J. Cardiovasc. Surg.* (Torino) 2004;45:381-384.

In: Off-Pump Coronary Artery Bypass Grafting
Editors: S.G. Raja and M. Amrani

ISBN 978-1-62081-575-5

Chapter 21

COMPLICATIONS UNIQUE TO OFF-PUMP CORONARY ARTERY BYPASS GRAFTING

Jacob Bergsland[1] and Emir Mujanovic[2]
[1]Cardiac Surgeon, The Intervention Centre, Oslo University Hospital, Oslo, Norway and Medical Director, BH HeartCentre, Tuzla, Bosnia and Herzegovina
[2]Chief of Surgery, BH Heart Centre, Tuzla, Bosnia and Herzegovina

ABSTRACT

Coronary artery bypass grafting has been performed predominantly with the use of cardiopulmonary bypass and cardioplegic arrest, which allows optimization of the surgical field and consistent placement of grafts. However, the use of cardiopulmonary bypass is associated with numerous complications. A surgical technique avoiding cardiopulmonary bypass should, in theory, reduce the incidence of such complications and lead to improved patient outcomes. This assumption has rekindled interest in performing off-pump coronary artery bypass surgery. The use of off-pump bypass grafting to avoid the detrimental effects of extracorporeal circulation demonstrates great promise in reducing pump-related complications. However, with new techniques come new challenges. Off-pump coronary artery bypass grafting is technically more demanding. Avoidance of the cardiopulmonary bypass circuit has been linked to the development of a hypercoagulable state postoperatively. Complications related to the management of the ascending aorta and target vessels during the performance of beating heart surgery are also being reported. Moreover, despite increasing experience in a number of centers, hemodynamic collapse does occur during off-pump bypass, requiring rapid institution of cardiopulmonary bypass. This chapter provides an overview of complications unique to off-pump coronary artery bypass grafting and outlines strategies to avoid and deal with these complications.

Introduction

Coronary artery bypass grafting was first performed in the animal laboratory by Alexis Carrell and reported more than 100 years ago. Interestingly the procedure was performed off pump, using an arterial graft. CABG did not "take off" as a regular procedure before the development of a reliable cardiopulmonary bypass (CPB) machine in the 1950's. The procedure subsequently developed by Favalaro and others, utilized grafting with saphenous vein grafts, while circulation was supported by CPB, became one of the most performed operations in the Western world. CABG became the basis of a whole industry; this stimulated development of improved CPB circuits, better instruments, improved suture materials and other disposables and an extensive scientific literature developed documenting and defining the benefit of CABG compared to alternative therapies.

CABG was the inspiration for numerous quality assurance initiatives introduced by public and non-governmental agencies. It can thus be stated that CABG has been an important procedure not only for patients with coronary artery disease (CAD), but for medical development and quality assurance overall.

Carrell, in his experimental studies in dogs did not use CPB while grafting the subclavian artery to a coronary vessel. The Russian surgeon Kolosev [1-3] developed off-pump coronary artery bypass (OPCAB) grafting in animals as well as clinically. The reason for using CPB was not obvious to these investigators, since the coronary arteries are located on the surface of the heart, and therefore easily visible. The problem of course was the heart's motion and the difficulty in connecting vessels as small as 1.5 mm to a moving target. Despite these difficulties, the South American surgeons Buffolo and Benneti [4,5] demonstrated excellent results of OPCAB surgery in large series of patients. The problem of cardiac motion was dealt with by having good assistants, using excellent techniques and skilled anesthesiologists.

In the late 1980's and early 90's increasingly sophisticated techniques and advances in technology made it possible to standardize the OPCAB procedure. However, with new techniques come new challenges. Over the past two decades several complications more or less unique to OPCAB have been recognized. This chapter focuses on these complications and briefly discusses tips and tricks to avoid the pitfalls and complications associated with OPCAB.

Complications Related to Hemostasis and Coagulation

Bleeding

Bleeding is one of the most dreaded and common complications of coronary bypass surgery. It occurs irrespective of whether or not CPB has been used. However, it is more common and serious following CABG performed with CPB [6]. CPB is known to activate the fibrinolytic system and damages thrombocytes. These effects are less pronounced with OPCAB resulting in less blood loss. At the same time it is important to mention that surgical bleeding should be suspected early in OPCAB instead of reliance on correction of suspected defects in the coagulation system.

Graft Thrombosis

Several studies have shown evidence of impaired graft patency in OPCAB compared to CABG with CPB and arrested heart [7,8]. Possible technical reasons for this will be discussed later. There is, however, increasing evidence for the need for using a more aggressive antithrombotic regimen in OPCAB [9-12]. Although it has not been conclusively proven that hypercoagulabilty exists after OPCAB [13], yet the rationale for an aggressive antiplatelet regimen is probably to ensure decreased platelet deposition in areas of endothelial damage.

Deep Vein Thrombosis

Deep vein thrombosis is not uncommon following CABG and may be more common in OPCAB. Aggressive antithrombotic regimens should therefore be utilized to prevent venous thrombotic events [14].

Hemodynamic Complications

Development of Unstable Hemodynamics

Maintenance of stable hemodynamics is essential during OPCAB. One of the most frequent complications of the procedure is hypotension, myocardial ischemia and hemodynamic collapse. This may require initiation of emergency CPB, and in case of cardiac arrest, internal cardiac massage and several minutes of inadequate organ perfusion. Conversion from OPCAB to CPB under such circumstances has been shown to cause serious complications [15]. In one series with conversions performed for serious hemodynamic instability 6 out of 9 patients suffered serious ischemic complications postoperatively [16]. Controlled elective conversion to CPB, without collapse, is usually not serious [17] and the operation may continue with CPB on the beating heart or if necessary with cardioplegic arrest. Most conversions are caused by myocardial ischemia and it is recommended to perform grafting on the beating heart with CPB support to prevent further global ischemia caused by aortic cross clamping. To avoid conversion, meticulous and close observation of the patient, the heart and hemodynamics is necessary throughout the procedure.

Planning the Operation and Avoiding Instability

In the following section most of the discussion will be related to OPCAB performed through median sternotomy unless mentioned otherwise. A brief description of special complications of OPCAB performed through alternate surgical approaches is included at the end of the chapter.

To avoid complications during OPCAB the surgeon has to plan the operation carefully and review all available information. In on-pump surgery a more "assembly" line approach may be taken, since the order in which grafts are performed is more or less unimportant except in cases of acute coronary obstruction. As long as the graftable vessels and the use of conduits are defined, the order of grafting is not important. In OPCAB the graft order may be essential. In unstable patients a stenosed left anterior descending (LAD) artery is usually bypassed first, since this vessel is approached with minimal dislocation of the heart. If all vessels except LAD are totally occluded, bypassing the LAD may be risky, causing ischemia and it is usually recommended to bypass an obstructed RCA first, thereby supplying LAD through collaterals during grafting.

Complications during Induction of Anesthesia

OPCAB is a "new" procedure for cardiac surgeons who were trained during the time when CABG was almost exclusively performed with CPB. During on-pump CABG manipulation of the heart prior to cannulation is minimal and subsequently the whole procedure is supported by CPB. Complications during on-pump CABG are frequently caused by CPB itself or by inadequate myocardial protection resulting in difficult weaning from CPB at the end of the procedure. Most cardiac surgeons have experienced the so-called "crashing onto CPB or similar" when the patient gets acutely unstable during induction of anesthesia or opening of the chest. Such instability may be caused by ischemia, hypovolemia etc and is more dangerous in OPCAB. An experienced anaesthesiologist is therefore essential. A well planned induction regimen and maintenance of necessary medical therapy for the cardiac condition is crucial at this point [17].

Complications from Cardiac Positioning

Grafting of the various coronary territories during OPCAB procedures necessitates positioning of the heart to achieve optimal exposure in order to perform anastomosis with minimum effort. The main methods of positioning are deep pericardial sutures, the so-called Lima Stitch and various myocardial suction devices used to pull the apex in different directions to present the various vessels. The positioning using these techniques usually does not cause severe hemodynamic disturbances [18].

Deep Pericardial Sutures or Lima Stitch

The stitches are placed through the pericardium and used to pull and thereby rotate the heart. Although uncommon, careless placement of such stitches has been reported to damage, the phrenic nerve, esophagus and even the descending aorta. More commonly the stitches are placed too superficially and may tear out during grafting, causing sudden loss of the appropriate position.

Suction Cups

Suction cups may cause hematoma of the myocardium and if placed on an important collateral coronary vessel supplying the myocardium can compromise coronary perfusion with resultant ischemia and hemodynamic collapse.

Traction on Mammary Grafts during Positioning

In on-pump CABG, the left internal mammary (LIMA) to LAD graft is usually performed last. This makes it unnecessary to use a generous length of the conduit. On the other hand, in OPCAB, the LAD is grafted first to supply blood to the anterior wall, with minimal cardiac displacement. During positioning for grafting the other vessels, if the conduit is short, elevation of the heart will cause tension on the LIMA with resultant damage to the anastomosis. If the tension is less, the anastomosis may remain intact, but the tension may decrease or interrupt the flow in the graft causing ischemia of the anterior wall.

TECHNICAL COMPLICATIONS DURING THE GRAFTING PROCEDURE

Graft Patency and Quality of Anastomosis

Grafting the coronaries is generally considered somewhat more difficult using OPCAB technique. Stabilization is seldom total and continuous cardiac contractions usually continue to produce a slight motion during the procedure. This is usually controllable by the skillful surgeon assisted by an experienced assistant. The positioning of the heart is limited by the need to maintain optimal hemodynamics and by the method of positioning. The LAD and right coronary artery (RCA) and their branches are generally easily exposed while excellent exposure of the circumflex ant its marginal branches may be more difficult. Excellent instrumentation and suture material is essential in OPCAB surgery. Positioning of the needle and its manipulation during penetration of the tissues are more critical than in on-pump CABG, because the motion of the heart and imperfect needle motion may cause large holes or tears in endothelial surfaces. This may set up a circle of prothrombosis and graft occlusion. Anastomosis on moving target vessel combined with the possibility of other technical imperfections leaves the possibility of graft occlusion immediately or in the postoperative phase. Following successful tackling of the learning curve and increasing experience concerns regarding graft patency can be safely addressed.

Identification of Obstructed Grafts

The main method of assuring the patency of the coronary grafts is excellent technique and intraoperative graft verification. Although we believe that graft verification should be utilized in all coronary artery surgery procedures, it is essential in OPCAB. The use of graft verification with a simple method such as transit-time flowmetry (TTFM) makes it possible to secure close to 100% graft patency at the end of the surgical procedure.

Use of Shunts

Prevention of ischemia during grafting may be prevented by insertion of intracoronary shunts during grafting. We have demonstrated the effect of such shunts. Prior to shunt insertion bleeding from the incised coronary artery is frequently controlled by snares compressing the proximal coronary. Shunts may damage the endothelium and potentially set up for graft thrombosis or accelerated arteriosclerosis. Our own experience has not shown any evidence of such problems (19). Various complications of shunts have been demonstrated. Shunts, especially if constructed of stiff plastic material, may cause dissection of the native coronary, which will usually set off graft occlusion. Shunts made of softer plastic material may be caught by a suture resulting in difficulty in removing it. Shunts may be kinked and non-functioning during the grafting procedure and cause a false sense of security for the surgeon who may trust that the patient is protected from ischemia .

We have found that a well-placed and functioning intracoronary shunt represents good insurance against cardiac ischemia and hemodynamic instability (19). It is most important for the LAD, which supplies the important anterior wall. Ischemia in the LAD distribution is a not uncommon and serious issue and may cause hemodynamic collapse. Occlusion of RCA during grafting may cause third degree AV-block and hemodynamic instability. Such block may be managed by temporary pacing but we prefer using a shunt. Although the intracoronary shunt may have limited flow due to small internal diameter, we find that the flow is usually adequate to prevent complications.

Use of Coronary Snares

The use of proximal (and sometimes distal) snaring is an alternative to the use of shunt, but does not supply flow through the graft site during anastomosis and may cause ischemia. The snares have also been shown to cause damage to the native vessels and predisposes for future obstruction or stenosis [19]. The least attractive method of managing the opened coronary vessel during grafting is to leave the vessel open to air. This will decrease the pressure in the native coronary to close to zero and therefore make the corresponding myocardium ischemic. If it is impossible to insert a shunt gentle snaring may be the method of choice, since collaterals will then maintain a certain level of pressure in the native vessel.

Constant monitoring of potential ischemia is mandatory. At present transesophageal echocardiography is the most suitable method since it provides real-time strain recordings that give the surgeon instant information about developing ischemia (19).

Prevention of Graft Problems

To prevent complications during performance of the coronary grafts we have found that avoidance of snares, use of intracoronary shunt and immediate post-graft flow measurement using TTFM contribute to achieving optimal results [19-21]. Construction of a well functioning LIMA to LAD anastomosis is a critical step in the OPCAB procedure; therefore confirmation of the patency and functionality of this graft is essential before other grafts are performed.

Complications Caused by Stabilizing Devices

Mechanical stabilization of the target coronary vessel was the main technical development that made OPCAB a reality. Although the surgeons from Brazil as well as our own group were able to perform coronary grafting without stabilization it was difficult, and the question of patency both early and at midterm was a concern. Gundry clearly demonstrated lowered graft patency in OPCAB in his 1989 publication (7). Mechanical stabilization changed the paradigm, and the proper use of the stabilizing devices remains critical.

Pressure Stabilizers

A multitude of stabilizers have been developed, but they can be divided into two main types: pressure stabilizers and suction stabilizers. Pressure stabilizers are usually low profile and exert stabilization by simple pressure on the myocardium next to the coronary artery vessel to be grafted. Complications can occur from such stabilizers when inadequate pressure is applied. This may cause motion of the heart relative to the stabilizers and abrasion of the underlying myocardium with subsequent bleeding from the surface of the heart, which occasionally may be difficult to control. More commonly small venous branches may be torn; suturing may usually control this type of bleeding.

If too much pressure is applied, hemodynamics may be compromised or the coronary may be functionally occluded resulting in ischemia. In such cases a shunt may not help since the occlusion may occur proximal to the shunt. It is therefore essential that the stabilizers be applied carefully, avoiding obstruction of the coronary being grafted or important side branches.

Suction Stabilizers

Suction stabilizers limit the need for pressure on the myocardium. On the other side, suction stabilizers are usually higher profile and may make the suturing more difficult. Hematomas and bleeding may occur if excessive suction is applied.

With all stabilizers position may be suddenly lost if positioning is not secure. This has been known to cause disruption of the surgical procedure and in some cases cardiac perforation by the prongs of the device.

Complications Due to Manipulation of the Aorta

Dissection of Aorta

One of the advantages of the OPCAB technique is reduced manipulation of the aorta making embolization less likely since neither cannulation nor cross clamping is necessary. As long as saphenous vein grafts are utilized, partial clamping is commonly used. CPB makes it possible to instantly change and control the aortic pressure thereby decreasing the tearing forces in the aorta. In OPCAB pressure control is more difficult, and if the partial clamp is applied while the pressure is high, dissection of the aorta might occur [22,23]. Expert anesthetic management may decrease the chance of such damage. Also a number of new devices have been developed to make partial clamping of aorta unnecessary. A brief description of these devices is presented later.

Embolization

We have demonstrated that stroke rates decrease in OPCAB [24], most likely secondary to decreased manipulation and instrumentation of the aorta. The inability to palpate and examine the aorta with low blood pressure, as can easily be done when CPB is used, may make it easier to overlook major aortic plaques during OPCAB. This may be one of the reasons that stroke rates have not been consistently reduced compared to on-pump CABG. Epi-aortic scanning [25], use of other imaging methods and use of non-clamp techniques for proximal anastomosis may reduce the embolization from the aorta [26]. Total arterial OPCAB revascularization with aortic non-touch technique has shown to result in the lowest stroke rates following CABG.

Complications Due to Alternative Surgical Approaches

MIDCAB or LAST Procedures

The MIDCAB operation represents an attractive alternative for revascularization of the LAD. It has lost popularity due to the increasingly efficient percutanous stenting procedures. The procedure still is an attractive alternative for the revascularization of isolated totally obstructed, symptomatic LAD disease.

The operation is relatively difficult and the harvesting of the LIMA may be challenging. The LIMA is usually not harvested in its full length and may therefore be short since the LAD is generally grafted quite distally. Avulsion of the LIMA at the anastomotic site has been reported [27,28]. Other complications reported from this procedure include chylothorax secondary to damage to the thoracic duct and herniation of the heart due to the opening of the pericardium. Phrenic nerve damage has also been reported.

The endoscopic harvesting of LIMA combined with minimally invasive or robotic creation of the LIMA to LAD anastomosis represents an attractive option for surgeons familiar with thoracoscopic cardiac surgery.

Left Thoracotomy Approach to the Circumflex Coronary Artery

This approach is attractive in previous revascularized patients where the main problem is related to the circumflex coronary [29,30]. A left thoracotomy offers excellent exposure to the circumflex artery. The proximal anastomosis is usually performed to the descending thoracic aorta. The main complications of such an operation are related to the difficulty assessing graft length [31] and unexpected severity of aortic atherosclerosis which may cause early obstruction or massive distal embolization. Hemodynamic instability and need for conversion to CPB may be challenging from a left thoracotomy approach and may require femoral arterial and venous cannulation which may be difficult or even impossible unless the patient is properly positioned. Diffuse arteriosclerosis may also be a major problem in such cases.

Complications from the Use of Anastomotic Devices

The development of proximal and distal anastomotic devices was supposed to greatly facilitate OPCAB performed by traditional or thoracoscopic / robotic approaches [32]. Such devices have unfortunately been found to have their own specific complications. A proximal anastomotic device that does not require partial clamping of the aorta could potentially decrease the amount of embolization when saphenous veins are attached to the aorta. However, it has been reported that thrombosis inside the connector is common and that embolization does not decrease when the device is utilized [33,34]. This occurs in the OPCAB setting in which such a connector would be most valuable [35]. Although connectors with improved design have shown to achieve better results [36], their use has not become widespread.

Hypothermia

OPCAB, especially when performed with sternotomy, may rapidly lead to significant hypothermia particularly if the operating room is cold and the operation lasts over a prolonged period. We experienced significant hypothermic episodes during our early implementation of the OPCAB program in Buffalo before starting to use active warming of infusion solutions and surface warming of the skin. The efficacy of surface warming has been obvious to us and proven in controlled studies [37]. Management of patient temperature is also relevant because of its importance in the avoidance of bleeding.

Conclusion

The performance of CABG without CPB is an old idea, which was revived in the early 90's and gained variable popularity around the world. Some centers have adopted OPCAB as the primary surgical method of revascularization, while other groups never adopted or abandoned attempts to introduce the procedure.

It seems clear to these authors that OPCAB performed by an expertly trained team of anesthetic and surgical personnel, can produce the best results for patients in need of surgical revascularization. The need to follow a systematic approach is necessary and OPCAB must not be performed as standard CABG by just eliminating CPB.

Although the benefits of OPCAB may be small in low risk and younger patients, the benefits in older patients with diffuse arteriosclerosis or other risk factors, may indeed be significant. A systematic approach is then however essential and avoidance of serious complications a must. Using a selective approach i.e. the application of OPCAB only in high-risk patients is probably unwise, because the team will be inadequately trained and routines less established.

Conversion to CPB in OPCAB is undesirable and associated with poor outcomes. Especially poor are the results of what we label "double conversion", where patients scheduled to have on-pump CABG are found to have intraoperative contraindication(s) to CPB. When such patients are then operated with OPCAB, but due to technical problems or lack of experience converted back to on-pump CABG, results are often disastrous.

In our opinion, OPCAB represents the best option for surgical coronary revascularization. Ideally the operation should be performed with arterial grafts and without manipulation of the aorta. In case aorta must be manipulated, epi-aortic scanning should be performed. Grafts must routinely be checked intraoperatively for patency by TTFM or other suitable technique.

An expert team is necessary, and evidence based protocols must be used for perioperative management if the full potential of OPCAB should be realized.

REFERENCES

[1] Kolesov, E. V. Preoperative checking of IMA(s): to do or not to do? *Eur. J. Cardiothorac. Surg*. 2000;17:190-1.

[2] Kolesov, V. I., Kolesov, E. V. Twenty years' results with internal thoracic artery-coronary artery anastomosis. *J. Thorac. Cardiovasc. Surg*. 1991;101:360-1.

[3] Olearchyk, A. S., Vasilii I. Kolesov, A pioneer of coronary revascularization by internal mammary-coronary artery grafting. *J. Thorac. Cardiovasc. Surg*. 1988;96:13-8.

[4] Benetti, F. Off pump coronary surgery in Argentina. *Sem. Thorac. Cardiovasc. Surg*. 2002;14:328-33.

[5] Buffolo, E., Branco, J. N., Gerola, L. R., Aguiar, L. F., Teles, C. A., Palma, J. H., et al. Off-pump myocardial revascularization: critical analysis of 23 years' experience in 3,866 patients. *Ann. Thorac. Surg*. 2006;81:85-9.

[6] Raja, S. G., Dreyfus, G. D. Impact of off-pump coronary artery bypass surgery on postoperative bleeding: current best available evidence. *J. Card. Surg*. 2006;21:35-41.

[7] Gundry, S. R., Romano, M. A., Shattuck, O. H., Razzouk, A. J., Bailey, L. L. Seven-year follow-up of coronary artery bypasses performed with and without cardiopulmonary bypass. *J. Thorac. Cardiovasc. Surg*. 1998:1273-7.

[8] Khan, N. E., De Souza, A., Mister, R., Flather, M., Clague, J., Davies, S., et al. A randomized comparison of off-pump and on-pump multivessel coronary-artery bypass surgery. *N Eng. J. Med*. 2004;350:21-8.

[9] D'Ancona, G., Donias, H. W., Karamanoukian, R. L., Bergsland, J., Karamanoukian, H. L. OPCAB therapy survey: off-pump clopidogrel, aspirin or both therapy survey. *Heart Surg. Forum*. 2001;4:354-8.

[10] Mujanovic, E., Nurkic, M., Caluk, J., Terzic, I., Kabil, E., Bergsland, J. The effect of combined clopidogrel and aspirin therapy after off-pump coronary surgery. *Innovations*. 2009;4:265-8.

[11] Vavuranakis, M., Latsios, G., Aggelis, D., Bosinakou, I., Karambelas, I., Tousoulis, D., et al. Randomized comparison of the effects of ASA plus clopidogrel versus ASA alone on early platelet activation in acute coronary syndromes with elevated high-sensitivity C-reactive protein and soluble CD40 ligand levels. *Clin. Therap*. 2006;28:860-71.

[12] Vallely, M. P., Bannon, P. G., Bayfield, M. S., Hughes, C. F., Kritharides, L. Quantitative and temporal differences in coagulation, fibrinolysis and platelet activation after on-pump and off-pump coronary artery bypass surgery. *Heart Lung Circ*. 2009;18:123-30.

[13] Poston, R., Gu, J., Brown, J., Gammie, J., White, C., Manchio, J., et al. Hypercoagulability affecting early vein graft patency does not exist after off-pump coronary artery bypass. *J. Cardiothorac. Vasc. Anesth*. 2005;19:11-8.

[14] Ambrosetti, M., Salerno, M., Zambelli, M., Mastropasqua, F., Tramarin, R., Pedretti, R. F. Deep vein thrombosis among patients entering cardiac rehabilitation after coronary artery bypass surgery. *Chest* 2004;125:191-6.

[15] Soltoski, P., Salerno, T., Levinsky, L., Schmid, S., Hasnain, S., Diesfeld, T., et al. Conversion to cardiopulmonary bypass in off-pump coronary artery bypass grafting: its effect on outcome. *J. Card. Surg*. 1998;13:328-34.

[16] Mujanovic, E., Kabil, E., Hadziselimovic, M., Softic, M., Azabagic, A., Bergsland, J. Conversions in off-pump coronary surgery. *Heart Surg. Forum*. 2003;6:135-7.

[17] Kessler, P., Aybek, T., Neidhart, G., Dogan, S., Lischke, V., Bremerich, D. H., et al. Comparison of three anesthetic techniques for off-pump coronary artery bypass grafting: general anesthesia, combined general and high thoracic epidural anesthesia, or high thoracic epidural anesthesia alone. *J. Cardiothorac. Vasc. Anesth*. 2005;19:32-9.

[18] D'Ancona, G., Karamanoukian, H., Ricci, M., Kawaguchi, A., Bergsland, J., Salerno, T. Myocardial revascularization on the beating heart after recent onset of acute myocardial infarction. *Heart Surg. Forum*. 2001;4:74-9.

[19] Bergsland, J., Lingaas, P. S., Skulstad, H., Hol, P. K., Halvorsen, P. S., Andersen, R., et al. Intracoronary shunt prevents ischemia in off-pump coronary artery bypass surgery. *Ann. Thorac. Surg*. 2009;87:54-60.

[20] D'Ancona, G., Karamanoukian, H. L., Ricci, M., Schmid, S., Bergsland, J., Salerno, T. A. Graft revision after transit time flow measurement in off-pump coronary artery bypass grafting. *Eur. J. Cardiothorac. Surg*. 2000;17:287-93.

[21] D'Ancona, G., Karamanoukian, H. L., Salerno, T. A., Schmid, S., Bergsland, J. Flow measurement in coronary surgery. *Heart Surg. Forum*. 1999;2:121-4.

[22] Tabry, I. F., Costantini, E. M. Acute aortic dissection early after off-pump coronary surgery: true frequency underestimated? *Tex. Heart Inst. J*. 2009;36:462-7.

[23] Chavanon, O., Carrier, M., Cartier, R., Hebert, Y., Pellerin, M., Page, P., et al. Increased incidence of acute ascending aortic dissection with off-pump aortocoronary bypass surgery? *Ann. Thorac. Surg*. 2001;71:117-21.

[24] Bergsland, J., Hasnain, S., Lajos, T. Z., Salerno, T. A. Elimination of cardiopulmonary bypass: a prime goal in reoperative coronary artery bypass surgery. *Eur. J. Cardiothorac. Surg*. 1998;14:59-62.

[25] Zingone, B., Rauber, E., Gatti, G., Pappalardo, A., Benussi, B., Dreas, L., et al. The impact of epiaortic ultrasonographic scanning on the risk of perioperative stroke. *Eur. J. Cardiothorac. Surg*. 2006;29:720-8.

[26] Douglas, J. M., Jr., Spaniol, S. E. A multimodal approach to the prevention of postoperative stroke in patients undergoing coronary artery bypass surgery. *Am. J. Surg*. 2009;197:587-90.

[27] Viel, G., Balmaceda, U., Sperhake, J. P. Avulsion of the left internal mammary artery graft after minimally invasive coronary surgery: fatal complication or medical error? A case report. *Med. Sci. Law* 2009;49:60-4.

[28] McMahon, J., Bergsland, J., Arani, D. T., Salerno, T. A. Avulsion of the left internal mammary artery after minimally invasive coronary bypass. *Ann. Thorac. Surg*. 1997;63:843-4.

[29] Grosner, G., Lajos, T. Z., Schimert, G., Bergsland, J. Left thoracotomy reoperation for coronary artery disease. *J. Card. Surg*. 1990;5:304-8.

[30] Lajos, T. Z., Akhter, M., Bergsland, J., Grosner, G., Lewin, A. N., Salerno, T. A., et al. Limited access left thoracotomy for reoperative coronary artery disease: on or off pump. *J. Card. Surg*. 2000;15:291-5.

[31] St. Goar, F. G., Fann, J. I., Komtebedde, J., Foster, E., Oz, M. C., Fogarty, T. J., et al. Endovascular edge-to-edge mitral valve repair: short-term results in a porcine model. *Circulation* 2003;108:1990-3.

[32] Bonilla, L. F., Sullivan, D. J. New approaches for vascular anastomoses. *Current Interv. Cardiol. Rep*. 2001;3:44-9.

[33] Skjelland, M., Bergsland, J., Lundblad, R., Lingaas, P. S., Rein, K. A., Halvorsen, S., et al. Cerebral microembolization during off-pump coronary artery bypass surgery with the Symmetry aortic connector device. *J. Thorac. Cardiovasc. Surg*. 2005;130:1581-5.

[34] Skjelland, M., Michelsen, A., Brosstad, F., Svennevig, J. L., Brucher, R., Russell, D. Solid cerebral microemboli and cerebrovascular symptoms in patients with prosthetic heart valves. *Stroke* 2008;39:1159-64.

[35] Bergsland, J., Hol, P. K., Lingas, P. S., Lundblad, R., Rein, K. A., Andersen, R., et al. Intraoperative and intermediate-term angiographic results of coronary artery bypass surgery with Symmetry proximal anastomotic device. *J. Thorac. Cardiovasc. Surg*. 2004;128:718-23.

[36] Puskas, J. D., Halkos, M. E., Balkhy, H., Caskey, M., Connolly, M., Crouch, J., et al. Evaluation of the PAS-Port Proximal Anastomosis System in coronary artery bypass surgery (the EPIC trial). *J. Thorac. Cardiovasc. Surg*. 2009;138:125-32.

[37] Kim, J. Y., Shinn, H., Oh, Y. J., Hong, Y. W., Kwak, H. J., Kwak, Y. L. The effect of skin surface warming during anesthesia preparation on preventing redistribution hypothermia in the early operative period of off-pump coronary artery bypass surgery. *Eur. J. Cardiothorac. Surg*. 2006;29:343-7.

In: Off-Pump Coronary Artery Bypass Grafting
Editors: S.G. Raja and M. Amrani
ISBN 978-1-62081-575-5

Chapter 22

STRATEGIC FORCES INFLUENCING THE ADOPTION OF OFF-PUMP CORONARY ARTERY BYPASS GRAFTING

Michael Simmons,[1] Dinesh Kurian[2] and Robert S. Poston[3]

[1]Research Associate, University of Arizona College of Medicine, Tucson, AZ, US
[2]Research Associate, Boston University, Boston, MA, US
[3]Chief Division of Cardiothoracic Surgery,
Jack G. Copeland Endowed Chair of Cardiovascular Surgery,
Michael Drummond Distinguished Professor of Cardiovascular and Thoracic Surgery,
University of Arizona, Tucson, AZ, US

ABSTRACT

Despite increasing competition from percutaneous interventions and other novel methods of non-surgical coronary revascularization, coronary artery bypass grafting (CABG) remains one of the most definitive and durable treatments for coronary artery disease, especially for patients with extensive and diffuse disease. In recent years the CABG procedure itself has undergone innovation and evolution. Off-pump coronary artery bypass (OPCAB) grafting is one such innovation. The available evidence from a large number of randomized clinical trials, nonrandomized clinical trials, propensity-matched analyses, and experimental data suggests that outcomes are comparable between off-pump and on-pump CABG and that OPCAB may have disctinct advantages for specific patient populations, but skepticism still exists about the safety and efficacy of the off-pump technique, preventing universal adoption of OPCAB grafting. This chapter examines the strategic forces influencing the adoption of off-pump, limited-access, and robotic-assisted CABG.

INTRODUCTION

The late 1990's saw an increased interest in performing off-pump coronary artery bypass (OPCAB) surgery. Proponents of the technique pointed to early excellent results from experts and touted it as a better way to perform coronary artery bypass. The suggestion was that operating without the use of the cardiopulmonary bypass pump mitigates post-operative morbidities such as cerebral dysfunction, systemic inflammatory response, and perioperative myocardial depression [1]. Accordingly, OPCAB performance rates steadily increased until they peaked at about 30% of all CABG performed in the US annually.

More recently, there has been a growing sense that OPCAB has failed to deliver on its promise of being the next great innovation in cardiovascular surgery. Well-planned and powered studies such as the ROOBY study [2,3], which concluded in 2008, compared OPCAB to on-pump, conventional coronary artery bypass surgery (CCAB). This study demonstrated strong evidence that long-term outcomes were improved with CCAB including a greater completeness of revascularization and superior one-year graft patency. While surgical experience with OPCAB may have played a role in the results of the ROOBY study [3,4], the results were generally accepted as not favorable to OPCAB and the proportion of these cases performed in the US subsequently declined to around 15%.

While the clinical debate about these techniques remains ongoing, the future of OPCAB is tied to how pertinent stakeholders determine its value in comparison to CCAB. A modern healthcare definition of value for a surgical procedure is the quotient of improved outcomes it yields divided by the difference in costs [5]. A consensus of the surgical literature suggests that OPCAB provides discrete clinical benefits over CCAB, particularly for high risk patients, as well as documented cost advantages [6,7]. While this would seem to confirm that OPCAB provides added value, the lack of wide spread adoption for this procedure suggests that other market forces are playing an important role.

A five-forces analysis of competitive environment is a standard tool used in investigating new procedures and/or products in other commercial industries [8]. Applying this framework to OPCAB reveals a procedure characterized by important weaknesses including a high threat of substitutes amongst competitors as well as suppliers and buyers with significant bargaining power. Its strengths are its appeal to specific segments of the myocardial revascularization market and important (albeit moderate) barriers to entry from competitors due to its learning curve.

Off-pump techniques can also be used during minimally invasive, robot-assisted coronary artery bypass surgery (RCAB) [9-11]. Although the long-term clinical outcomes following RCAB remain to be established, many studies support its economic value, showing suitable short-term outcomes [12] and improved resource utilization [13]. An important question for RCAB is the strategic strength of this procedure within the myocardial revascularization market. The five-forces analysis of RCAB shows that in comparison to OPCAB, it heightens barriers to entry for surgical competitors, targets additional key segments of the revascularization market that might not otherwise be considered for surgical referral, and fosters positive-sum competition—a form of competition that expands the industry's profit-potential and is characteristic of healthy markets. Moreover, the use of RCAB in concert with percutaneous revascularization techniques (i.e. hybrid procedure) encourages cooperation with supplier segments by capitalizing on complementary services that they provide. As a result, RCAB has the potential to deliver on the unfulfilled promises of OPCAB as a major innovation within cardiovascular surgery because of these market forces.

ANALYSIS OF THE COMPETITIVE ENVIRONMENT OF OPCAB

A five forces analysis is a framework proposed by Porter for analyzing the strategic position of a particular product or service within the competitive milieu of its industry [8]. The five competitive forces are (1) the threat of new entrants; (2) the threat of substitutes; (3) the bargaining power of suppliers; (4) the bargaining power of buyers; and (5) rivalry amongst existing competitors (Figure 1). Several definitions are necessary to apply this framework to the OPCAB industry:

- Providers of OPCAB: cardiothoracic surgeons
- Suppliers: cardiologists
- Substitutes: CCAB, percutaneous techniques performed by interventional cardiologists
- Buyers: patients, insurance providers

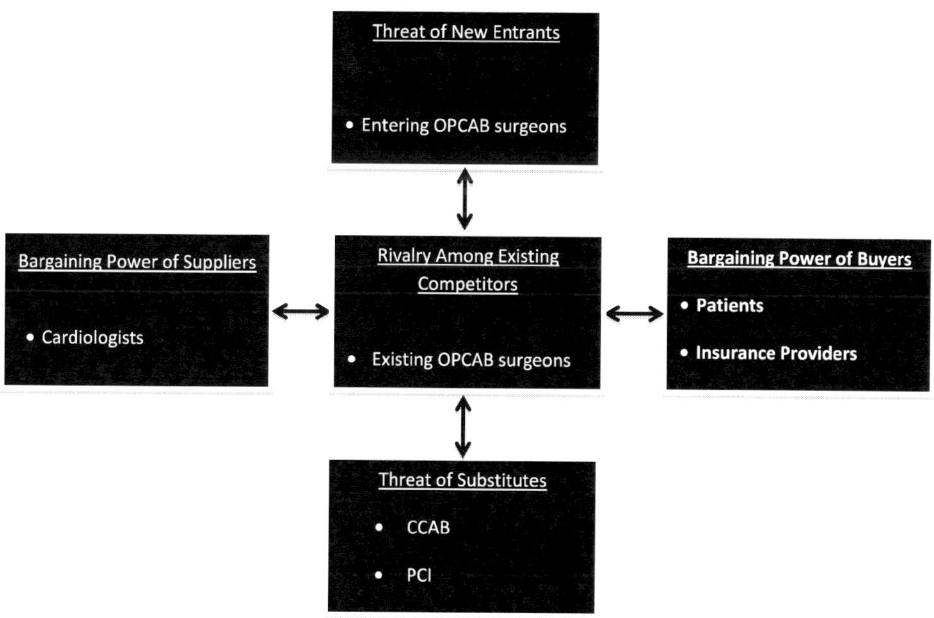

CCAB = conventional coronary artery bypass grafting ; OPCAB = off-pump coronary artery bypass grafting ; PCI = percutaneous coronary intervention.

Figure 1. The five competitive forces shaping the OPCAB industry.

I. Threat of New Entrants

Graduates of cardiac surgery fellowships and existing cardiac surgeons who wish to perform this procedure are new entrants. They can be hindered from developing careers in

OPCAB by important entry barriers, which provide advantages to incumbent surgeons, including: (1) demand-side benefits of scale; (2) the leverage of the learning curve; and (3) first-mover advantage [8].

Demand-side benefits of scale. Evidence suggests that experienced OPCAB surgeons yield superior outcomes than those with less experience. As a result, experience with this procedure provides a surgeon with appeal to patients and referring providers, often influencing demand. In situations where a surgeon's annual volume correlates with increased demand for OPCAB, this creates a barrier to entry referred to as demand-side benefits of scale. Demand-side benefits of scale discourage entry by limiting referrals to newcomers.

Leverage of the learning curve. A steep learning curve provides a sustainable advantage for the earliest entrant into industries where learning is kept proprietary. Knowledge about learning processes in cardiac surgery is made public for ethical reasons. However, surgeons that are learning OPCAB do not possess equivalent skill in handling complex, higher-risk cases or for patients requiring more than three grafts [14]. Poor outcomes can result from the learning curve for this procedure. Recent requirements for public reporting of CABG results put the developing program at a major disadvantage given the possibility of bad outcomes while learning on patients referred for bypass surgery that have increasingly high risk profiles [15,16]. Established OPCAB surgeons, on the other hand, have greater confidence to provide their service to a wider segment of the current market, creating an even greater barrier to entry.

First-mover advantages. Incumbent surgeons that were the first to provide OPCAB within a region often enjoy first-mover advantages over secondary entrants. Being the first to provide a novel procedure within a catchment area helps establish relationships with interested providers that might not otherwise have considered referring to the surgeon's hospital. Once established, these relationships can be hard to disrupt. Incumbents further reinforce this advantage by setting working relationships with hospital and surgery staff that efficiently deliver this service and by promoting brand identity and word-of-mouth reputation as the experts in this procedure. This status provides disproportionate access to patients that seek out options for their healthcare. These "quality seeking" patients are often well-educated [17], low-risk for surgical complications and have insurance plans that pay higher percentages of charges than other patient segments. These low-risk patients are the most suitable types of patients for learning OPCAB. However, they are often not available to surgeons that are not the first movers within a region.

It should be noted that OPCAB is a stagnant industry. In the past 10 years, the total proportion of patients with coronary artery disease that have been treated with CABG has declined from around 400,000/year to 220,000/year with only 15% of those cases performed off-pump. Moreover, recent evidence supports CCAB as an adequate and possibly superior substitute for OPCAB [2]. This is likely to reduce the threat of new entrants because the resources required to complete the learning curve are hard to justify in light of the marginal strategic benefit provided by an OPCAB program. In order to maintain market share under these circumstances, incumbents tend to strengthen the barriers to entry in the face of falling demand by emphasizing all of their advantages (and disadvantages of potential competitors) to consumers and suppliers.

II. Threat of Substitutes

Substitutes for OPCAB are the various alternate ways of performing myocardial revascularization, including CCAB and percutaneous coronary intervention (PCI). OPCAB in general has pros and cons in relation to these other options but may have a distinctive advantage in women, patients with high-grade atherosclerosis, and elderly patients with high levels of co-morbidities [4,18,19]. Many surgeons focus OPCAB only on patient segments that stand to benefit most, a strategy that greatly narrows the range of acceptable substitutes for OPCAB and is consistent with the principles of healthy market competition [20]. However, the technical complexity of OPCAB makes it difficult for many surgeons to maintain excellent results when performing this procedure only on a small subset of their most challenging cases. These surgeons prefer to utilize OPCAB on all cases unless there is an important reason to use cardiopulmonary bypass (e.g. hemodynamic instability) so that their skills and the comfort level of the team are well-rehearsed.

III. Bargaining Power of Suppliers

Cardiologists are powerful suppliers for two reasons: (1) they credibly compete with OPCAB surgeons through offering PCI; and (2) they do not depend heavily on OPCAB surgeons for revenue.

Interventional cardiologists provide significant competition to OPCAB even in segments of patients that have established mortality benefits from CABG compared to PCI. Recent focus on patient-centered care reinforces the cardiologists' right to offer and the patients' right to choose any acceptable option if it better meets the unique personal needs of the patient and their family. The reality of cardiologists providing the preferred intervention for most patients with coronary artery disease and serving as the gatekeeper for surgical referrals provides them with substantial bargaining power over OPCAB surgeons. It should be noted, however, that cardiologists have a professional obligation to refer patients for OPCAB when there is a clear health benefit for doing so. OPCAB surgeons benefit strategically from emphasizing the unique applicability of off-pump surgery to women, patients with high-grade atherosclerosis, and elderly patients with high levels of co-morbidities. This education of referring providers often occurs during local outreach efforts.

IV. Bargaining Power of Buyers

The US healthcare industry has a split system of buyers; patients are the true "customers" who provide consent regarding providers and treatment sought, and insurance providers make the actual payment for services. The bargaining power of these two related buyer segments in relation to the OPCAB industry is currently in favor of insurance providers. However, this balance of power is changing as individual patients gain access to understandable information about medical services and clinical outcomes of the various options and providers available to them.

Insurance providers. Insurance providers function as an intermediary between patients, who often cannot pay the total cost of their operation up-front, and surgeons, who rarely receive out-of-pocket payment directly from patients for their services. This role allows insurance companies to function as gatekeepers and price setters. Insurance providers have negatively influenced the growth of OPCAB by establishing payment policies that do not reflect the unique benefits of OPCAB over CCAB regardless of patient comorbidities. As a result, it is easy for companies to cut OPCAB surgeons from their provider networks if they do not agree to the same contract terms as CCAB. The greater technical skill required to complete OPCAB successfully in high-risk patients is not recognized by reimbursement strategies.

Patients. Until recently, many patients have been uninformed or under-informed on the nuances of medical treatment options. In addition, decisions regarding surgical coronary arterial revascularization are often made under duress. These patients constitute a weak buyer group with potentially compromised autonomy. It is a commonly accepted ethical principle that individuals with compromised autonomy are entitled to protection [21]. CABG surgeons have an ethical obligation to protect vulnerable patients through such means as the public reporting of outcomes through the Internet and letting patients know that this information is available. Providing this information gives strength to patients as a buyer group while promoting healthy competition based on quality [20]. The elderly are a rapidly growing Internet user group that is highly interested in accessing health information online [17,22]. Since OPCAB procedures have specific appeal to elderly populations, public reporting on the Internet could help raise patient interest in the procedure in the future.

V. Rivalry amongst Existing Competitors

The rivalry of cardiac surgeons competing with other cardiac surgeons is understood by its *intensity* and *basis of competition* [8]. The intensity is often high because CABG volumes and the proportion of cases performed via OPCAB have been declining and groups that perform OPCAB are often equal in size and/or influence. These circumstances create a "zero-sum rivalry" where surgeons are only able to increase their case-load volume by poaching potential cases from other surgeons. Few patients are willing to travel great distances for OPCAB surgery, which serves to keep the competition local and aggravate the rivalry. OPCAB providers can alter the *basis* on which they compete with each other and CCAB surgeons by participating in public reporting of their outcomes [8]. When certain groups attempt to meet the needs of unique patient populations that benefit the most from OPCAB and raise awareness that this option is available, this fosters healthy, "positive-sum" competition amongst cardiac surgeons to be able to report the best outcomes.

RCAB Competitive Positioning

Performing OPCAB with robotic assistance (RCAB) allows for the use of a sternal-sparing incision. This approach is highly attractive to patients, which enhances its competitive positioning within the industry compared to OPCAB via a sternotomy in two main ways:

1 RCAB heightens barriers to entry, giving surgeons an even greater first-mover advantage than OPCAB via a sternotomy;
2 RCAB repositions the competitive field compared to PCI, thus altering the bargaining power of an influential supplier and creating the potential for positive-sum competition.

Barriers to Entry

Learning curve. Numerous studies have demonstrated a demanding learning curve for RCAB that can last through as many as 100 cases [23-26]. In addition, this type of high-profile innovation provokes important organizational challenges that require close attention in order to create sustainable success. These complex challenges increase the barriers to entry for RCAB in comparison to OPCAB, enhancing its first-mover advantage. Another issue is that patients who are low-risk for CABG are more likely to discuss options with their providers regarding different surgeons, as opposed to high-risk patients who may be forced to make decisions and accept the *status quo* under duress. Established RCAB providers generally attract greater numbers of these patients because of their experience. This leaves subsequent surgeons wishing to learn RCAB with few low-risk surgery opportunities, further complicating their learning curve and making it difficult to establish a practice in this area (Figure 2).

Supply-side economies of scale. The acquisition costs of a robot and additional expenses from the learning curve for RCAB can be a substantial barrier to entry, especially in light of declining reimbursement for CABG in the last decade. Such expense can be difficult for cardiac programs to justify unless it fits the center's global strategy. After getting through the learning curve period, we have found that RCAB initiates superior reimbursement from insurance companies from two sources:

1 Improved payer mix. By appealing to younger patient populations that are actively employed and seeking out their best options, RCAB attracts patients who generally have private insurance (Blue Cross, UnitedHealth, etc.). These insurers reimburse providers with a higher percentage of charges for their services than Medicare—the most common insurer of aged populations.
2 Pay for performance. RCAB can bring greater reimbursement from Medicare because it raises patient satisfaction levels, which Medicare awards through a new value-based purchasing program that was initiated on 7/1/2011. In addition, it allows surgeons to avoid costly never-events such as sternal infection that are not reimbursed and have estimated hospital costs that range from $20K to $80K per patient [27]. Since RCAB spares the sternum entirely, this risk is eliminated in these cases.

Competitive Positioning Relative to Cardiologists

CABG for triple vessel coronary artery disease has demonstrated superiority over PCI in terms of major adverse cardiac or cerebrovascular events (MACCE) at one year [28,29].

Despite this finding, CABG rates have significantly decreased in lieu of complex multi-vessel PCI over the past decade [30]. A variety of factors help explain these trends, but an obvious thesis is that patients prefer less invasiveness and the faster recovery associated with PCI.

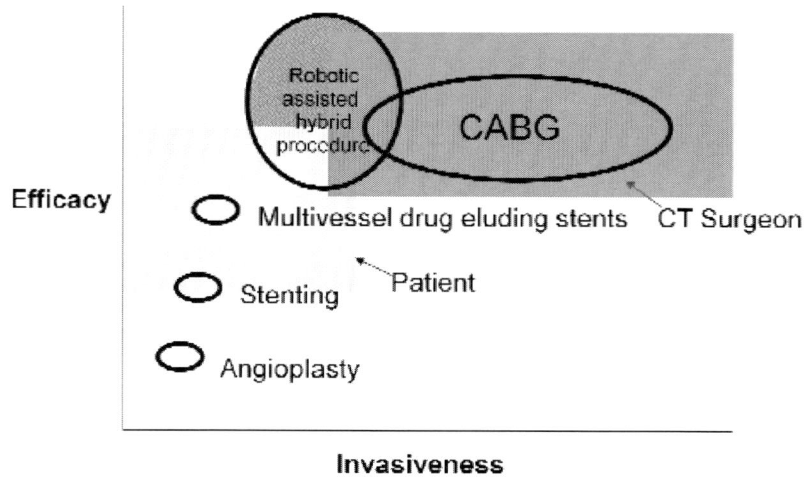

Figure 2. Patient/surgeon comfort zones. Although angioplasty and stenting are not as effective as CABG in treating multi-vessel CAD, the procedures are still very appealing to patients because of their high efficacy/invasiveness ratio. RCAB also appeals to patients because it delivers similar efficacy to CABG at a much lower level of invasiveness.

Such strong patient preference for less invasive treatment options prevents the referral of many patients for cardiac surgery even in specific cases where it might have significant clinical merit over multivessel PCI [31,32] By enabling the left internal thoracic artery (LITA) to be grafted onto the left anterior descending coronary artery (LAD), RCAB spares the sternum while providing the most optimal long-term treatment for LAD stenosis [33,34]. When such a procedure is available, cardiologists may feel a greater professional obligation to thoroughly discuss alternatives to PCI because the assumption that patients would not be interested in knowing about surgical alternatives prior to undergoing PCI becomes more difficult to defend.

In addition to improving the chances that patients will be provided a more thorough discussion of their available options, RCAB encourages cooperation with cardiologists by promoting a new form of collaboration called the hybrid procedure. For this approach, both RCAB and PCI are used to address a patient with multi-vessel CAD. Hybrid procedures exploit the long-term revascularization benefit of the LIMA to LAD graft, and then utilize stents to substitute for saphenous vein grafting of non-LAD targets, which have been demonstrated to have an incidence of total occlusion at 1 year as high as 30-40% [35]. Initial studies of the hybrid procedure have demonstrated that it is a feasible and cost-effective form of revascularization that may lead to significantly fewer complications and allow for faster recovery [36-38].

The hybrid procedure provides strategic advantages that are not available to surgeons that only perform OPCAB via sternotomy. While the hybrid approach can be used with CABG procedures performed via full sternotomy, the strongest rationale for this strategy is to extend the benefits of RCAB to a larger number of patients than would be possible without PCI. The hybrid procedure allows RCAB surgeons to mitigate some of the disadvantage of having to compete with the gatekeepers of the patients for referrals. By creating a partnership through the hybrid procedure, RCAB surgeons may enjoy a stronger referral relationship with cardiologists than other cardiac surgeons because the hybrid procedure can increase the cardiologists' profitability potential. Involvement in hybrid cases can distinguish cardiologists within their own field just like RCAB distinguishes surgeons in the OPCAB industry. These benefits come at the price of accepting some reliance on RCAB surgeons. The ultimate result of this relationship is that RCAB surgeons gain bargaining power with cardiologists, while both surgeon and cardiologist alike benefit from offering an effective and distinctive service that patients value.

Positive-Sum Competition

An encouraging aspect of RCAB is that it fosters positive-sum competition with PCI for addressing the healthcare needs of patients in a manner that CABG via sternotomy was not able to do. Obese individuals [39], diabetic individuals, and selected patients who have undergone previous cardiac surgery [40] demonstrate significant clinical advantages of avoiding a full sternotomy. Actively employed individuals with 1-2 vessel disease are among the populations to which RCAB has the most appeal because of the improvements in recovery time. We have seen these patients demonstrate the willingness to travel significant distances to undergo RCAB. This extends the benefit of positive-sum competition to well outside the typical catchment area served by any given hospital.

Survival and early recovery. Although data on clinical outcomes are preliminary, RCAB appears to offer the same or improved early outcomes for mortality and morbidity and identical graft patency [41] compared to OPCAB, with no worsening in results when employing cardiopulmonary bypass via peripheral access [42] (Table 1). Both quality of life in the early phase after surgery and time to return to normal functional status are found to be considerably improved by RCAB [43]. Of note, patients who required conversion to sternotomy CABG did not show any difference in outcomes to patients originally assigned to the sternotomy group [41]. At one year, patient satisfaction and the risk of major adverse cardiac and cerebrovascular events are improved in RCAB patients [12], though totally endoscopic coronary artery bypass (a sub-segment of RCAB) demonstrated a lower rate of graft patency [44].

Differences in cost. Although the additional parts required to use the surgical robot may pose higher up-front costs, there is considerable opportunity to save on costs down the road. Direct costs for RCAB may be higher than sternotomy CABG (approx. $1,000), and the costs will often be higher during the learning curve (typically owing to longer operative time – approx. $5,000) [13]. Nevertheless, subsequent to completion of the learning curve, costs will be saved indirectly through decreased length of stay in the ICU, decreased length of stay on the hospital wards, and decreased use of blood products. Even after factoring in costs of robotic parts and PCI resources for the hybrid procedure, RCAB offers a favorable value proposition. Reductions in never events such as mediastinitis allow hospitals to capture a greater proportion of the reimbursement as contribution. More efficient bed utilization allows hospitals to increase their operational efficiency. Furthermore, the increase in patient satisfaction has value, as hospitals can avoid costly methods to improve satisfaction by the same amount via other strategies.

Table 1. A comparative outcomes measures framework comparing robotic assistance coronary artery bypass (RCAB) to full sternotomy coronary artery bypass grafting (CABG)

RCAB	Sternotomy CABG
Survival	
Same as Sternotomy CABG	Same as RCAB
Degree of recovery	
Identical graft patency to Sternotomy CABG	Identical graft patency to RCAB
Time to recovery	
Shorter time to recovery (2 to 3 weeks)	Typically, one-two months to return of normal activities
Disutility of care	
Improved cosmesis Decreased incidence of mediastinitis Reduced physiological and anatomical manipulation	Midline sternal scarring Risk for mediastinitis
Sustainability of recovery	
No difference in three year survival	No three year survival advantage
Long term consequencies of care	
Improved patient satisfaction Little available research on long term consequences such as cognitive changes	More available research on long term consequences such as cognitive changes

CONCLUSION

The OPCAB industry is characterized by relatively low barriers to entry, high threat of substitutes, strong suppliers and strong buyers. Its strengths rest in how it targets differentiated patient populations. RCAB is an adaptation of OPCAB that expands upon the patient value proposition of OPCAB while strategically enhancing the surgeons' competitive positioning within the myocardial revascularization industry. By offering the promise of improved patient outcomes, as well as more efficient resource utilization, RCAB has the potential to offer value to the field of cardiac revascularization.

REFERENCES

[1] Peterson, E. D., Mark, D. B. Off-Pump Bypass Surgery—Ready for the Big Dance? *JAMA* 2004;291:1897-9.

[2] Shroyer, A. L., Grover, F. L., Hattler, B., et al. On-pump versus off-pump coronary-artery bypass surgery. *N Engl. J. Med.* 2009;361:1827-37.

[3] Peterson, E. D. Innovation and comparative-effectiveness research in cardiac surgery. *New England Journal of Medicine* 2009;361:1897-9.

[4] Puskas, J. D., Edwards, F. H., Pappas, P. A., et al. Off-pump techniques benefit men and women and narrow the disparity in mortality after coronary bypass grafting. *Ann. Thorac. Surg*. 2007;84:1447-56.

[5] Porter, M. E. What is value in health care? *N Engl. J. Med.* 2010;363:2477-81.

[6] Schultz, S. C., Woodward, S., Ebra, G. Resource utilization in off-pump versus conventional coronary artery bypass grafting in a community hospital: a comparative analysis using propensity scoring. *Heart Surg. Forum*. 2011;14:E81-6.

[7] Sellke, F. W., DiMaio, J. M., Caplan, L. R., et al. Comparing on-Pump and off-pump coronary artery bypass grafting. *Circulation* 2005;111:2858-64.

[8] Porter, M. E. The five competitive forces that shape strategy. *Harvard Business Review* 2008;86:78-93.

[9] Damiano, R. J., Jr., Ehrman, W. J., Ducko, C. T., et al. Initial United States clinical trial of robotically assisted endoscopic coronary artery bypass grafting. *J. Thorac. Cardiovasc. Surg*. 2000;119:77-82.

[10] Carpentier, A., Loulmet, D., Aupecle, B., et al. [Computer assisted open heart surgery. First case operated on with success]. Comptes rendus de l'Academie des sciences Serie III, *Sciences de la vie* 1998;321:437-42.

[11] Modi, P., Rodriguez, E., Chitwood, W. R., Jr. Robot-assisted cardiac surgery. *Interact. CardioVasc. Thorac. Surg*. 2009;9:500-5.

[12] Sellke, F. W., Chu, L. M., Cohn, W. E. Current state of surgical myocardial revascularization. *Circ. J.* 2010;74:1031-7.

[13] Poston, R. S., Tran, R., Collins, M., et al. Comparison of economic and patient outcomes with minimally invasive versus traditional off-pump coronary artery bypass grafting techniques. *Ann. Surg*. 2008;248:638-46.

[14] Karagounis, A., Asimakopoulos, G., Niranjan, G., Valencia, O., Chandrasekaran, V. Complex off-pump coronary artery bypass surgery can be safely taught to cardiothoracic trainees. *Interact. Cardio Vasc. Thorac. Surg*. 2006;5:222-6.

[15] Parry, M., Arthur, H., Brooks, D., Groll, D., Pavlov, A. Measuring function in older adults with co-morbid illnesses who are undergoing coronary artery bypass graft (CABG) surgery. *Archives of gerontology and geriatrics* 2011 Jun. 28. [Epub ahead of print]

[16] Bridgewater, B., Grayson, A. D., Brooks, N., et al. Has the publication of cardiac surgery outcome data been associated with changes in practice in northwest England: an analysis of 25,730 patients undergoing CABG surgery under 30 surgeons over eight years. *Heart* 2007;93:744-8.

[17] Keenan, T. A. Patient Responsibility in Health Care: *An AARP Bulletin Survey*. 2011.

[18] Huffmyer, J., Raphael, J. The current status of off-pump coronary bypass surgery. *Curr. Opin. Anaesthesiol*. 2011;24:64-9.

[19] Puskas, J. D., Thourani, V. H., Kilgo, P., et al. Off-Pump coronary artery bypass disproportionately benefits high-risk patients. *Ann. Thorac. Surg*. 2009;88:1142-7.

[20] Porter, M. E., Teisberg, E. O. Redefining competition in health care. *Harv. Bus. Rev*. 2004;82:64-76, 136.

[21] Protection of human subjects; Belmont Report: notice of report for public comment. *Fed. Regist*. 1979;44:23191-7.

[22] Chu, A., Mastel-Smith, B. The outcomes of anxiety, confidence, and self-efficacy with Internet health information retrieval in older adults: a pilot study. *CIN* 2010;28:222-8.

[23] Oehlinger, A., Bonaros, N., Schachner, T., et al. Robotic endoscopic left internal mammary artery harvesting: what have we learned after 100 cases? *Ann. Thorac. Surg.* 2007;83:1030-4.

[24] Bonaros, N., Schachner, T., Wiedemann, D., et al. Closed chest hybrid coronary revascularization for multivessel disease - current concepts and techniques from a two-center experience. *Eur. J. Cardiothorac. Surg.* 2011;40:783-7.

[25] Novick, R. J., Fox, S. A., Kiaii, B. B., et al. Analysis of the learning curve in telerobotic, beating heart coronary artery bypass grafting: a 90 patient experience. *Ann. Thorac. Surg.* 2003;76:749-53.

[26] Desai, P. H., Tran, R., Steinwagner, T., Poston, R. S. Challenges of telerobotics in coronary bypass surgery. *Expert Rev. Med. Devices* 2010;7:165-8.

[27] Hollenbeak, C. S., Murphy, D. M., Koenig, S., Woodward, R. S., Dunagan, W. C., Fraser, V. J. The clinical and economic impact of deep chest surgical site infections following coronary artery bypass graft surgery. *Chest* 2000;118:397-402.

[28] Serruys, P. W., Morice, M. C., Kappetein, A. P., et al. Percutaneous coronary intervention versus coronary-artery bypass grafting for severe coronary artery disease. *N Engl. J. Med.* 2009;360:961-72.

[29] Marui, A., Kimura, T., Tanaka, S., Furukawa, Y., Kita, T., Sakata, R. Significance of off-pump coronary artery bypass grafting compared with percutaneous coronary intervention: a propensity score analysis. *Eur. J. Cardiothorac. Surg.* 2011 Jun. 13. [Epub ahead of print]

[30] Epstein, A. J., Polsky, D., Yang, F., Yang, L., Groeneveld, P. W. Coronary revascularization trends in the United States, 2001-2008. *JAMA* 2011;305:1769-76.

[31] Ribichini, F., Taggart, D. Implications of new ESC/EACTS guidelines on myocardial revascularization for patients with multivessel coronary artery disease. *Interact. Cardio Vasc. Thorac. Surg.* 2011;12:663-6.

[32] Kolh, P., Wijns, W., Danchin, N., et al. Guidelines on myocardial revascularization. *Eur. J. Cardiothorac. Surg.* 2010;38:S1-S52.

[33] Diegeler, A., Thiele, H., Falk, V., et al. Comparison of stenting with minimally invasive bypass surgery for stenosis of the left anterior descending coronary artery. *N Engl. J. Med.* 2002;347:561-6.

[34] Hueb, W. A., Soares, P. R., Almeida de Oliveira, S., et al. Five-Year Follow-Up of the Medicine, Angioplasty, or Surgery Study (MASS) : A Prospective, Randomized Trial of Medical Therapy, Balloon Angioplasty, or Bypass Surgery for Single Proximal Left Anterior Descending Coronary Artery Stenosis. *Circulation* 1999;100:II-107-II-13.

[35] Lee, M. S., Park, S.-J., Kandzari, D. E., et al. Saphenous vein graft intervention. *JACC: Cardiovascular Interventions* 2011;4:831-43.

[36] De Cannière, D., Jansens, J. L., Goldschmidt-Clermont, P., Barvais, L., Decroly, P., Stoupel, E. Combination of minimally invasive coronary bypass and percutaneous transluminal coronary angioplasty in the treatment of double-vessel coronary disease: Two-year follow-up of a new hybrid procedure compared with "on-pump" double bypass grafting. *Am. Heart J.* 2001;142:563-70.

[37] Kon, Z. N., Brown, E. N., Tran, R., et al. Simultaneous hybrid coronary revascularization reduces postoperative morbidity compared with results from

conventional off-pump coronary artery bypass. *J. Thorac. Cardiovasc. Surg.* 2008;135:367-75.

[38] Narasimhan, S., Srinivas, V. S., DeRose, J. J., Jr. Hybrid coronary revascularization: a review. *Cardiol. Rev.* 2011;19:101-7.

[39] Wiedemann, D., Schachner, T., Bonaros, N., et al. Does obesity affect operative times and perioperative outcome of patients undergoing totally endoscopic coronary artery bypass surgery? *Interact. Cardiovasc. Thorac. Surg.* 2009;9:214-7.

[40] Martens, T. P., Hefti, M. M., Kalimi, R., Smith, C. R., Argenziano, M. Robot-assisted off-pump minimally invasive reoperative coronary artery bypass grafting: case report. *Heart Surg. Forum.* 2004;7:E533-4.

[41] Atluri, P., Kozin, E. D., Hiesinger, W., Joseph Woo, Y. Off-pump, minimally invasive and robotic coronary revascularization yield improved outcomes over traditional on-pump CABG. *Int. J. Med. Robot* 2009;5:1-12.

[42] Argenziano, M., Katz, M., Bonatti, J., et al. Results of the prospective multicenter trial of robotically assisted totally endoscopic coronary artery bypass grafting. *Ann. Thorac. Surg.* 2006;81:1666-75.

[43] Bonaros, N., Schachner, T., Wiedemann, D., et al. Quality of life improvement after robotically assisted coronary artery bypass grafting. *Cardiology* 2009;114:59-66.

[44] Jegaden, O., Wautot, F., Sassard, T., et al. Is there an optimal minimally invasive technique for left anterior descending coronary artery bypass? *J. Cardiothorac. Surg.* 2011;6:37.

SECTION 3: CONTROVERSIES

In: Off-Pump Coronary Artery Bypass Grafting
Editors: S.G. Raja and M. Amrani
ISBN 978-1-62081-575-5

Chapter 23

SHUNT OR SNARE FOR OFF-PUMP CORONARY ARTERY BYPASS GRAFTING

Naresh Trehan,[1] Rajneesh Malhotra[2] and Udgeath Dhir[3]
[1]Chairman and Managing Director, Medanta Heart Institute, The Medicity, Gurgaon, India
[2]Director, Department of Cardiac Surgery, Medanta Heart Institute, The Medicity, Gurgaon, India
[3]Consultant Cardiac Surgeon, Department of Cardiac Surgery, Medanta Heart Institute, The Medicity, India

ABSTRACT

To avoid the harmful effects of cardiopulmonary bypass, off-pump coronary artery bypass (OPCAB) grafting is being increasingly used as an effective alternative to conventional coronary artery bypass grafting. Technological advancement has made off-pump coronary artery bypass safe and feasible. During OPCAB grafting, local vascular control of the target vessel and a bloodless field are crucial. Intraluminal shunts and snares are two modalities for vascular control during OPCAB grafting. Intraluminal shunts aim to achieve hemostasis at the arteriotomy site, provide a relative bloodless field, and allow antegrade flow to provide myocardial protection. On the other hand, snares provide bloodless surgical field with a state of relative ischemia during anastomosis. Debate is still unsettled whether to shunt or snare the target vessels during OPCAB grafting. This chapter provides an overview of the current evidence for and against the use of shunts and snares and attempts to resolve the controversy.

To raise new questions and new possibilities and to review old problems from a new angle requires creative imagination and marks real advance in Science.

Introduction

The continuous effort to improve clinical outcome and competition with non surgical methods of myocardial revascularization has led the cardiac surgical fraternity to critically scrutinize and evolve off -pump coronary artery bypass (OPCAB) grafting. Introduction of OPCAB grafting was associated with genuine concerns such as handling the heart for proper exposure of target vessel, adequate stabilization of the heart, vascular control and quality of distal anastomosis.

A dry and stable field is an essential prerequisite for precise distal coronary anastomosis which is a major goal of coronary artery bypass grafting (CABG). Technological advances over the past two decades have resolved the issue of stability [1-4]. However, the issue of how to best achieve vascular control and a dry operating field still remains unsettled. Snaring and intraluminal shunts (ILS) are the currently the two most common techniques used for vascular control.

Proponents of ILS claim their advantages in terms of providing a relatively bloodless field, hemodynamic stability and providing distal perfusion [5,6]. ILS help in construction of distal anastomosis by exposing the margins of artery and prevention of sewing of posterior wall. Though they were introduced in 1975 [7] their efficacy and safety has only been accepted in recent years.

Proponents of 'snaring' have their own rationale. Snares provide absolute bloodless field and endothelial damage is avoided. Secondarily the temporary ischemia during snaring does not cause significant metabolic changes. [8]

In order to resolve the controversy regarding "snaring" or "shunting", we objectively analyze the evidence from human studies for safety and efficacy of these two strategies for vascular control during OPCAB grafting.

Clinical Benefits

The clinical benefit of shunting was first documented by Luchetti et al. [9]. They evaluated the wall motion score index and ejection fraction (EF) using transesophageal echocardiography and found shunting to be beneficial in terms of hemodynamic stability. Similarly Menon et al. [10] found reduced ischemia and preserved left ventricular (LV) function when ILS were used.

Yeatman et al. [11] randomized 20 patients, each to shunting and snaring groups, who underwent elective CABG and had triple vessel disease with EF > 40%. Exclusion criteria included recent myocardial infarction (MI), emergency operations and reoperation. They demonstrated superiority of intraluminal shunting as there was marked deterioration in ventricular performance in snared vessels. In shunting group recovery was complete after 5 minutes of reperfusion but recovery was delayed in snared group. However there was no difference in mortality, perioperative MI, need for inotropes or intensive care unit (ICU) stay between the groups. Clearly, results of this study suggest that ILS provide benefit by way of better hemodynamics, preserved LV function and less myocardial ischemia. Shunting has protective effect against stunning while recovery is delayed in snaring group. There was not much difference in clinical outcomes as the LV function was near normal in both the groups.

Definitely there would be impact of ILS in patients with low EF, congestive heart failure, emergency or redo operations or any compromised state.

Endothelial Injury

Manipulation of human coronary arteries during off-pump operations leads to endothelial denudation and plaque rupture. In OPCAB surgery it occurs with snares [12], applications of bulldogs [13], mist – blower [14], and papaverine [15] solutions. Despite the aforementioned benefits intraluminal shunts may denude the endothelium and cause vessel damage, thrombosis or subsequent stenosis [16]. Several studies have been published to address the impact of coronary shunting and snaring on endothelial injury.

It is useful to consider the potential mechanism of injury in the two techniques. In general, snaring involves encircling target vessels with elastic silicone tapes or polypropylene sutures buttressed with silicone tubing and wrapped with tourniquets to obtain hemostasis at the arteriotomy site. These sutures are placed deep into the myocardium with the aim that the subjacent epimyocardial tissue acts as a buffer between the snare and the vessel wall. Still, there is an almost circumferential compression being exerted on all the layers of the vessel wall. Perrault et al. [17] did not find a difference in the device application groups compared with arteriosclerotic controls in the relaxation to serotonin. Gerola and associates [18] however, have shown that snaring causes compression and buckling of elastic lamellae with medial fractures in atherosclerotic arteries. The application of snare can cause embolization of atheromatous fragments, cause infarction [20], create fistula between adjacent structures [21] or induce lesions at site of application [22].

With ILS, damage to endothelium could occur as a result of brushing of the endothelium, leading to its denudation upon ILS insertion. That is perhaps unavoidable. Alternatively, the bulbous ends of the ILS could exert pressure on the wall, leading to endothelial ischemia if too large a shunt is used. Potentially, coronary artery dissection is possible, although this has not yet been reported. There are no effects on the medial and adventitial layers.

From the available data, it is clear that both techniques can damage the vessel wall. Each technique has its own mechanism of injury. The intraluminal shunt may damage endothelial and subendothelial layers, whereas snaring could affect all the layers of the wall. However, the significance of any of the observed effects in dysfunctional coronary arteries is yet to be established.

Flow Dynamics

The advantage of shunt over snaring is that shunting allows distal perfusion during anastomosis and that provides some amount of myocardial protection. Studies designed to measure the flow through an ILS are difficult to perform. The ILS is inserted distal to a stenotic lesion, the severity of which varies in each case. In the laboratory, too, creation of discrete coronary lesions is difficult. Techniques for measuring regional myocardial metabolism and regional myocardial blood flow (RMBF) in real time, distal to ILS insertion, are not available.

To overcome these difficulties, Kamiya and colleagues [23] investigated the efficacy of the ILS in a theoretical model based on fluid mechanics. Based on the assumption that the intracoronary pressure would be equal both upstream and downstream of the ILS and assuming blood to be a Newtonian fluid, they used equations derived from physics to quantitate flow, in situations of laminar and turbulent flow, before and after ILS insertion. They derived "flow ratio," the ratio of postattachment to preattachment flow. They found that with laminar flow, the flow ratio is proportional to the sixth power of the inner diameter of the ILS; for turbulent flow, flow ratio is proportional to the third power of the inner diameter of the ILS. They found that although commercially available ILS come in sizes of 1 mm to 4 mm, corresponding to coronary artery diameters, in reality their inner diameters are much smaller and, hence, flow ratios are small. Thus, after ILS insertion, coronary flow decreases to 2% to 14% of preattachment flow during turbulent flow and to less than 0.1% in laminar flow. It has been shown that flow is laminar proximal to a coronary stenosis and turbulent distally, which is where an ILS is placed. Therefore, it appears that the ILS would carry only 2% to 14% of blood forward. Muraki and coworkers [24] in a different model have shown a fall in RMBF to 30% of baseline under normotensive conditions, and a fall to 10% during hypotensive episodes.

Shunting no doubt allows forward flow but a meager amount. Nevertheless there is no electrocardiographic or biochemical evidence of ischemia. There are certain protective mechanisms, which include formation of collaterals, possible hibernation of myocardium and distal placement of arteriotomy which limits the amout of myocardium at risk.

Depending on the mass of myocardium 40-60ml of blood is required for myocardial protection [25]. Grunenfelder et al.[26] have shown that at pressure of 75 mmHg flow through 1.5 mm was 40ml/min. Under hypotensive conditions with pressure less than 40 mmHg flow dropped to 50% of baseline with shunt less than 2 mm and to 70% with larger shunt. Thus 1.5-2mm shunts provide adequate myocardial protection. Gurbuz et al. [27] randomly assigned two groups of patients undergoing OPCAB into snare or shunt group and found troponin I levels higher in the snare group.

How much is the barest minimum of blood flow to prevent myocardial ischemia? Unfortunately, there is no definite answer to this question. As discussed nicely by Levinson [28], prevention of ischemia may not require much flow at all. In the early days of angioplasty, failed procedures with ischemia were managed by passing a Stack catheter distally. This autoperfusion catheter was a fine multiperforate tube, and hence, flows were small. But even these small flows were enough in most cases to buy the time needed to perform emergency surgical revascularization. The ILS may be compared with the Stack catheter, and therefore, the small amount of flow allowed may be adequate for the prevention of ischemia.

SHUNT SIZE

The size of shunt is of utmost importance. Surgeons are biased for bigger size, more distal perfusion and more clear operative field. However, improved distal perfusion and visisbility comes at the price of increased endothelial injury. Wippermann [29] and Hangler [30] studied various shunt sizes. The biggest limitation of both the Wippermann [29] and the

Hangler [30] studies lies in their selection of shunt size. While Hangler inserted shunts that were "leak proof," in Wippermann's study, the ILS was "slightly oversized" to the coronary artery. Thus, significant endothelial loss was to be expected both from the brushing effect at insertion as well as from pressure on the wall of the artery. That cannot be recommended as the method of using an ILS. Most OPCAB grafting surgeons who use ILS would not attempt to "match" shunt and coronary artery size.

Demeria et al. [31] addressed this issue in laboratory setting. In a study performed in normal pig coronary arteries, they compared coronary morphology and endothelial reactivity after the insertion of ILS of three different sizes with the aim of oversizing, undersizing or using an ILS congruent to the artery diameter. They also assessed the amount of bleeding at the anastomosis site. They found severe decreases in coronary reactivity and a total disappearance of the endothelium with an oversized shunt that provided perfect hemostasis. No significant endothelium loss or dysfunction was noted with a drastically undersized shunt, but continuous bleeding was noted. When a congruent shunt was used (2-mm shunt for 2.2-mm vessel), only selective endothelial dysfunction involving Gi-protein–mediated relaxation was deranged. Further, 50% of the endothelium was preserved. There was intermittent bleeding, but the authors considered that anastomosis could still be done (Table 1). Thus oversized shunts are out of question. In the above study the undersized shunt was 62% of coronary diameter and congruent was 90%. In clinical setting we can follow the middle path by selecting the shunt which is 75% of the size of target vessel, which would suffice the needs of adequate hemostasis, little endothelial damage and adequate distal flow.

Table 1. Impact of shunt size on hemostasis, coronary reactivity and endothelial loss

Variable	Over sized	Under Sized	Congruent
Hemostasis	Perfect	Imperfect	Intermittent
Coronary reactivity	Markedly decreased	Non dysfunction	Selective involving Gi-protein mediated relaxation
Endothelial loss	Total disappearance	Not significant	50% preservation

Graft Patency

One of the major concerns with the use of shunts as well as snares is the impact on graft patency secondary to endothelial damage and denudation. Bergsland et al. [32] performed angiographic study to address this issue. In this study twenty-seven patients were randomly assigned to shunt and 29 to no shunt. There were no differences between groups with regard to demographics or risk factors, except for more smokers in the shunt group. In 3 patients, shunt insertion was unsuccessful, and the graft was performed as in the no-shunt group. Two shunts had a diameter of 1.25 mm, 14 had a diameter of 1.50 mm, 7 had a diameter of 1.75 mm, and 1 had a diameter of 2.00 mm. All no-shunt patients were treated without shunt. Forty-eight patients, 24 randomized to no-shunt and 24 to shunt, had on-table angiograms. Three of the latter were grafted without shunt. One patient in each group had dissection of the distal left internal mammary artery (LIMA); both were repaired by revising the anastomosis and had normal repeat angiograms. All grafts in the shunt group were Fitzgibbon grade A, whereas there were 4 grade B grafts in the no-shunt group ($p = 0.06$). Of the 4 no-shunt anastomoses with Fitzgibbon grade B, 3 became normal on postoperative angiograms, but 1 lesion in the distal LIMA was present on postoperative angiogram and required intervention.

Fifty-three patients underwent postoperative angiography. Twenty-three lesions were demonstrated in the area of the LIMA to LAD anastomosis or in the native vessel close to the anastomosis. Fifteen of the lesions were not present on preoperative angiography. The lesions were more common proximal to the anastomosis than distal: proximal 9 of 53; distal 2 of 53 ($p = 0.03$). There was no difference between the two groups. Average severity of the new lesions was 44% (SD 17%). Both distal lesions were retrospectively seen to be present on the on-table angiogram, as were 4 of 11 proximally located new lesions. Five new proximal lesions were not seen on on-table angiogram; in 2 cases, comparison between on-table and postoperative angiogram was not possible.

There was a trend toward more anastomotic lesions in no-shunt patients, both at on-table angiography and postoperatively in the distal LIMA, indicating that shunt may be helpful in avoiding technical mistakes. Other investigators have also demonstrated equal or improved angiographic results in shunted patients [10].

Conclusion

There is growing evidence for the benefits of using shunts in terms of better clinical outcome [33], reduced ischemia [34] and enhanced graft patency [32]. A properly sized shunt with hydrophilic surface, improved flow characteristics, improved flexibility, and hemostasis should be used to ensure good visualization of the anastomotic site so as to perform a technically precise anastomosis on a beating heart. Snares cause circumferential compression of media and adventitia which can b minimized with the use of shunts. At present "risk benefit" analysis definitely favors the use of ILS during OPCAB surgery.

References

[1] Akpinar, B., Güden, M., Sagbas, E., et al. Off-pump coronary artery bypass grafting with use of the octopus 2 stabilization system. *Heart Surg. Forum* 2000;3:282-6.

[2] Jansen, E. W., Borst, C., Lahpor, J. R., et al. Coronary artery bypass grafting without cardiopulmonary bypass using the octopus method: results in first one hundred patients. *J. Thorac. Cardiovasc. Surg*. 1998;116:60-7.

[3] Dullum, M. K., Resano, F. G. Xpose: a new device that provides reproducible and easy access for multivessel beating heart bypass grafting. *Heart Surg. Forum* 2000;3:113-7.

[4] Ricci, M., Karamanoukian, H. L., Di Ancona, G., Bergsland, J., Salerno, T. A. Exposure and mechanical stabilization in off pump coronary artery bypass grafting via sternotomy *Ann. Thorac. Surg*. 2000;70:1736-40.

[5] Baumgartner, F. J., Cheissari, A., Capouya, E. R., Panagiotides, G. P., Katouzian, A., Yokoyama, T. Technical aspects of total revascularization in off pump coronary bypass via sternotomy approach. *Ann. Thorac. Surg*. 1999;67:1653-8.

[6] Rivetti, R. A., Gandra, S. M. Initial experience using an intraluminal shunt during revascularization on the beating heart. *Ann. Thorac. Surg*. 1997;63:1742-7.
[7] Trapp, W. G., Bisarya, R. Placement of coronary artery bypass graft without oxygenator. *Ann. Thorac. Surg*. 1975;19:1-9.
[8] Luccheti, V., Caputo, M., Suleiman, M. S., et al. Beating heart coronary revascularization without metabolic myocardial damage. *Eur. J. Cardiothorac. Surg*. 1998;14:443-444.
[9] Lucchetti, V., Capasso, F., Caputo, M., et al. Intra coronary shunt prevents left ventricular function impairment during beating heart coronary revascularization. *Eur. J. Cardiothorac. Surg*. 1999;15:255-9.
[10] Menon, A. K., Albes, J. M., Oberhoff, M., Karsh, K. R., Ziemer, G. Occlusion versus shunting during MIDCAB : effect on left ventricular function and quality of anastomosis. *Ann. Throac. Surg*. 2002;73:1418-23.
[11] Yeatman, M., Caputo, M., Narayan, P., et al. Intracoronary shunts reduce transient intraoperative myocardial dysfunction during off-pump coronary operations. *Ann. Thorac. Surg*. 2002;73:1411-7.
[12] Hangler, H. B., Pfaller, K., Aniretter, H., Dapunt, O. E., Bonatti, J. O. Coronary endothelial injury after local occlusion on the human beating heart. *Ann. Thorac. Surg*. 2001;71:122-7.
[13] Fonger, J. D., Yang, X. M., Chen, R. A., Handershild, C. C., Shemin, R. J. Impaired relaxation of human mammary artery after temporay clamping. *J. Thorac. Cardiovasc. Surg*. 1992;104:966-71.
[14] Okasaki, Y., Takarabe, K., Murayama, J., et al. Coronary endothelial damage during off pump CABG related to coronary clamping and gas insufflations. *Eur. J. Cardiothorac. Surg*. 2001;19:834-9.
[15] Rubens, F. D., Labow, R. S., Meek, E., et al. Papaverine solutions cause loss of viability of endothelial cells. *J. Cardiothorac. Surg*. (Torino). 1998;39:193-9.
[16] Dygert, J. H., Thatte, H. S., Kumbhani, D. J., et al. Intracoronary shunt-induced endothelial cell damage in porcine heart. *J. Surg. Res*. 2006;131:168-174.
[17] Perrault, L. P., Desijardins, N., Nicker, C., et al. Effects of occlusion devices for minimally invasive coronary artery bypass surgery on coronary endothelial function of atherosclerotic arteries. *Heart Surg. Forum* 2000;3:287-92.
[18] Gerola, L. R., Moura, L. A., Leao, L. E., et al. Arterial wall damage caused by snaring of the coronary arteries during off-pump revascularization. *Heart Surg. Forum* 2000;3:103-6.
[19] Izzat, M. B., Yim, A. P., El Zufari, M. H. Snaring of a coronary artery causing distal atheroma embolization. *Ann. Thorac. Surg*. 1998, 66:1806-8.
[20] Splittgerber, F. H., Minale, C. Septal myocardial infarction: a complication of coronary artery stay sutures. *Ann. Thorac. Surg*. 1993;56:400-1.
[21] Tanemoto, K. T., Kuroki, K., Kanaoka, Y., Murakami, T. Septal branch right ventricular fistula: a complication in coronary artery snaring. *Ann. Thorac. Surg*. 1999;68:246-8.
[22] Alessandrini, F., Gaudino, M., Glieca, F., et al. Lesions of the target vessel during minimally published in 1996: endothelial effects of hemostatic devices for continuous cardioplegia or minimally invasive operations. Updated in 1999. *Ann. Thorac. Surg*. 1999;68:1118-20.

[23] Kamiya, H., Watanabe, G., Kanamori, T. Flow simulation of the intracoronary shunt tube for off-pump coronary arthery bypass. *Eur. J. Cardiothorac. Surg*. 2003;23:665-9.

[24] Muraki, S., Morris, C. D., Budde, J. M., et al. Preserved myocardial perfusion during simulated off-pump coronary arthery bypass grafting. *J. Thorac. Cardiovasc. Surg*. 2002;23:53-62.

[25] De Muinck, E. D., Verkerke, B. J., Rakhorst, G., Lie, K. I., Myocardial protection during coronary angioplasty with autoperfusion and forced perfusion: an in vitro comparision. *Int. J. Artif. Organs* 1994;17:83-7.

[26] Grunenfelder, J., Comber, M., Lachat, M., et al. Validation of intracoronary shunt flow measurements for offpump coronary bypass operations. *Heart Surg. Forum* 2004;7:26-30.

[27] Gurbuz, A., Emrecan, B., Yilik, L., et al. Intracoronary shunt reduces postoperative troponin leaks: a prospective randomized study. *Eur. J. Cardiothorac. Surg*. 2006;29:186-9.

[28] Levinson, M. M. Editorial commentary. *Heart Surg. Forum* 2004;7:E11-2.

[29] Wippermann, J., Albes, J. M., Bruhin, R., et al. Choronic ultrastrucural effects of temporary intraluminal shunts in a porcine off-pump model. *Ann. Thorac. Surg*. 2004;78:543-8.

[30] Hangler, H. B., Pfaller, K., Ruttmann, E., et al. Effects of intracoronary shunts on coronary endothelial coating in the human beating heart. *Ann. Thorac. Surg*. 2004:77:776-80.

[31] Demaria, R. G., Fortier, S., Malo, O., Carrier, M., Perrault, L. P. Influence of intracoronary shunt size on coronary endothelial effects of hemostatic device OPCAB. *Heart Surg. Forum* 2002;5(Suppl.):165.

[32] Bergsland, J., Lingaas, P. S., Skulstad, H., et al. Intracoronary shunt prevents ischemia in off-pump coronary artery bypass surgery. *Ann. Thorac. Surg*. 2009;87:54-60.

[33] Collison, S. P., Aggarwal, A., Trehan, N. Controversies in the use off intraluminal shunts during off-pump coronary artery bypass grafting surgery. *Ann. Thorac. Surg*. 2006;82:1559-66.

[34] Emmiler, M., Kocagullari, C. U., Ela, Y., Cekirdekci, A. Influence of intracoronary shunt on myocardial damage: a prospective randomized study. *Eur. J. Cardiothorac. Surg*. 2008;35:1000-4.

In: Off-Pump Coronary Artery Bypass Grafting
Editors: S.G. Raja and M. Amrani

ISBN 978-1-62081-575-5

Chapter 24

Endoscopic Versus Open Vein Harvesting for Coronary Artery Bypass Grafting

Maral Ouzounian[1], Celeste MacPherson[1] and Imtiaz S. Ali[2]
[1]Division of Cardiac Surgery, Dalhousie University, Halifax, Nova Scotia, Canada
[2]Division of Cardiac Surgery, Libin Cardiovascular Institute of Alberta, University of Calgary, Calgary, Alberta, Canada

Abstract

Recently developed minimally invasive endoscopic vein harvesting (EVH) techniques have largely replaced traditional longitudinal open vein harvest (OVH) for coronary artery bypass grafting (CABG).

The past decade has seen a rapid uptake in the use of EVH in many centers, although controversy remains regarding vein graft quality and the impact of EVH on long-term graft patency and clinical outcomes. EVH has been demonstrated to improve short-term wound-related outcomes, including wound infections, post-operative pain, mobility, length of hospital stay, and patient satisfaction. This chapter will review the technical aspects of EVH including the impact of the learning curve and the technical details of EVH harvesting on vein graft quality. The literature regarding the effect of harvesting technique on graft quality, as determined by histological evaluation, angiographic graft patency, and clinical outcomes will also be evaluated.

Introduction

The long saphenous vein (SV) remains the most commonly used conduit for coronary artery bypass grafting (CABG). Minimally invasive endoscopic vein harvesting (EVH) techniques have been developed and have largely replaced traditional longitudinal open vein harvest (OVH). The introduction of EVH in 1996[1] was an important contribution to the overall goal of cardiac surgery to be less invasive and to promote earlier recovery for the patient undergoing CABG. Indeed, in 2005, the consensus panel of the International Society of Minimally Invasive Cardiothoracic Surgery (ISMICS) recommended EVH as the standard of care for patients requiring SV grafts for coronary revascularization, and EVH techniques are currently used in over 70% of cardiac surgery centers in the United States [2]. Despite the rapid uptake of the technique over the past decade, certain controversies remain regarding conduit quality and long-term patency results with EVH. The benefits of EVH to leg-wound associated morbidity have been consistently demonstrated and extensively reported [2-9]. Avoiding the need for a long incision has led to a significant reduction of donor-site wound healing disturbances, including serious wound infections, and has resulted in less pain, shorter hospital stay, fewer readmissions to hospital, and improved patient satisfaction [10,11]. This chapter will review the technical aspects of EVH and will summarize the literature regarding wound-related morbidity as well as graft quality and durability.

The EVH Procedure

Technical Aspects

Several disposable and reusable EVH systems with and without carbon dioxide insufflation are available, including the most frequently used disposable systems: VasoView by Maquet, VirtuoSaph by Terumo, and ClearGlide by Sorin. After proper positioning of the patient, the location of the vein is identified by the operator through gentle "milking" of the vein, while feeling the thrill with the other hand. If the operator is unable to palpate the vein, osseous landmarks are used for localization. Through a three cm incision just above the medial aspect of the knee, 35 cm of the upper leg greater SV may be harvested. If the entire 70 cm length of vein is needed, the options are to repeat the procedure through the same incision in the other direction, or to begin the harvesting procedure 2-3 cm above the medial malleolus followed by a second incision just above the knee to harvest the vein to the groin. After the vein is identified, a balloon tip trocar is inserted into the incision and the tunnel is inflated with carbon dioxide. The conical dissection cone is advanced toward the groin on the anterior surface of the vein under videoscopic visualization. Circumferential blunt dissection of the vein is completed along the posterior and lateral aspects throughout its length, after which the collateral branches are isolated and divided with bipolar electrocautery. Vein trauma is minimized by constant visualization, proper counter-traction, and careful hemostasis. Proximal saphenous vein ligation is performed through a separate "stab and grab" incision at the extremity of the tunnel. Once the vein is extracted, the proximal end is cannulated and gently dilated to avoid endothelial trauma. The branches are doubly clipped and avulsions are repaired with fine monofilament suture material. The vein is gently flushed to remove any clots that may have accumulated. Finally, the tunnel is evacuated of residual blood and after wound closure the leg is wrapped with a compression bandage for at least 12 hours.

Optimizing Vein Quality

Brown and colleagues used optical coherence tomography (OCT) for intraoperative assessment of the entire tract of the harvested SV to investigate the effect of preheparinization and sealed carbon dioxide insufflation on intraluminal clot burden[12]. Preheparinization before EVH (either a 5000-IU bolus or full-dose heparin to achieve an activated clotting time >300 seconds) resulted in significant reductions in clot fraction and clot volume.

Additionally, significant reductions in clot burden were observed after EVH with an open CO_2 insufflation system without preheparinization. An open CO_2 system may be achieved by using either the ClearGlide system or, as is performed at our institution, the VasoView device without balloon inflation, such that CO_2 insufflation is used to facilitate visualization, but without a sealed tunnel. These findings support the hypothesis that clot formation during EVH is the result of stagnant blood that is not anticoagulated being allowed to remain within a collapsed vein.

There was no difference in this study among the three intervention groups: (a) low-dose and (b) full-dose preheparinization and (c) an open CO_2 insufflation system without preheparinization. Although this study was not powered to determine whether intraluminal clot strands predispose to graft failure, we believe that care should be taken to standardize and optimize vein quality during EVH and that preheparinization and/or an open CO_2 insufflation system should be used to reduce clot burden. In a similar study, Burris et al. demonstrated significantly higher endothelial integrity and lower tissue factor activity in veins that were not distended with saline compared to those that were distended using syringe injection with no method of controlling the distending pressure[13].

Learning Curve

A significant institutional and personal learning curve exists upon adoption of the EVH technique. Macroscopic lesions, such as holes or torn side branches requiring suture repairs, occur 3-5 times more often after EVH than after open harvest, and concern exists regarding the overall reduced ability of abiding by "no-touch" principles and preserving the vasa vasorum when handling vascular tissue endoscopically[9] [14].

Desai and colleagues compared veins harvested by an open technique to those harvested by EVH performed by experienced versus novice technicians using OCT to image veins intraoperatively and computed tomographic angiography (CTA) to assess graft patency on post-operative day five[15]. They found that technicians inexperienced with EVH (<100 cases of experience) were far more likely to provoke deep vessel injury when compared with those with more than 900 cases of experience. Furthermore, when the number of discrete injures exceeds a threshold of 4, the risk of early graft failure rises by more then 50% (67% versus 96% graft patency at 5 days; p=0.05).

In this well-designed study, intimal injury diagnosed by OCT correlated with endothelial disruption on histological examination and the expression of tissue factor activity on the luminal surface, supporting the hypothesis that focal injury with disruption of the endothelium can provoke an occlusive thrombus and loss of the graft. Vein graft quality is dependent on technician experience, and careful attention must be paid to assuring safe and reliable training of technicians at the beginning of their learning curve.

Complications

EVH is in general a safe procedure, although minor complications such as skin burns, tunnelitis, hematomas, and seromas may occur. There are several complications that relate to the use of CO_2 insufflation, including severe hypercapnia, subclinical CO_2 embolization (10.4%), and massive CO_2 embolization (0.22%)[16,17].

Monitoring with a capnograph and arterial blood gases is imperative, as the rate of mechanical ventilation should be adjusted to manage moderate elevations of arterial pCO_2. An important preventive measure to avoid this rare but dreaded complication is maintaining the CO_2 insufflation pressure lower than the central venous pressure. One group recently evaluated the hemodynamic effects during EVH for off-pump CABG (OPCAB) and found that EVH was associated with a tolerable range of hypercarbia that did not have any adverse effects on hemodynamics[18].

	Design	Citation	Treated	Control	NTotal	Effect	Lower	Upper	PValue
	Non-Random	Allen 00	7 / 225	99 / 585	810	.158	.072	.345	.000
	Non-Random	Bitondo 01	9 / 133	26 / 92	225	.184	.082	.416	.000
	Non-Random	Brandt 03	8 / 741	31 / 1168	1909	.400	.183	.876	.018
	Non-Random	Coppoolse 99	28 / 1400	33 / 300	1700	.165	.098	.278	.000
	Non-Random	Croutch 99	9 / 180	55 / 388	568	.319	.154	.660	.001
	Non-Random	Davis 98	18 / 110	30 / 99	209	.450	.232	.873	.017
	Non-Random	Felisky 02	24 / 340	99 / 380	720	.216	.134	.346	.000
	Non-Random	Galbraith 00	21 / 77	44 / 135	212	.776	.418	1.438	.419
	Non-Random	Horvath 98	4 / 31	1 / 29	60	4.148	.435	39.521	.185
	Non-Random	Isgro 99	9 / 103	29 / 105	208	.251	.112	.562	.000
	Non-Random	Kan 99	3 / 60	12 / 59	119	.206	.055	.774	.012
	Non-Random	Li 98	1 / 50	14 / 106	156	.134	.017	1.050	.027
	Non-Random	Lutz 01	3 / 88	13 / 85	173	.195	.054	.713	.007
	Non-Random	Marty 00	1 / 22	4 / 18	40	.167	.017	1.651	.093
	Non-Random	Meyer 00	0 / 9	0 / 5	14	.579	.010	33.502	.790
	Non-Random	Morris 98	2 / 27	5 / 24	51	.304	.053	1.741	.164
	Non-Random	Pagni 98	5 / 50	4 / 40	90	1.000	.250	3.998	1.000
	Non-Random	Patel 01	2 / 100	12 / 100	200	.150	.033	.687	.006
	Non-Random	Rodrigus 00	27 / 131	5 / 27	158	1.142	.396	3.295	.805
Fixed	**Non-Random (19)**		**181 / 3877**	**516 / 3745**	**7622**	**.295**	**.242**	**.360**	**.000**
Random	**Non-Random (19)**		**181 / 3877**	**516 / 3745**	**7622**	**.314**	**.225**	**.438**	**.000**
	Random	Allen 98, 03	2 / 51	11 / 58	109	.174	.037	.829	.016
	Random	Schurr 02	2 / 80	6 / 60	140	.231	.045	1.187	.058
	Random	Yun 05	7 / 95	20 / 103	198	.330	.133	.821	.014
Fixed	**Random (3)**		**11 / 226**	**37 / 221**	**447**	**.270**	**.133**	**.550**	**.000**
Random	**Random (3)**		**11 / 226**	**37 / 221**	**447**	**.270**	**.133**	**.550**	**.000**
Fixed	**Combined (22)**		**192 / 4103**	**553 / 3966**	**8069**	**.293**	**.242**	**.355**	**.000**
Random	**Combined (22)**		**192 / 4103**	**553 / 3966**	**8069**	**.306**	**.228**	**.412**	**.000**

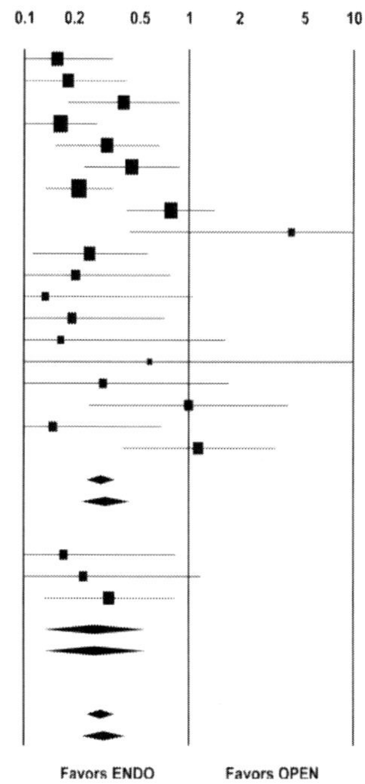

Figure 1. Wound complications following EVH vs. OVH. Reproduced with permission from Cheng et al. *Innovations* 2005 [7].

Wound-Related Outcomes

Wound Healing

The incidence of wound complications following traditional OVH ranges from 2-25%, resulting in significant economic and clinical burden. A meta-analysis of eleven randomized controlled trials reported a significant reduction in wound infection using an endoscopic technique (OR 0.22, 95% CI; 0.14–0.37, p<0.00001), for a number needed to treat of fourteen[5]. In another large meta-analysis, the ISMICS Consensus Group reviewed 36 randomized and non-randomized trials of 9632 patients undergoing saphenous vein harvest and found a 69% reduction in the overall risk of all wound complications by EVH (OR 0.31, 95% CI 0.23-0.41, p<0.0001; Figure 1)[7].

Similarly, they found a reduction in the risk of wound infections (OR 0.23, 95% CI 0.20–0.53; P < 0.0001) as well as the need for surgical wound intervention (OR 0.16, 95% CI 0.08–0.29; p<0.0001) following endoscopic harvest. The reduction in donor-site infections mainly occurs because of preserved tissue perfusion and a lower likelihood of creating vital tissue flaps than with open saphenectomy. This may be of particular importance in patients with diabetes, obesity, and peripheral vascular disease in whom EVH has eliminated the excessive risk observed with traditional OVH [19,20].

Non-infective wound healing disturbances of hematoma, edema, skin necrosis, wound dehiscence, drainage, and seroma are also significantly reduced with EVH [4].

Postoperative Pain, Mobility, and Patient Satisfaction

Several studies have demonstrated improved quality of life indices, including postoperative pain, time to mobilization, and patient satisfaction following EVH. The incidence of pain (23.1% versus 6.7%), neuralgia (24.3% versus 7.1%), and patient satisfaction (49% versus 75%) was significantly improved with EVH compared with OVH [7]. Using a visual analogue scale, patients undergoing EVH rated their experience of pain two points lower on a 0-10 scale throughout the entire postoperative period and labeled themselves pain-free days earlier than their OVH counterparts [6,21,22].

A number of studies have reported earlier mobility for patients undergoing EVH as well as improved mobility at hospital discharge and six weeks after surgery [22,23]. Patient satisfaction with the cosmetic result is initially higher with EVH than after traditional harvest, although the cosmetic outcome is equivalent six weeks after surgery[22].

Hospital Length of Stay and Costs

Earlier mobilization of patients and a reduction of wound complications may result in a reduction of recovery time and therefore hospital length of stay (LOS). The results in small series have not been consistent, although two meta-analyses have reported a reduction in hospital LOS by EVH with a weighted mean difference ranging from -0.85 to -1.04 days; 95% CI −1.92 to −0.16[4,7]. In an economic analysis of cost-effectiveness, Rao and colleagues calculated health related quality of life utility estimates and reported that EVH was more cost-effective than OVH[24]. However, costs of outpatient visits, readmissions, and wound treatments were not included in this study.

Outcomes Related to Graft Quality and Durability

Histological Evaluation

Despite differences in tissue handling between the techniques, earlier studies failed to demonstrate a difference in the endothelial and conduit integrity of veins harvested with EVH compared to open harvest [6,22,25-27]. However, in a small but elegant recent study using multiphoton imaging, immunofluorescence, and biochemical techniques, Rousou and colleagues observed that EVH has a detrimental effect on the structure and function of the vein endothelium [28]. Lower levels of cellular viability, more membrane damage, reduced calcium mobilization, and reduced nitric oxide production were demonstrated after EVH compared to open harvest. It is possible, as the authors assert, that these results differ from previously published findings because more sensitive techniques were used to indicate endothelial function.

It should be noted, however, that the technician harvesting veins in this report only had experience with 110 EVH cases, and that a VasoView system with sealed CO_2 insufflation was employed, with no mention of preheparinization. These observations warrant larger trials with standardized EVH techniques in order to confirm the findings and to determine whether the level of endothelial dysfunction observed translates to reduced graft patency rates and patient outcomes.

Graft Patency

Only a small number of studies are available that provide insight to the implications of histological vein injury on graft patency. Two small randomized controlled trials did not show any difference in patency rates by coronary angiography between patients undergoing EVH or OVH[9,29]. Follow-up was less than a year, however, and the trials may have been underpowered. In a third study, Davis and colleagues compared results of contrast-enhanced CT and found similar patency rates at a mean of 3.7 years after EVH compared to patients that had undergone OVH 0.7 years earlier [30].

Clinical Outcomes

The few studies investigating the mid- and long-term impact of endoscopic vein harvesting on clinical outcomes following CABG are summarized in Table 1. In a secondary analysis of 3000 patients from the PREVENT IV trial, Lopes and colleagues found an association of EVH with higher rates of vein graft failure (46.7% vs. 38.0%, $p<0.001$) and adverse clinical outcomes including mortality (HR 1.52; $p=0.005$)[31]. This study was designed to assess ex vivo treatment of vein grafts with edifoligide, and patients were not randomly assigned to harvest procedure.

In the absence of randomization, outcomes cannot be definitively attributed to harvest technique. Furthermore, the study was conducted at 107 sites between 2002 and 2003, and a number of technical factors were not standardized, including technician experience, institutional EVH volume, and details of the harvest technique.

Zenati and colleagues also published a secondary analysis of a randomized trial, the Randomized On/Off Bypass (ROOBY) trial, designed to evaluate differences in clinical outcomes between patients undergoing on- and off-pump CABG[32]. Of the 2203 patients recruited into the original trial, 1471 (66.8%) had conduit data recorded and 894 (40.6%) had angiographic follow-up at 1 year. These latter two groups formed the basis of the subgroup analysis, in which the authors found inferior rates of vein graft patency and increased repeat revascularization rates in the EVH group. This study has similar limitations to the subgroup analysis of the PREVENT IV trial: (a) Learning curve. Both studies were recruiting patients in the early part of the last decade, when EVH uptake in the US was low (<10%).

The variability in experience levels, the effect of the learning curve, and the potentially low number of cases per institution or practitioner should be considered when interpreting these findings; (b) Technical details. Data regarding technical details during conduit harvest and intraoperative flow characteristics were unfortunately not recorded during these studies and may have an effect on graft patency; and (c) Selection bias. The primary purpose of these studies was not to compare vein harvest techniques. Surgeons were encouraged to use whichever harvesting technique they preferred, and a selection bias may exist with unmeasured confounders affecting surgeons' decision to use an EVH approach.

In contrast to these two studies demonstrating adverse clinical outcomes with EVH, four studies have reported no increase in adverse events following EVH [8, 33-35]. The earliest study was reported by Allen and colleagues who found similar five-year freedom from death, myocardial infarction, or recurrent angina between the two groups (75% vs. 74%, p=0.85), although the number of patients in each group of this randomized study was small (EVH, n=54, OVH, n=58)[33]. In an observational study of 5,825 patients of whom 34% had EVH, our group found no association with midterm adverse outcomes including death and readmission to hospital for a cardiac cause after a mean follow-up of 2.6 years (HR 0.93, p=0.22). In a small retrospective study, Kirmani and colleagues found no difference in the rates of freedom from angina, readmission, or need for further anti-anginals between the two groups [35]. Finally, the Northern New England Cardiovascular Study Group also reported a large observational study of 8,524 patients of whom 52.5% underwent CABG with EVH between 2001 and 2004[34]. Using both conventional multivariate regression models as well as a propensity-matched analysis, they observed a significant association of EVH with reduced mortality (HR 0.74; p=0.007) and a non-significant association with increased risk of repeat revascularization (HR 1.29; p=0.092). Interestingly, the rates of EVH increased markedly from 34% to 75% during the study period, leading the authors of an accompanying editorial to comment "OVH may not be dead and buried, but it is certainly moving in that direction"[36].

Future Prospects

As we attempt to improve immediate and long-term outcomes of our patients following surgical revascularization for coronary artery disease, the choice and method of conduit harvest is an important consideration. EVH has become the technique of choice for harvesting the long saphenous vein in many centers, and the bulk of the literature supports the safety of this strategy with respect to graft patency, long-term mortality, and cardiac outcomes. The lack of unanimity in the literature is not surprising given the wide range of EVH techniques and operator experience in the reported studies. Although a large randomized trial would yield a more definitive answer, such a trial may not be feasible given patient, surgeon, and institutional preference for EVH in many centers and the clear benefit of EVH in improving wound-related, short-term outcomes. Utilization of EVH in the US alone exceeds 100,000 cases per year, largely because of patient demand for minimally invasive techniques.

Table 1. Studies examining the impact of EVH on mid- and long-term clinical outcomes

Authors, year	Method	N	Follow up	Outcomes	Results
Allen et al., 2003 [33]	RCT	54 EVH 58 OVH	5 years	Death, MI, recurrent angina	75% vs. 74%, p=0.85
Lopes et al., 2009 [31]	Prospective, non-randomized	1753 EVH 1247 OVH	3 years	Death, MI, repeat revascularization	20.2% vs. 17.4%, p=0.04
Ouzounian et al., 2010 [8]	Retrospective	2004 EVH 3821 OVH	2.6 years	Death, readmission to hospital for cardiac cause	HR 0.93, p=0.22
Kirmani et al., 2010 [35]	Case-control	89 EVH 182 OVH	17 m 38 m	Death, freedom from angina, readmission, new anti-anginals	p=NS for each outcome
Dacey et al., 2011 [34]	Retrospective	4480 EVH 4062 OVH	4 years	Death Repeat revascularization	HR 0.74, p=0.007 HR 1.29, p=0.092
Zenati et al., 2011 [32]	Prospective, non-randomized	341 EVH 553 OVH	1 year	Death Revascularization Myocardial infarction	0.3% vs. 0.4%, p>.99 6.7% vs. 3.4%, p=0.03 1.8% vs. 2.0%, p>.99

Despite the fact that EVH is clearly here to stay, the technique should be optimized and standardized to improve surgical outcomes. Compromised endothelial integrity may be the primary determinant in the pathogenesis of thrombosis, intimal hyperplasia, and atherosclerosis within the saphenous vein graft [37]. To this end, techniques that reduce intraluminal clot formation and endothelial injury should be studied and applied. To date, pre-heparinization, avoidance of sealed CO_2 insufflation, avoidance of overdistension of the extracted vein graft, and an experienced operator have been shown to improve conduit quality. The learning curve has been demonstrated to be a significant concern, and acquiring and maintaining EVH skill safely will be an important quality improvement challenge. Quality assurance using intraoperative imaging techniques such as OCT may be beneficial, particularly during the early stages of an operator's learning curve. OCT imaging would provide high-resolution assessment of vessel integrity throughout the entire harvested SVG, and could guide selection of the optimal segment of conduit for revascularization. Continued analysis of conduit quality is important, but also mandates stringent follow up to determine its impact on graft patency and clinical outcomes. The surgical community should systematically monitor and report long-term clinical outcomes to assure safety and optimal results following coronary revascularization with EVH.

References

[1] Lumsden AB, Eaves FF, 3rd, Ofenloch JC, Jordan WD. Subcutaneous, video-assisted saphenous vein harvest: report of the first 30 cases. *Cardiovasc. Surg*. 1996;4:771-776.

[2] Allen K CD, Cohn W, Connolly M, et al. Endoscopic vascular harvest in coronary artery bypass grafting surgery: a consensus statement of the International Society of Minimally Invasive Cardiothoracic Surgery (ISMICS) 2005. Innovations: Technology and Techniques in *Cardiothoracic and Vascular Surgery* 2005;1:51-60.

[3] Accord R, Maessen J. Endoscopic vein harvesting for coronary bypass grafting: a blessing or a trojan horse? *Cardiol. Res. Pract*. 2011:813512.

[4] Athanasiou T, Aziz O, Al-Ruzzeh S, et al. Are wound healing disturbances and length of hospital stay reduced with minimally invasive vein harvest? A meta-analysis. *Eur. J. Cardiothorac. Surg*. 2004;26:1015-1026.

[5] Athanasiou T, Aziz O, Skapinakis P, et al. Leg wound infection after coronary artery bypass grafting: a meta-analysis comparing minimally invasive versus conventional vein harvesting. *Ann. Thorac. Surg*. 2003;76:2141-2146.

[6] Bonde P, Graham AN, MacGowan SW. Endoscopic vein harvest: advantages and limitations. *Ann. Thorac. Surg*. 2004;77:2076-2082.

[7] Cheng DAK, Cohn W, Connolly M, et al. Endoscopic vascular harvest in coronary artery bypass grafting surgery: a meta-analysis of randomized trials and controlled trials. Innovations: Technology and Techniques in *Cardiothoracic and Vascular Surgery*. 2005;1:61-74.

[8] Ouzounian M, Hassan A, Buth KJ, et al. Impact of endoscopic versus open saphenous vein harvest techniques on outcomes after coronary artery bypass grafting. *Ann. Thorac. Surg*. 2010;89:403-408.

[9] Yun KL, Wu Y, Aharonian V, et al. Randomized trial of endoscopic versus open vein harvest for coronary artery bypass grafting: six-month patency rates. *J. Thorac. Cardiovasc. Surg*. 2005;129:496-503.

[10] Allen KB, Griffith GL, Heimansohn DA, et al. Endoscopic versus traditional saphenous vein harvesting: a prospective, randomized trial. *Ann. Thorac. Surg*. 1998;66:26-31.

[11] Davis Z, Jacobs HK, Zhang M, Thomas C, Castellanos Y. Endoscopic vein harvest for coronary artery bypass grafting: technique and outcomes. *J. Thorac. Cardiovasc. Surg*. 1998;116:228-235.

[12] Brown EN, Kon ZN, Tran R, et al. Strategies to reduce intraluminal clot formation in endoscopically harvested saphenous veins. *J. Thorac. Cardiovasc. Surg*. 2007;134:1259-1265.

[13] Burris N SK, Brown J, Kwon M, et al. Incidence of residual clot strands in saphenous vein grafts after endoscopic harvest. Innovations: Technology and Techniques in *Cardiothoracic and Vascular Surgery* 2006;1:323-327.

[14] Dreifaldt M, Souza DS, Loesch A, et al. The "no-touch" harvesting technique for vein grafts in coronary artery bypass surgery preserves an intact vasa vasorum. *J. Thorac. Cardiovasc. Surg*. 2011;141:145-150.

[15] Desai P, Kiani S, Thiruvanthan N, et al. Impact of the learning curve for endoscopic vein harvest on conduit quality and early graft patency. *Ann. Thorac. Surg*. 2011;91:1385-1391.

[16] Chiu KM, Chen CL, Chu SH, Lin TY. Endoscopic harvest of saphenous vein: a lesson learned from 1,348 cases. Surg Endosc 2008;22:183-187.

[17] Leissner KB, Woo A, Ortega R, Stanley GD. Endoscopic saphenous vein harvest: severe hypercarbia. *J. Cardiothorac. Vasc. Anesth*. 2006;20:759-760.

[18] Kim SH KD, Yoon TG, Lim JA, Woo NS, Kim TY. Haemodynamic effects during endoscopic vein harvest of the saphenous vein for off-pump coronary artery bypass grafting surgery. *Eur. J. Anaesthesiol*. 2009;26:969-973.

[19] Allen KB, Heimansohn DA, Robison RJ, et al. Risk factors for leg wound complications following endoscopic versus traditional saphenous vein harvesting. *Heart. Surg. Forum* 2000;3(4):325-330.

[20] Nasso G, Anselmi A, De Filippo CM, et al. Evaluation of less invasive method for saphenous vein harvest in patients with type II diabetes. *J. Cardiovasc. Med*. (Hagerstown) 2007;8:511-516.

[21] Coppoolse R, Rees W, Krech R, et al. Routine minimal invasive vein harvesting reduces postoperative morbidity in cardiac bypass procedures. Clinical report of 1400 patients. *Eur. J. Cardiothorac. Surg*. 1999;16 Suppl 2:S61-66.

[22] Kiaii B, Moon BC, Massel D, Langlois Y, et al. A prospective randomized trial of endoscopic versus conventional harvesting of the saphenous vein in coronary artery bypass surgery. *J. Thorac. Cardiovasc. Surg*. 2002;123:204-212.

[23] Patel AN, Hebeler RF, Hamman BL, et al. Prospective analysis of endoscopic vein harvesting. Am. J. Surg. 2001;182:716-719.

[24] Rao C, Aziz O, Deeba S, et al. Is minimally invasive harvesting of the great saphenous vein for coronary artery bypass surgery a cost-effective technique? *J. Thorac. Cardiovasc. Surg*. 2008;135:809-815.

[25] Alrawi SJ, Balaya F, Raju R, Cunningham JN, Jr., Acinapura AJ. A comparative study of endothelial cell injury during open and endoscopic saphenectomy: an electron microscopic evaluation. *Heart Surg. Forum* 2001;4:120-127.

[26] Crouch JD, O'Hair DP, Keuler JP, et al. Open versus endoscopic saphenous vein harvesting: wound complications and vein quality. *Ann. Thorac. Surg.* 1999;68:1513-1516.

[27] Fabricius AM, Diegeler A, Doll N, Weidenbach H, Mohr FW. Minimally invasive saphenous vein harvesting techniques: morphology and postoperative outcome. *Ann. Thorac. Surg.* 2000;70:473-478.

[28] Rousou LJ, Taylor KB, Lu XG, et al. Saphenous vein conduits harvested by endos copic technique exhibit structural and functional damage. *Ann. Thorac. Surg.* 2009;87:62-70.

[29] Perrault LP, Jeanmart H, Bilodeau L, et al. Early quantitative coronary angiography of saphenous vein grafts for coronary artery bypass grafting harvested by means of open versus endoscopic saphenectomy: a prospective randomized trial. *J. Thorac. Cardiovasc. Surg*. 2004;127:1402-1407.

[30] Davis Z, Garber D, Clark S, et al. Long-term patency of coronary grafts with endoscopically harvested saphenous veins determined by contrast-enhanced electron beam computed tomography. *J. Thorac. Cardiovasc. Surg.* 2004;127:823-828.

[31] Lopes RD, Hafley GE, Allen KB, et al. Endoscopic versus open vein-graft harvesting in coronary-artery bypass surgery. *N. Engl. J. Med.* 2009;361:235-244.

[32] Zenati MA, Shroyer AL, Collins JF, et al. Impact of endoscopic versus open saphenous vein harvest technique on late coronary artery bypass grafting patient outcomes in the ROOBY (Randomized On/Off Bypass) Trial. *J. Thorac. Cardiovasc. Surg.* 141:338-344.

[33] Allen KB, Heimansohn DA, Robison RJ, Schier JJ, Griffith GL, Fitzgerald EB. Influence of endoscopic versus traditional saphenectomy on event-free survival: five-year follow-up of a prospective randomized trial. *Heart Surg. Forum* 2003;6:E143-145.

[34] Dacey LJ, Braxton JH, Jr., Kramer RS, et al. Long-term outcomes of endoscopic vein harvesting after coronary artery bypass grafting. *Circulation* 2011;123:147-153.

[35] Kirmani BH, Barnard JB, Mourad F, Blakeman N, Chetcuti K, Zacharias J. Mid-term outcomes for Endoscopic versus Open Vein Harvest: a case control study. *J. Cardiothorac. Surg.* 2010;5:44.

[36] Aranki SF, Shopnick B. Demise of open vein harvesting. *Circulation* 2011;123:127-128.

[37] Thatte HS, Khuri SF. The coronary artery bypass conduit: I. Intraoperative endothelial injury and its implication on graft patency. *Ann. Thorac. Surg.* 2001;72:S2245-2252.

In: Off-Pump Coronary Artery Bypass Grafting
Editors: S.G. Raja and M. Amrani
ISBN 978-1-62081-575-5

Chapter 25

DUAL ANTIPLATELET THERAPY AFTER OFF-PUMP CORONARY ARTERY BYPASS GRAFTING

***Alexander Kulik*[1] *and Marc Ruel*[2]**
[1]Cardiovascular Surgeon, Lynn Heart and Vascular Institute
Boca Raton Regional Hospital, Charles E. Schmidt College of Medicine
Florida Atlantic University, Boca Raton, FL, US
[2]Cardiac Surgeon and Cardiac Surgery Research Chair
University of Ottawa Heart Institute
Cellular and Molecular Medicine and Epidemiology
University of Ottawa, Clinical and Translational Research
University of Ottawa, Ottawa, ON, Canada

ABSTRACT

Antiplatelet therapy is critical for the management of coronary artery disease. For patients undergoing coronary artery bypass graft (CABG) surgery, controversy remains regarding the optimal postoperative antiplatelet regimen to maintain graft patency and reduce ischemic complications. With respect to on-pump CABG, considerable evidence is available to support the use of aspirin, to be administered within 48 hours after surgery and continued indefinitely. To ensure adequate platelet inhibition early after surgery, doses greater than 100 mg daily should be used if aspirin is the sole antiplatelet agent given. On the other hand, following off-pump coronary artery bypass (OPCAB) surgery, there is a common perception that antiplatelet therapy with aspirin alone is likely to be insufficient. Several studies have documented that OPCAB is associated with a postoperative hypercoagulable state, and OPCAB patients have reduced platelet sensitivity to aspirin after surgery. In the context of these prothrombotic conditions, dual antiplatelet therapy with clopidogrel and aspirin after OPCAB is suggested to maintain graft patency. However, this recommendation is based on weak evidence and has yet to be confirmed in a well-conducted randomized trial. Future studies exploring the use of the new antiplatelet agents, prasugrel and ticagrelor, will be of interest to identify the optimal antiplatelet regimen after on-pump and off-pump coronary surgery. This chapter provides a review of the literature to evaluate the risks and benefits of aspirin and clopidogrel therapy after CABG, with a specific focus on OPCAB to examine the rationale for postoperative dual antiplatelet therapy.

INTRODUCTION

Antiplatelet therapy, including the administration of aspirin and clopidogrel, remains the mainstay of treatment for patients with coronary artery disease [1]. Following coronary artery bypass graft surgery (CABG), inhibition of platelet function is essential to help maintain graft patency and prevent major adverse cardiovascular events. Over 30 years of experience has accrued with the use of antiplatelet agents after cardiac surgery [2]. However, controversy exists regarding the optimal postoperative antiplatelet regimen. After CABG, the benefits of preventing graft thrombosis must be balanced against the risks of bleeding complications associated with platelet inhibition.

First discovered in 1897, aspirin irreversibly inhibits platelet cyclooxygenase-1. By decreasing thromboxane-A2 production, aspirin prevents platelet aggregation, reducing the risk of stroke, myocardial infarction (MI) and vascular death in patients with ischemic heart disease [3,4]. Essentially all patients undergoing CABG are candidates for long-term aspirin therapy. Nevertheless, even when used appropriately, aspirin is sometimes ineffective in terms of platelet inhibition early after surgery [5,6]. This phenomenon, termed "aspirin resistance", adversely affects postoperative vein graft patency [7], contributing to early graft occlusion rates as high as 20% reported in some studies [8]. Aspirin alone may also be insufficient to prevent early graft failure following off-pump coronary artery bypass (OPCAB), an operation that can lead to a hypercoagulable state [9-16]. In this context, more intense antiplatelet therapy, including the use of clopidogrel, has been suggested to improve postoperative graft patency and clinical outcomes after CABG.

Clopidogrel is a thienopyridine antiplatelet agent that inhibits the $P2Y_{12}$ adenosine diphosphate receptor at the platelet surface, thereby preventing platelet aggregation [17]. In contrast to ticlopidine, another thienopyridine that had been shown to improve graft patency [18-19], clopidogrel is sevenfold more potent and free of ticlopidine's unfavorable side effect profile that included neutropenia and rash [20]. Clopidogrel irreversibly modifies the platelet adenosine diphosphate (ADP) receptor, and platelets which are exposed to clopidogrel are inhibited for the remainder of their lifespan (7-10 days) [20]. Combining aspirin therapy with clopidogrel leads to potent synergistic antithrombotic effects [21], and clear benefits have been demonstrated in several landmark coronary artery disease trials studying the impact of dual antiplatelet therapy [22-23].

After CABG however, less is known regarding the benefits and risks associated with combining aspirin with clopidogrel [2]. Moreover, newer antiplatelet agents, such as prasugrel and ticagrelor, have recently been introduced [24-26], increasing the number of therapeutic options available for postoperative platelet inhibition. In this context, we reviewed the literature regarding the use of antiplatelet therapy after CABG, with a particular focus on OPCAB surgery. We summarized the risks and benefits associated with postoperative aspirin and clopidogrel, and specifically examined the rationale for administering dual antiplatelet therapy after OPCAB.

Aspirin Therapy after On-Pump CABG

Aspirin and Graft Patency after CABG

Considerable research has been performed to evaluate the impact of aspirin therapy on graft patency in the period following CABG. Over the years, several doses, regimens, and initiation times have been studied. The first randomized trials on the subject were conducted in the late 1970's, demonstrating that aspirin was safe for use in the postoperative period. However, no benefit was seen in terms of graft patency in these early studies, likely because of limited trial enrollment. Moreover, the antiplatelet regimen was administered late in the postoperative period, typically 3 or more days after surgery [27-29]. In the first reported study published in 1979, no improvement was seen with respect to clinical outcomes or early angiographic patency in a trial of 50 patients randomized to either aspirin and dipyridamole, warfarin, or no antithrombotic therapy after CABG [27].

Thereafter, the focus of postoperative trials shifted to the assessment of aspirin administration in the early hours after surgery. Chesebro et al., at the Mayo Clinic, conducted a controlled trial comparing graft patency in 407 patients randomized to placebo or the combination of aspirin and dipyridamole beginning as early as 7 hours after surgery. Within one month of surgery, vein graft patency was significantly higher in patients treated with antiplatelet therapy (98% versus 90%, aspirin and dipyridamole versus placebo, $P<0.0001$) [30]. In a subsequent report, the authors noted an improvement in vein graft patency with antiplatelet therapy one year following surgery (89% versus 77%, aspirin and dipyridamole versus placebo, $P<0.0001$). Antiplatelet therapy was also shown to prevent the development of late vein graft occlusions in those patients whose grafts were documented as patent at the 1-month time-point (6% versus 14% late occlusion rate, aspirin and dipyridamole versus placebo, $P=0.02$) [31].

While the combination of aspirin and dipyridamole was shown to be beneficial, a number of other antithrombotic regimens have also been tested in randomized trials. Compared to placebo, aspirin alone has been shown to improve vein graft patency [32], with one placebo-controlled study documenting an improvement in patency from 68% to 90% with the use of postoperative aspirin [33].

Other investigations have evaluated the addition of warfarin to antiplatelet therapy, yielding conflicting and mostly negative results [34-38].

In one of the largest and most thorough post-CABG antiplatelet studies, the Veterans Administration Cooperative Study randomized 772 CABG patients to one of five antiplatelet regimens: 1) aspirin 325 mg per day; 2) aspirin 325 mg three times per day; 3) aspirin 325 mg plus dipyridamole 75 mg three time per day; 4) sulfinpyrazone 267 mg three times per day; and 5) placebo three times per day. All therapies were given for one year and started 48 hours before CABG except aspirin which, when selected, was given in one dose of 325 mg 12 hours before surgery. Within 60 days of surgery, 555 patients (1781 grafts) underwent angiographic graft assessment, revealing the following graft patency rates: aspirin once per day, 93.5%; aspirin three times per day, 92.3%; aspirin and dipyridamole, 91.9%; and sulfinpyrazone, 90.2%. Compared to the patency rate of placebo (85.2%), Goldman et al. reported that all aspirin-containing therapeutic regimens significantly improved graft patency ($P<0.05$) [39].

In a subsequent report of 1-year graft patency assessed in 406 patients (1,315 grafts), the graft occlusion rate was 15.8% in all of the aspirin groups combined, compared with 22.6% for the placebo group (P=0.03). Thus, early postoperative aspirin administered for one year, regardless of dose, improved 60-day and one-year graft patency [40]. Surprisingly however, angiographic patency was not improved when aspirin was used beyond the one-year time-point after CABG, as compared with placebo [41].

With several trials featuring varied treatment protocols published in the literature, Fremes et al. reviewed the impact of antiplatelet and anticoagulant therapy on vein graft patency in a meta-analysis of 17 randomized trials. Summarizing the data, the authors reported that aspirin significantly prevented graft occlusion as compared with placebo [aspirin with or without dipyridamole versus placebo odds ratio (OR): 0.60; 95% confidence interval (CI): 0.51, 0.71; P<0.0001].

On the other hand, combining dipyridamole with aspirin provided no additional benefit compared to aspirin alone (aspirin plus dipyridamole versus aspirin alone OR: 0.94; 95%CI: 0.72, 1.24; P=0.71), and warfarin did not improve graft patency compared to aspirin (aspirin versus warfarin OR: 0.95; 95%CI: 0.62, 1.44; P=0.87). The authors further noted that a low (100 mg) to medium (325 mg) dose of daily aspirin was more effective and safer than a high dose (975 mg). While preoperative administration provided no additional benefit, the ideal time for initiation of aspirin appeared to be within 6 hours after CABG.

All together, the authors recommended indefinite aspirin use postoperatively in doses of 100-325 mg daily [42]. Subsequently, Lim et al. performed a meta-analysis of 5 randomized controlled trials to compare the efficacy of low dose (50-100 mg daily) and medium dose (300-325 mg daily) aspirin therapy following CABG. Compared to low dose aspirin, there was a trend towards an improvement in graft patency in favor of medium dose aspirin (relative risk ratio: 0.74; 95%CI: 0.52, 1.06; P=0.10).

Although statistical significance was not achieved, the authors advocated for the use of aspirin at a medium dose of 325 mg daily due to its excellent safety profile and minimal increase in cost [43]. This finding is in agreement with the results of a study by Zimmermann et al. which demonstrated that low-dose aspirin (100 mg) is insufficient to effectively inhibit platelet function after CABG, since patients develop resistance to the antiplatelet effect of aspirin in the early postoperative period [6].

Aspirin and Clinical Outcomes after CABG

In addition to the graft benefits associated with aspirin, several observational studies have shown that aspirin is associated with improved clinical outcomes after CABG. Published in 2002, Mangano et al. evaluated the impact of aspirin administration within 48 hours following surgery in a study involving 70 centers in 17 different countries. Among 5,022 patients who survived the first 48 hours after surgery, aspirin (up to 650 mg daily) was administered to 59.7%.

In their analysis, the authors reported that postoperative aspirin therapy within 48 hours of surgery was associated with a 68% reduction in the incidence of postoperative death (1.3% versus 4.0%, aspirin versus no aspirin, P<0.001). Aspirin was also associated with a 48% reduction in the incidence of MI (2.8% versus 5.4%, P<0.001), a 50% reduction in the incidence of stroke (1.3% versus 2.6%, P=0.01), a 74% reduction in the incidence of renal failure (0.9% versus 3.4%, P<0.001), and a 62% reduction in the incidence of bowel infarction (0.3% versus 0.8%, P=0.01) [44].

In another study assessing the impact of long-term postoperative aspirin therapy, Johnson et al. found that CABG patients who consistently took aspirin over a 4-year period after surgery had significantly better long-term survival compared to those who did not (relative risk of death 0.58; 95%CI: 0.47, 0.70) [45].

Risks of Aspirin after CABG

While the benefits associated with aspirin after CABG are considerable, the risks of bleeding complications with its administration in the postoperative period are relatively low.

A number of randomized controlled studies have confirmed that aspirin is safe for use following CABG. Gavaghan et al. performed a double-blind randomized controlled study comparing aspirin 324 mg or placebo given within 1 hour of CABG. Duringthe first 24 hours after surgery, the chest tube blood loss and the red cell transfusion requirements were similar between the groups, and there was no significant difference in the reopening rates [46].

Comparable findings were reported in the Mayo Clinic study where either placebo or the combination of aspirin and dipyridamole was administered 7 hours after CABG in 407 patients. Chest tube bleeding was similar between the two groups [30]. In a subsequent multi-center study involving 1112 CABG patients, Sanz et al. found similar reopening rates (average 3.9%) among patients who were randomized to either aspirin, aspirin plus dipyridamole, or placebo, starting 7 hours after surgery [32].

Finally, in the observational study by Mangano et al. involving 5,022 CABG patients, the authors reported that aspirin administration within 48 hours of surgery did not increase the risk of hemorrhage, gastritis, infection, or impaired wound healing (OR for adverse events: 0.63; 95%CI: 0.54, 0.74) [44]. Overall, the literature reports that aspirin therapy is well tolerated early after CABG.

Postoperative Aspirin and Current Guidelines

In keeping with the published observational and randomized trial data, the current guidelines recommend that aspirin be administered within 48 hours after CABG [47]. Ideally, doses close to 325 mg daily should be used (if aspirin is the sole antiplatelet agent given) in order to provide sufficient platelet inhibition early after surgery [6, 43]. Aspirin should then be continued indefinitely because of its beneficial effects in terms of preventing subsequent clinical events [4]. Surprisingly, these recommendations are not consistently followed. Highlighting a missed opportunity for secondary prevention, several studies have reported that up to 20% of patients are not prescribed aspirin after surgery or they discontinue therapy in the months and years following CABG [48-49].

ANTIPLATELET THERAPY AFTER OFF-PUMP CABG

Graft Patency Concerns Following Off-Pump CABG

The use of cardiopulmonary bypass (CPB) during CABG has several deleterious effects on the body, including the activation and consumption of clotting factors and platelets, and the initiation of a systemic inflammatory response [50, 51]. To avoid the morbidity associated with CPB, off-pump coronary revascularization emerged as a popular alternative to conventional CABG in the mid-1990's. Advantages of the OPCAB approach have been demonstrated in several studies, including less blood loss, lower transfusion requirements, shorter length of stay, and a reduction in morbidity and mortality [52-55]. Despite the surging interest in OPCAB, it soon became apparent that off-pump surgery could contribute to a higher graft failure rate. By avoiding CPB, off-pump surgery results in improved hemostasis by averting the platelet and fibrinolytic defects associated with bypass. On the other hand, the clotting disorders and platelet dysfunction induced by CPB may have desirable effects by protecting anastomosis patency and preventing graft thrombosis. With reports documenting a relative hypercoagulable or prothrombotic state after off-pump surgery, questions were raised whether antiplatelet therapy with aspirin alone would be sufficient for patients following OPCAB.

In one of the first studies to assess graft patency after OPCAB, Gundry et al. compared the long-term clinical and angiographic outcomes of 107 off-pump patients to 112 on-pump patients who had surgery between 1989 and 1990. After 7-years of follow-up, the authors noted that twice as many patients in the OPCAB group required re-catheterization (30% versus 16%, OPCAB versus on-pump CABG, P=0.01). The graft patency rate was lower in the OPCAB group (34% versus 72%, OPCAB versus on-pump CABG, P=0.0004), leading to a greater need for repeat revascularization amongst OPCAB patients (20% versus 7%, OPCAB versus on-pump CABG, P=0.009) [56]. Subsequently, Kim et al. compared the 1-year graft patency of 122 OPCAB patients to 65 conventional CABG patients. Angiography at 1-year demonstrated a vein graft patency rate of 67.9% in the OPCAB group compared to 88.3% in the on-pump CABG group (P<0.001) [10].

Coagulation and Platelet Function after OPCAB

To identify factors contributing to the higher OPCAB graft failure rate, several research groups then compared platelet function and clotting disturbances in the perioperative period after on- and off-pump surgery. Upon review of coagulation studies from 22 OPCAB patients, Mariani et al. noted that procoagulant activity (represented by prothrombin factors 1 and 2) was significantly elevated on the first postoperative day after off-pump surgery [9]. Subsequently, Casati and colleagues compared multiple hematologic parameters from patients undergoing on-pump and off-pump bypass. These authors reported a profound decrease in platelet count and an increase in fibrinolytic activity after on-pump surgery. Off-pump surgery, on the other hand, caused more activation of fibrinogen and acute phase reactants, consistent with the deposition of thrombus at surgical sites of injury. Compared to on-pump CABG, OPCAB led to increased platelet counts [11]. Similar findings were noted by Quigley et al. in a comparison of coagulation function after on- and off-pump surgery. Based on their evaluation using thromboelastography, the authors identified a state of hypercoagulability within the first 3 days after off-pump surgery. While there was an increase in coagulation activity after OPCAB, the authors reported a decrease in coagulation activity after on-pump CABG [14].

Other studies have pointed towards platelet function contributing to the increased risk of thrombotic events after OPCAB. Whereas diminished platelet function is seen early after on-pump surgery [50], Bidstrup et al. noted platelet activity to significantly increase immediately following OPCAB [13]. Similar results were reported by Bednar et al. in a comparison of 80 on- and off-pump patients. Based on P-selectin expression, platelet activity was noted to significantly increase after off-pump surgery, with greater activity seen after OPCAB compared to conventional CABG with CPB. Among patients recovering from OPCAB, the authors found that aspirin had less of an effect in terms of inhibiting platelet aggregation [16]. These results are important in the context of the strong link that has been demonstrated between higher platelet activity (i.e. P-selectin expression) in patients with coronary artery disease and the risk of thrombotic complications [57-59].

The association between platelet function and graft thrombosis after OPCAB was subsequently evaluated in a study by Poston et al. These authors performed a series of coagulation and platelet tests in 76 OPCAB patients, and graft patency was assessed by computed tomography (CT) angiography. Early graft failure was noted in 8 patients. Compared to patients who had functioning grafts, patients with early graft failure had significantly greater aspirin resistance, based on platelet thrombelastography and aggregometry testing 3 days after OPCAB [15].

Rationale for Dual Antiplatelet Therapy after OPCAB

All together, the studies noted above confirmed that a hypercoagulable state exists early after OPCAB. Further, concerns were raised regarding the decrease in platelet sensitivity to aspirin following off-pump surgery. The activation of acute phase reactants and local tissue injury associated with major surgery, without the coagulation and platelet derangements induced by CPB, are believed to shift the balance toward more postoperative thromboembolic complications after OPCAB compared to conventional CABG [12]. As such, several authors have suggested that patients undergoing OPCAB should be treated with a more aggressive perioperative anticoagulation and antiplatelet regimen [9, 10, 12, 15, 16]. With the growing awareness of the prothrombotic milieu following OPCAB, Emory University, one of the leading off-pump centers, instituted a policy change in 2003 to treat all OPCAB patients with both clopidogrel and aspirin after surgery for the duration of 3 months [60].

Compared to aspirin alone, dual therapy with aspirin and clopidogrel inhibits both platelet aggregation as well as platelet activity based on P-selectin expression [61]. In a small randomized trial comparing the combination of clopidogrel 75 mg with aspirin 150 mg daily to aspirin 150 mg alone, Nielsen et al. confirmed that patients who received dual antiplatelet therapy achieved greater platelet inhibition based on thromboelastography studies 30 days after OPCAB [62]. Clopidogrel on its own, however, appears to be insufficient as a sole antiplatelet agent early after CABG. Unlike aspirin, clopidogrel does not appreciably inhibit platelet aggregation during the first 5 postoperative days after coronary surgery [63], and it is not until days 9-28 after CABG that the antiplatelet effects of clopidogrel (at daily doses of 75 mg) become apparent [64].

ASPIRIN AND CLOPIDOGREL THERAPY AFTER ON- AND OFF-PUMP CABG

Dual Antiplatelet Therapy after CABG – Post-Hoc Analyses

Although a consensus was growing regarding the need for dual antiplatelet therapy after OPCAB, no clinical data had yet become available regarding the impact of clopidogrel following coronary surgery. The potential clinical benefits of postoperative clopidogrel were evaluated for the first time as part of *post-hoc* sub-group analyses from the CURE and CREDO multi-center cardiology trials.

In the CURE study, 12,562 patients presenting with acute coronary syndromes without ST-segment elevation were randomized to aspirin alone or aspirin plus clopidogrel for 3-12 months. Theprimary outcome (cardiovascular death, nonfatal MI or stroke) occurred in 9.3% of patients treated with aspirin plus clopidogrel compared to 11.4% in patients treated with aspirin alone (relative risk reduction: 20%; 95%CI: 10.0, 28.0; P<0.001) [22].

In the subgroup of patients who ultimately underwent CABG after enrollment in the trial, there was a trend favoring aspirin plus clopidogrel in a reduction of the primary outcome (14.5% versus 16.2%, aspirin plus clopidogrel versus aspirin alone; relative risk: 0.89; 95%CI: 0.71, 1.11). However, that benefit was entirely preoperative while the patients were awaiting surgery, and no benefit for clopidogrel was demonstrated for CURE patients following CABG [65].

Subsequently, in the CREDO trial, 2,116 patients with symptomatic coronary artery disease and objective evidence of ischemia were randomized to aspirin plus clopidogrel or aspirin alone for 12 months after coronary angiography and PCI. TheCREDO trial observed an overall 26.9% relative risk reduction (95%CI: 3.9%, 44.4%) in the composite end-point at one year (death, MI, and stroke) with clopidogrel and aspirin compared to aspirin alone (8.6% versus 11.8%, P=0.02) [23]. Of the 83 patients that underwent CABG after angiography (no PCI), there was a modest albeit non-significant reduction in 1-year events with clopidogrel (12.2% versus 14.3%, clopidogrel and aspirin versus aspirin alone; relative risk reduction: 16.7%; P=0.78) [66]

Dual Antiplatelet Therapy after CABG – Observational Studies

With a suggestion that dual antiplatelet therapy may be beneficial following CABG, several observational studies were then performed, with a focus on both on- and off-pump patients. In one of the first reports, Ibrahim et al. compared the mid-term graft patency of 62 OPCAB patients who received either 75-160 mg aspirin daily or the combination of aspirin with clopidogrel 75 mg daily. Postoperative angiography within 1-year demonstrated a trend in favor of improved saphenous vein graft patency for patients treated with dual antiplatelet therapy (87% versus 66%, aspirin plus clopidogrel vs. aspirin alone, P=0.19) [67]. Thereafter,

Gurbuz et al. performed an observational study to assess the impact of clopidogrel administration on the short-term outcomes of 591 off-pump CABG patients. Allpatients received aspirin after surgery, and a select group of 186 patients also received clopidogrel postoperatively. After adjusting for clinical factors in multivariate analysis, postoperative clopidogrel was associated with less symptom recurrence (hazard ratio [HR]: 0.3; 95%CI: 0.15, 0.99; P<0.0001) as well as fewer major adverse cardiac events, including fatal or non-fatal MI or coronary reintervention (HR: 0.2; 95%CI: 0.10, 0.45; P<0.0001) [68].

Two recent observational studies have used administrative databases to evaluate the potential benefits of clopidogrel administration after on-pump and off-pump CABG. In a report by Kim et al. published in 2009, the early clinical outcomes of 3,268 patients who received both clopidogrel and aspirin early after CABG (with or without CPB) were compared to 11,799 patients who were treated with aspirin alone using the University Health System Consortium database. Employing multivariate logistic regression and propensity-score analysis, the authors found that compared with aspirin alone, dual antiplatelet therapy was associated with lower in-hospital mortality (1.0% versus 1.8%; adjusted OR: 0.50; 95%CI: 0.25, 0.99). However, there was no difference in the rate of ischemic events (1.3% versus 1.5%; adjusted OR 0.99; 95%CI: 0.59, 1.64), and surprisingly, bleeding events were significantly lower in the group that received both aspirin and clopidogrel (4.2% versus 5.2%; adjusted OR: 0.70; 95%CI: 0.51, 0.97). This raised important concerns that selection bias may have severely limited the analysis [69]. Similar findings were reported by Sørensen et al. who evaluated the efficacy of clopidogrel after CABG using administrative data from 3,545 patients in Denmark. With multivariate and propensity-score analysis, the authors reported a lower risk of death (adjusted HR: 0.34; 95%CI: 0.20, 0.61) in patients who received clopidogrel after surgery. However, clopidogrel did not significantly reduce the incidence of recurrent MI, cardiovascular death, or the need for repeat revascularization in this study [70]. This suggests that, within this cohort, clopidogrel may have been administered preferentially to healthier patients believed to have greater long-term survival [71].

Dual Antiplatelet Therapy after CABG – Clinical Trials

To date, 4 clinical trials have evaluated the impact of clopidogrel on the process of vein graft disease and graft occlusion after CABG. However, none of these studies were designed to specifically focus on patients undergoing OPCAB surgery, and most enrolled a mix of both on- and off-pump patients. In the first study published in 2009, C. Gao and colleagues performed a non-randomized trial involving 197 CABG patients, 37% of whom underwent off-pump surgery. Patients were assigned postoperatively to either clopidogrel 75 mg daily (N=102) or clopidogrel 75 mg plus aspirin 100 mg daily (N=95), based on a weekly alternating treatment scheme. This trial was neither blinded nor placebo-controlled. One month and 1 year after surgery, vein graft patency was assessed by CT angiography. No significant difference was seen comparing isolated clopidogrel treatment to dual antiplatelet therapy after CABG (1 month: 98.1% versus 98.2%, P=0.73; 1 year: 93.5% versus 96.3%, P=0.25; clopidogrel versus clopidogrel plus aspirin) [72]. Subsequently, Sun et al. published a placebo-controlled trial that used partial blinding comparing the combination of postoperative clopidogrel 75 mg plus aspirin 81 mg daily to aspirin 81 mg alone among 100 patients undergoing on-pump CABG. At 30 days, graft patency was assessed using CT angiography, which was performed in 79 patients. No difference was seen in terms of graft patency between the 2 groups, either amongst all grafts (92.9% versus 95%, aspirin versus aspirin and clopidogrel, P=0.43), or vein grafts alone (93.2% versus 93.5%, aspirin versus aspirin and clopidogrel, P=0.92) [73].

In the largest trial that has been performed on the subject, G. Gao et al. randomized 249 patients undergoing CABG (58% off-pump) to receive either clopidogrel 75 mg plus aspirin 100 mg daily or aspirin 100 mg alone starting within 48 hours of surgery. No blinding or placebo control was used in this trial. At 3 months, 90% of patients returned for graft patency assessment using CT angiography. Overallgraft patency was not significantly different between the 2 groups (89.7% versus 93.5%, aspirin versus aspirin and clopidogrel, P=0.07). However, vein graft patency was significantly improved in the combined treatment group compared to isolated aspirin treatment (85.7% versus 91.6%, aspirin versus aspirin and clopidogrel, P=0.04), suggesting that dual antiplatelet therapy may improve vein graft patency 3 months after CABG [74].

The 3 above noted trials all suffered from serious limitations, such as the absence of randomization, the lack of placebo controls, insufficient blinding, and the use of CT angiography to assess graft patency, as compared to conventional angiography which is the gold-standard. Most importantly, by using low-dose aspirin (100 mg or less) or administering clopidogrel on its own, these investigators may have provided insufficient platelet inhibition early after CABG to the control subjects. By under-treating one group, this created a bias in favor of the patients who received combination therapy, possibly contributing to the significant results reported by G. Gao et al. [74].

Using a different design, we recently reported our randomized double-blind placebo-controlled trial whereby isolated aspirin therapy at a dose of 162 mg daily was compared to dual antiplatelet therapy with aspirin 162 mg plus clopidogrel 75 mg daily. The majority of patients (96%) underwent on-pump CABG in our study. To evaluate graft patency, patients underwent conventional coronary angiography 1 year after surgery. Furthermore, each patient underwent intravascular ultrasound assessment of one randomly selected vein graft, since research had previously suggested that combined antiplatelet therapy could slow the process of saphenous vein graft disease [75-78].

Recently reported, we found that the combination of aspirin plus clopidogrel did not significantly reduce the development of vein graft intimal hyperplasia based on intravascular ultrasound 1 year after CABG, compared with aspirin alone. Although not powered for the outcome of graft function, overall graft patency (95.2% versus 95.5%, aspirin and clopidogrel versus aspirin, P=0.90) and vein graft patency (94.3% versus 93.2%, aspirin and clopidogrel versus aspirin, P=0.69) were not different between the groups at 1 year, and there was no difference in the incidence of cardiovascular events [79].

Our trial casts doubt on the potential benefit of dual antiplatelet therapy after on-pump CABG. While a larger study would be necessary to confirm our results, we doubt such a trial will be performed. Power calculations based on CASCADE suggested that a sample size of 8,000 grafts would be required to demonstrate an improvement in patency with clopidogrel treatment [71].

Risks of Dual Antiplatelet Therapy after CABG

Combining clopidogrel therapy with aspirin slightly increases the risk of bleeding complications compared to the use of aspirin alone. In the CURE trial that enrolled acute coronary syndrome patients, major bleeding events developed in 3.7% of subjects who received dual antiplatelet therapy, versus 2.7% in those who received only aspirin (P=0.001) [22]. Clearly, administering clopidogrel immediately before CABG substantially increases the risk of bleeding in the postoperative period [2, 80]. However, its use after surgery, including either on-pump or off-pump bypass, appears to be safe. In the OPCAB study by Gurbuz et al. involving 591 patients, the incidence of bleeding complications were comparable between patients treated with aspirin plus clopidogrel or aspirin alone (1.8% versus 3.3%, aspirin plus clopidogrel versus aspirin alone, P=0.8) [68]. Thereafter, the surgical group at Emory University evaluated their protocol of initiating antiplatelet therapy early after OPCAB, when the chest tube drainage was ≤50 mL/hour for 2 consecutive hours. The outcomes of 171 patients who received postoperative daily aspirin were compared to 193 patients who received daily aspirin and clopidogrel. The authors reported that no patient in the clopidogrel-treated group required reopening for bleeding. Moreover, the 24-hour chest tube drainage in the two groups was comparable, and there was no difference in the incidence of blood transfusion [81].

We subsequently confirmed these findings in an observational study of patients who had undergone either on-pump or off-pump surgery. Using a similar chest tube drainage protocol, antiplatelet therapy was initiated when the postoperative chest tube drainage was ≤50 mL/hour for 2 consecutive hours. A total of 63 patients received clopidogrel 75 mg and aspirin 81 mg daily, while 54 patients received aspirin 325 mg alone. The amount of chest tube drainage after patients received antiplatelet therapy was equivalent between the two groups, and clopidogrel administration was not associated with an increase in the incidence of reopening, transfusion, or the quantity of blood products transfused [82]. In the CASCADE trial, we found no difference in the incidence of major bleeding events at 1 year between patients who were randomized to aspirin and clopidogrel (1.8%) and those who received aspirin alone (0%, P=0.5) [79]. Therefore, when given according to a predefined postoperative protocol, early postoperative clopidogrel can safely be administered to on-pump and off-pump patients, without increasing the risk of bleeding complications.

Conclusion

Over the last thirty years, a number of observational and randomized controlled trials have been performed to evaluate the use of antiplatelet therapy after surgical coronary revascularization. Following on-pump CABG, considerable evidence is available to support the use of aspirin to be administered within 48 hours after surgery and continued indefinitely. To ensure adequate platelet inhibition early after surgery, doses close to 325 mg daily should be used if aspirin if the sole antiplatelet agent given [6,43]. On the other hand, after off-pump CABG, antiplatelet therapy with aspirin alone may be insufficient. Several observational studies have demonstrated that a hypercoagulable state occurs after OPCAB, and patients have reduced platelet sensitivity to aspirin following off-pump surgery. To maintain graft patency in the context of the prothrombotic conditions associated with OPCAB, the use of dual antiplatelet therapy with clopidogrel and aspirin is advised. Combination treatment appears to be the current standard of practice after off-pump surgery, but admittedly, these recommendations are based on low-quality evidence and mainly expert opinion. While the duration of combination therapy remains unclear, 1-3 months of dual antiplatelet therapy after OPCAB appears to be the norm.

To date, several small trials have evaluated the use of combination antiplatelet therapy after CABG, yielding mostly negative results. No trial has specifically focused on OPCAB patients. Therefore, the benefits of dual antiplatelet therapy with aspirin and clopidogrel after off-pump surgery have yet to be confirmed in a large randomized setting. Nevertheless, it remains doubtful that an adequately powered trial will ever be conducted given the necessary cost and large sample size.

Alternatively, attention may soon shift to 2 new recently introduced antiplatelet agents, prasugrel [24] and ticagrelor [25]. Compared to clopidogrel, these drugs appear to provide more consistent inhibition of the $P2Y_{12}$ receptor. Encouraging postoperative results have recently been reported [26]. However, data regarding the impact of these antiplatelet therapies on graft patency has yet to become available. Future studies exploring the use of prasugrel or ticagrelor after CABG will be of interest as we seek to find the ideal antiplatelet regimen for patients who, despite surgical revascularization, remain at lifelong risk for subsequent cardiovascular events.

REFERENCES

[1] Clappers N, Brouwer MA, Verheugt FW. Antiplatelet treatment for coronary heart disease. *Heart* 2007;93:258-65.

[2] Kulik A, Chan V, Ruel M. Antiplatelet therapy and coronary artery bypass graft surgery: perioperative safety and efficacy. *Expert Opin. Drug. Saf.* 2009;8:169-82.

[3] Fuster V, Dyken ML, Vokonas PS, Hennekens C. Aspirin as a therapeutic agent in cardiovascular disease. Special Writing Group. *Circulation* 1993;87:659-75.

[4] Collaborative meta-analysis of randomised trials of antiplatelet therapy for prevention of death, myocardial infarction, and stroke in high risk patients. *BMJ* 2002;324:71-86.

[5] Buchanan MR, Brister SJ. Individual variation in the effects of ASA on platelet function: implications for the use of ASA clinically. *Can. J. Cardiol.* 1995;11:221-7.

[6] Zimmermann N, Kienzle P, Weber AA, et al. Aspirin resistance after coronary artery bypass grafting. J. *Thorac. Cardiovasc. Surg.* 2001;121:982-4.

[7] Yilmaz MB, Balbay Y, Caldir V, et al. Late saphenous vein graft occlusion in patients with coronary bypass: possible role of aspirin resistance. *Thromb. Res.* 2005;115:25-9.

[8] Alexander JH, Hafley G, Harrington RA, et al. Efficacy and safety of edifoligide, an E2F transcription factor decoy, for prevention of vein graft failure following coronary artery bypass graft surgery: PREVENT IV: a randomized controlled trial. *JAMA* 2005;294:2446-54.

[9] Mariani MA, Gu YJ, Boonstra PW, Grandjean JG, van Oeveren W, Ebels T. Procoagulant activity after off-pump coronary operation: is the current anticoagulation adequate? *Ann. Thorac. Surg.* 1999;67:1370-5.

[10] Kim KB, Lim C, Lee C, et al. Off-pump coronary artery bypass may decrease the patency of saphenous vein grafts. *Ann. Thorac. Surg*. 2001;72:S1033-7.

[11] Casati V, Gerli C, Franco A, et al. Activation of coagulation and fibrinolysis during coronary surgery: on-pump versus off-pump techniques. *Anesthesiology* 2001;95: 1103-9.

[12] Kurlansky PA. Is there a hypercoagulable state after off-pump coronary artery bypass surgery? What do we know and what can we do? *J. Thorac. Cardiovasc. Surg*. 2003;126:7-10.

[13] Bidstrup BP, Scarrott H, Luque M. Platelet function after off pump coronary surgery. *Heart Surg. Forum* 2003;6:286-7.

[14] Quigley RL, Fried DW, Pym J, Highbloom RY. Off-pump coronary artery bypass surgery may produce a hypercoagulable patient. *Heart Surg. Forum*. 2003;6:94-8.

[15] Poston R, Gu J, Manchio J, Lee A, et al. Platelet function tests predict bleeding and thrombotic events after off-pump coronary bypass grafting. *Eur. J. Cardiothorac. Surg*. 2005;27:584-91.

[16] Bednar F, Osmancik P, Vanek T, et al. Platelet activity and aspirin efficacy after off-pump compared with on-pump coronary artery bypass surgery: results from the prospective randomized trial PRAGUE 11-Coronary Artery Bypass and REactivity of Thrombocytes (CABARET). *J.Thorac. Cardiovasc. Surg*. 2008;136:1054-60.

[17] Hollopeter G, Jantzen HM, Vincent D, et al. Identification of the platelet ADP receptor targeted by antithrombotic drugs. *Nature* 2001;409:202-7.

[18] Chevigne M, David JL, Rigo P, Limet R. Effect of ticlopidine on saphenous vein bypass patency rates: a double-blind study. *Ann. Thorac. Surg*. 1984;37:371-8.

[19] Limet R, David JL, Magotteaux P, Larock MP, Rigo P. Prevention of aorta-coronary bypass graft occlusion. Beneficial effect of ticlopidine on early and late patency rates of venous coronary bypass grafts: a double-blind study. *J. Thorac. Cardiovasc. Surg*. 1987;94:773-83.

[20] Quinn MJ, Fitzgerald DJ. Ticlopidine and clopidogrel. *Circulation* 1999;100:1667-72.

[21] Cadroy Y, Bossavy JP, Thalamas C, et al. Early potent antithrombotic effect with combined aspirin and a loading dose of clopidogrel on experimental arterial thrombogenesis in humans. *Circulation*. 2000;101:2823-8.

[22] Yusuf S, Zhao F, Mehta SR, et al. Effects of clopidogrel in addition to aspirin in patients with acute coronary syndromes without ST-segment elevation. *N. Engl. J. Med*. 2001;345:494-502.

[23] Steinhubl SR, Berger PB, Mann JT, 3rd, et al. Early and sustained dual oral antiplatelet therapy following percutaneous coronary intervention: a randomized controlled trial. *JAMA* 2002;288:2411-20.

[24] Wiviott SD, Braunwald E, McCabe CH, et al. Prasugrel versus clopidogrel in patients with acute coronary syndromes. *N. Engl. J. Med*. 2007;357:2001-15.

[25] Wallentin L, Becker RC, Budaj A,et al. Ticagrelor versus clopidogrel in patients with acute coronary syndromes. *N. Engl. J. Med*. 2009;361:1045-57.

[26] Held C, Asenblad N, Bassand JP, et al. Ticagrelor versus clopidogrel in patients with acute coronary syndromes undergoing coronary artery bypass surgery: results from the PLATO (Platelet Inhibition and Patient Outcomes) trial. *J. Am. Coll. Cardiol*. 2011;57:672-84.

[27] Pantely GA, Goodnight SH, Jr., Rahimtoola SH, et al. Failure of antiplatelet and anticoagulant therapy to improve patency of grafts after coronary-artery bypass: a controlled, randomized study. *N. Engl. J. Med.* 1979;301:962-6.

[28] McEnany MT, Salzman EW, Mundth ED, et al. The effect of antithrombotic therapy on patency rates of saphenous vein coronary artery bypass grafts. *J. Thorac. Cardiovasc. Surg* .1982;83:81-9.

[29] Sharma GV, Khuri SF, Josa M, Folland ED, Parisi AF. The effect of antiplatelet therapy on saphenous vein coronary artery bypass graft patency. *Circulation* 1983;68(3 Pt 2):II218-21.

[30] Chesebro JH, Clements IP, Fuster V, et al. A platelet-inhibitor-drug trial in coronary-artery bypass operations: benefit of perioperative dipyridamole and aspirin therapy on early postoperative vein-graft patency. *N. Engl. J. Med.* 1982;307:73-8.

[31] Chesebro JH, Fuster V, Elveback LR, et al. Effect of dipyridamole and aspirin on late vein-graft patency after coronary bypass operations. *N Engl. J. Med.* 1984;310:209-14.

[32] Sanz G, Pajaron A, Alegria E, et al. Prevention of early aortocoronary bypass occlusion by low-dose aspirin and dipyridamole. Grupo Espanol para el Seguimiento del Injerto Coronario (GESIC). *Circulation* 1990;82:765-73.

[33] Lorenz RL, Schacky CV, Weber M, et al. Improved aortocoronary bypass patency by low-dose aspirin (100 mg daily). Effects on platelet aggregation and thromboxane formation. *Lancet* 1984;1:1261-4.

[34] Brooks N, Wright J, Sturridge M, et al. Randomised placebo controlled trial of aspirin and dipyridamole in the prevention of coronary vein graft occlusion. *Br. Heart J.* 1985;53:201-7.

[35] Rajah SM, Salter MC, Donaldson DR, et al. Acetylsalicylic acid and dipyridamole improve the early patency of aorta-coronary bypass grafts. A double-blind, placebo-controlled, randomized trial. *J. Thorac. Cardiovasc. Surg.* 1985;90:373-7.

[36] Pfisterer M, Burkart F, Jockers G, et al. Trial of low-dose aspirin plus dipyridamole versus anticoagulants for prevention of aortocoronary vein graft occlusion. *Lancet* 1989;2:1-7.

[37] Pfisterer M, Burkart F, Jockers G, et al. Prevention of aortocoronary vein bypass graft occlusion: which antithrombotic treatment and for how long? *Thromb. Res. Suppl.* 1990;12:11-21.

[38] van der Meer J, Hillege HL, Kootstra GJ, et al. Prevention of one-year vein-graft occlusion after aortocoronary-bypass surgery: a comparison of low-dose aspirin, low-dose aspirin plus dipyridamole, and oral anticoagulants. The CABADAS Research Group of the Interuniversity Cardiology Institute of The Netherlands. *Lancet* 1993;342:257-64.

[39] Goldman S, Copeland J, Moritz T, et al. Improvement in early saphenous vein graft patency after coronary artery bypass surgery with antiplatelet therapy: results of a Veterans Administration Cooperative Study. *Circulation* 1988;77:1324-32.

[40] Goldman S, Copeland J, Moritz T, et al. Saphenous vein graft patency 1 year after coronary artery bypass surgery and effects of antiplatelet therapy. Results of a Veterans Administration Cooperative Study. *Circulation* 1989;80:1190-7.

[41] Goldman S, Copeland J, Moritz T, Henderson W, Zadina K, Ovitt T, Kern KB, Sethi G, Sharma GV, Khuri S, et al. Long-term graft patency (3 years) after coronary artery

surgery. Effects of aspirin: results of a VA Cooperative study. *Circulation* 1994;89:1138-43.

[42] Fremes SE, Levinton C, Naylor CD, Chen E, Christakis GT, Goldman BS. Optimal antithrombotic therapy following aortocoronary bypass: a meta-analysis. *Eur. J. Cardiothorac Surg*. 1993;7:169-80.

[43] Lim E, Ali Z, Ali A, et al. Indirect comparison meta-analysis of aspirin therapy after coronary surgery. *BMJ* 2003;327:1309.

[44] Mangano DT. Aspirin and mortality from coronary bypass surgery. *N. Engl. J. Med.* 2002;347:1309-17.

[45] Johnson WD, Kayser KL, Hartz AJ, Saedi SF. Aspirin use and survival after coronary bypass surgery. Am. Heart. J. 1992;123:603-8.

[46] Gavaghan TP, Gebski V, Baron DW. Immediate postoperative aspirin improves vein graft patency early and late after coronary artery bypass graft surgery. A placebo-controlled, randomized study. *Circulation* 1991;83:1526-33.

[47] Eagle KA, Guyton RA, Davidoff R, et al. ACC/AHA 2004 guideline update for coronary artery bypass graft surgery: a report of the American College of Cardiology/American Heart Association Task Force on Practice Guidelines (Committee to Update the 1999 Guidelines for Coronary Artery Bypass Graft Surgery). *Circulation* 2004;110:e340-437.

[48] Galea J, Manche A, Goiti JJ, Locke TJ, Wilkinson GA, Smith GH. Omission of aspirin in patients following coronary artery bypass graft surgery. *J. Clin. Pharm. Ther.* 1994;19:381-6.

[49] Bradshaw PJ, Jamrozik K, Gilfillan I, Thompson PL. Preventing recurrent events long term after coronary artery bypass graft: suboptimal use of medications in a population study. *Am. Heart J.* 2004;147:1047-53.

[50] Edmunds LH, Jr. Blood-surface interactions during cardiopulmonary bypass. *J. Card. Surg*. 1993;8:404-10.

[51] Edmunds LH, Jr., Colman RW. Thrombin during cardiopulmonary bypass. *Ann. Thorac. Surg*. 2006;82:2315-22.

[52] Cleveland JC, Jr., Shroyer AL, Chen AY, Peterson E, Grover FL. Off-pump coronary artery bypass grafting decreases risk-adjusted mortality and morbidity. *Ann. Thorac. Surg*. 2001;72:1282-8.

[53] Reston JT, Tregear SJ, Turkelson CM. Meta-analysis of short-term and mid-term outcomes following off-pump coronary artery bypass grafting. *Ann. Thorac. Surg* .2003;76:1510-5.

[54] Sellke FW, DiMaio JM, Caplan LR, et al. Comparing on-pump and off-pump coronary artery bypass grafting: numerous studies but few conclusions: a scientific statement from the American Heart Association council on cardiovascular surgery and anesthesia in collaboration with the interdisciplinary working group on quality of care and outcomes research. *Circulation* 2005;111:2858-64.

[55] Puskas JD, Kilgo PD, Lattouf OM, et al. Off-pump coronary bypass provides reduced mortality and morbidity and equivalent 10-year survival. *Ann. Thorac. Surg*. 2008;86(4):1139-46.

[56] Gundry SR, Romano MA, Shattuck OH, Razzouk AJ, Bailey LL. Seven-year follow-up of coronary artery bypasses performed with and without cardiopulmonary bypass. *J. Thorac. Cardiovasc. Surg*. 1998;115:1273-7.

[57] Tschoepe D, Schultheiss HP, Kolarov P, Schwippert B, Dannehl K, Nieuwenhuis HK, Kehrel B, Strauer B, Gries FA. Platelet membrane activation markers are predictive for increased risk of acute ischemic events after PTCA. *Circulation* 1993;88:37-42.

[58] Kabbani SS, Watkins MW, Ashikaga T, et al. Platelet reactivity characterized prospectively: a determinant of outcome 90 days after percutaneous coronary intervention. Circulation 2001;104:181-6.

[59] Blann AD, Nadar SK, Lip GY. The adhesion molecule P-selectin and cardiovascular disease. *Eur. Heart J.* 2003;24:2166-79.

[60] Puskas JD, Williams WH, Mahoney EM, et al. Off-pump vs conventional coronary artery bypass grafting: early and 1-year graft patency, cost, and quality-of-life outcomes: a randomized trial. *JAMA* 2004;291:1841-9.

[61] Klinkhardt U, Bauersachs R, Adams J, et al. Clopidogrel but not aspirin reduces P-selectin expression and formation of platelet-leukocyte aggregates in patients with atherosclerotic vascular disease. *Clin. Pharmacol. Ther.* 2003;73:232-41.

[62] Nielsen AB, Bochsen L, Steinbruchel DA. Hypercoagulability and platelet inhibition after OPCAB. Randomized intervention with clopidogrel. *Scand. Cardiovasc. J.* 2007;41:325-30.

[63] Lim E, Cornelissen J, Routledge T, et al. Clopidogrel did not inhibit platelet function early after coronary bypass surgery: A prospective randomized trial. *J. Thorac. Cardiovasc. Surg.* 2004;128:432-5.

[64] David JL, Limet R. Antiplatelet activity of clopidogrel in coronary artery bypass graft surgery patients. Thromb. Haemost. 1999;82:1417-21.

[65] Fox KA, Mehta SR, Peters R, et al. Benefits and risks of the combination of clopidogrel and aspirin in patients undergoing surgical revascularization for non-ST-elevation acute coronary syndrome: the Clopidogrel in Unstable angina to prevent Recurrent ischemic Events (CURE) Trial. *Circulation* 2004;110:1202-8.

[66] Saw J, Topol EJ, Steinhubl SR, et al. Comparison of long-term usefulness of clopidogrel therapy after the first percutaneous coronary intervention or coronary artery bypass grafting versus that after the second or repeat intervention. *Am. J. Cardiol.* 2004;94:623-5.

[67] Ibrahim K, Tjomsland O, Halvorsen D, et al. Effect of clopidogrel on midterm graft patency following off-pump coronary revascularization surgery. *Heart Surg. Forum* 2006;9:E581-856.

[68] Gurbuz AT, Zia AA, Vuran AC, Cui H, Aytac A. Postoperative clopidogrel improves mid-term outcome after off-pump coronary artery bypass graft surgery: a prospective study. *Eur. J. Cardiothorac. Surg.* 2006;29:190-5.

[69] Kim DH, Daskalakis C, Silvestry SC, et al. Aspirin and clopidogrel use in the early postoperative period following on-pump and off-pump coronary artery bypass grafting. *J. Thorac. Cardiovasc. Surg.* 2009;138:1377-84.

[70] Sorensen R, Abildstrom SZ, Hansen PR, et al. Efficacy of post-operative clopidogrel treatment in patients revascularized with coronary artery bypass grafting after myocardial infarction. *J. Am. Coll. Cardiol.* 2011;57:1202-9.

[71] Kulik A, Ruel M. Clopidogrel after coronary artery bypass graft surgery insufficient evidence. *J. Am. Coll. Cardiol.* 2011;58:1084-5.

[72] Gao C, Ren C, Li D, Li L. Clopidogrel and aspirin versus clopidogrel alone on graft patency after coronary artery bypass grafting. *Ann. Thorac. Surg.* 2009;88:59-62.

[73] Sun JC, Teoh KH, Lamy A, et al. Randomized trial of aspirin and clopidogrel versus aspirin alone for the prevention of coronary artery bypass graft occlusion: the Preoperative Aspirin and Postoperative Antiplatelets in Coronary Artery Bypass Grafting study. *Am. Heart. J.* 2010;160:1178-84.

[74] Gao G, Zheng Z, Pi Y, Lu B, Lu J, Hu S. Aspirin plus clopidogrel therapy increases early venous graft patency after coronary artery bypass surgery a single-center, randomized, controlled trial. *J. Am. Coll.* Cardiol. 2010;56:1639-43.

[75] Herbert JM, Tissinier A, Defreyn G, Maffrand JP. Inhibitory effect of clopidogrel on platelet adhesion and intimal proliferation after arterial injury in rabbits. *Arterioscler. Thromb.* 1993;13:1171-9.

[76] Harker LA, Marzec UM, Kelly AB, et al. Clopidogrel inhibition of stent, graft, and vascular thrombogenesis with antithrombotic enhancement by aspirin in nonhuman primates. *Circulation* 1998;98:2461-9.

[77] Hermann A, Weber AA, Schror K. Clopidogrel inhibits platelet adhesion and platelet-dependent mitogenesis in vascular smooth muscle cells. *Thromb. Res.* 2002;105:173-5.

[78] Kulik A, Le May M, Wells GA, Mesana TG, Ruel M. The clopidogrel after surgery for coronary artery disease (CASCADE) randomized controlled trial: clopidogrel and aspirin versus aspirin alone after coronary bypass surgery [NCT00228423]. Curr. Control Trials *Cardiovasc. Med.* 2005;6:15.

[79] Kulik A, Le May MR, Voisine P, et al. Aspirin plus clopidogrel versus aspirin alone after coronary artery bypass grafting: the clopidogrel after surgery for coronary artery disease (CASCADE) Trial. *Circulation* 2010;122:2680-7.

[80] Purkayastha S, Athanasiou T, Malinovski V, et al. Does clopidogrel affect outcome after coronary artery bypass grafting? A meta-analysis. *Heart* 2006;92:531-2.

[81] Halkos ME, Cooper WA, Petersen R, et al. Early administration of clopidogrel is safe after off-pump coronary artery bypass surgery. *Ann. Thorac. Surg.* 2006;81:815-9.

[82] Chan V, Kulik A, Bourke ME, Ressler L, Mesana TG, Ruel M. Clopidogrel is safe early after on- and off-pump coronary artery bypass surgery. *J. Card. Surg.* 2007;22:493-7.

In: Off-Pump Coronary Artery Bypass Grafting
Editors: S.G. Raja and M. Amrani
ISBN 978-1-62081-575-5

Chapter 26

OFF-PUMP CORONARY ARTERY BYPASS GRAFTING IN PATIENTS WITH IMPAIRED LEFT VENTRICULAR FUNCTION

Maximilian Y. Emmert and Volkmar Falk
Clinic for Cardiac Surgery, University Hospital Zurich, Zurich, Switzerland

ABSTRACT

Conventional CABG using cardiopulmonary bypass (CPB) and cardioplegic arrest has been the gold standard for surgical revascularization in patients with multivessel disease for many years. However, for patients with impaired left ventricular function (ILVF) surgical revascularization remains a challenge and numerous studies report worse outcomes.

ILVF is also acknowledged as a prognostic indicator in the EuroSCORE risk stratification system and the Society of Thoracic Surgeons score. ILVF is an independent risk-factor for worse outcome after cardiac surgery. In patients with ILVF the use of CPB is associated with an increased risk for postoperative mortality and morbidity. The deleterious effects of CPB such as capillary leak syndrome, systemic inflammatory syndrome in addition to aortic manipulation are well established. In the setting of ILVF ischemia during cardioplegic cardiac arrest may induce myocardial damage and enhance inflammatory activation leading to an impairment of cardiac function after reperfusion. Major risks of CPB and cardioplegic arrest in patients with LV dysfunction include global ischemia and myocardial stunning further damaging the ventricular function. In contrast, off-pump coronary artery bypass grafting (OPCAB) permits myocardial revascularisation without CPB and cardioplegic arrest potentially minimizing risks for patients with ILVF. While recent prospective, randomized trials primarily comparing low risk patients did not yield any potential benefit for OPCAB over on-pump CABG, numerous retrospective reports and registry data support the use of OPCAB for patients with ILVF. Although OPCAB may be beneficial for this subset of high-risk patients, the surgical management may be difficult.

The necessity for temporary stabilization and repetitive cardiac immobilisation and exposure may result in extended phases of hypotension and compromised cardiac output. As emergency conversion to on-pump surgery is associated with worse outcomes, OPCAB in patients with ILVF requires careful preoperative planning and intra-operative management. This chapter provides an overview about the management of patients with poor ejection fraction undergoing OPCAB.

INTRODUCTION

Conventional coronary artery bypass grafting (CABG) using cardiopulmonary bypass (CPB) and cardioplegic arrest has been the gold standard for surgical revascularization in patients with multivessel disease. Despite increasing age and risk profile of patients being referred for CABG, mortality and morbidity have remained constantly low1.

The guidelines of the American Heart Association (AHA) and of the European Society of Cardiology / European Association of Cardiothoracic Surgery (ESC/EACTS)) on CABG recommend surgical revascularization for patients with ILVF suffering from angina pectoris symptoms and presenting with either significant left main (or left main equivalent) stenosis, proximal left anterior descending (LAD) artery stenosis with 2 or 3 vessel disease [2-4].

Surgical revascularization in these patients remains a challenge and numerous studies seem to report worse outcomes in the setting of ILVF [5,6]. This is also reflected in the EuroSCORE, (www.euroscore.org) that gives a lot of weight to poor ventricular function as an independent risk-factor for worse outcome after cardiac surgery [7].

In patients with ILVF, the use of CPB may lead to worse outcomes [8,9]. These include excess of myocardial damage [10,11] and inflammatory activation [9] leading to a severe impairment of cardiac function[12]. Major risks of CPB and cardioplegic arrest in patients with ILVF include global ischemia, myocardial stunning [13] as well as endothelial dysfunction and impairment of vasodilatation [14]. This can lead to hemodynamic instability and low cardiac output requiring increased doses of inotropic support after on-pump surgery [15]. Aortic manipulation carries substantial risk of worse neurological outcome [16-18].

In contrast, off pump coronary artery bypass grafting (OPCAB) permits myocardial revascularisation without CPB and cardioplegic arrest and can potentially minimize these risks for patients ILVF19.

Prospective, randomized trials primarily comparing low risk patients did not display a potential benefit for OPCAB over on-pump CABG [20-22]. Numerous retrospective reports and registry data indicate significant advantages of OPCAB with regards to risk-adjusted morbidity[16'18'23-29] and importantly suggest OPCAB to disproportionally benefit high-risk patients including patients with ILVF[19'27'30].

The surgical management of these patients may present a challenge. The necessity for temporary stabilization, exposure and repetitive cardiac immobilisation can lead to extended phases of hemodynamic impairment which may result in dangerous situations requiring emergent conversion to [31-33] on-pump CABG. Therefore, OPCAB in patients with severe ventricular dysfunction requires careful preoperative planning and constant interaction between the surgeon and the anesthesiologist in order to optimise cardiac positioning, exposure, and hemodynamics [34].

Indications for Surgical Revascularization in Patients with Decreased Left Ventricular Function

Coronary artery disease is the major reason for heart failure (HF) and despite therapeutic advances, the prognosis for these patients is poor with a suggested mortality ranging from 5-30%. The indications for surgical revascularization in patients with ILVF is given when they suffer from angina pectoris symptoms and present with either significant left main disease (LMD), a LMD equivalent (proximal stenosis of both LAD and circumflex) or proximal LAD stenosis with 2- or 3- vessel disease.

In the STICH trial, the largest available prospective trial comparing medical therapy alone versus medical therapy plus surgical revascularization, the principal value of surgical revascularization in patients with ILVF was evaluated. While the intention-to-treat analysis did not find a significant difference between groups with regard to the death from any cause, the as-treated analysis showed a significant survival benefit for the group treated with medical therapy plus CABG. Similarly, the rates of death from cardiovascular causes and of death from any cause or hospitalization for cardiac causes were lower among patients who underwent CABG than among those who received medical therapy only[35].

Assessment of Myocardial Viability

The evaluation of myocardial viability has been suggested to be an important predictor for the outcome and long-term prognosis in patients with ILVF. It should be standardized and included in the preoperative work up as ILVF is not always irreversible. Numerous studies have demonstrated that the left ventricular function can improve and even normalize after CABG in patients with ischemic but viable myocardium [36]. The recent subgroup analysis on myocardial viability of the STICH trial demonstrated that the presence of viable myocardium is associated with a greater likelihood of survival in patients with ILVF. In contrast, surgical revascularization should be avoided on ventricles without viability as these patients will not benefit [37]. Hachamovitch and colleagues have further elucidated the importance of viability assessment with specific regards to the interaction between the degree of ischemia and fixed defects, the type of therapy (medical versus surgical), and the history of coronary artery disease (no previous myocardial infarction versus previous myocardial infarction) in predicting long-term survival [38]. In a retrospective design using Cox Proportional Hazard Modeling, 13969 patients who underwent adenosine or exercise stress single photon emission computed tomography (SPECT) myocardial perfusion scintigraphy were assessed. After risk-adjustment, a three-way interaction was identified between the detected ischemia, the type of therapy and the cardiovascular history in predicting long-term outcome and survival. This interaction identified an increasing survival benefit with revascularization in the setting of extensive ischemia for patients without prior MI, but not among patients with prior MI [38]. When excluding patients with more extensive scar from the analysis (>10% total myocardium fixed), with an increasing amount of ischemia, an increasing survival benefit for patients with and without prior MI treated with surgical revascularization was identified (Figure 1).

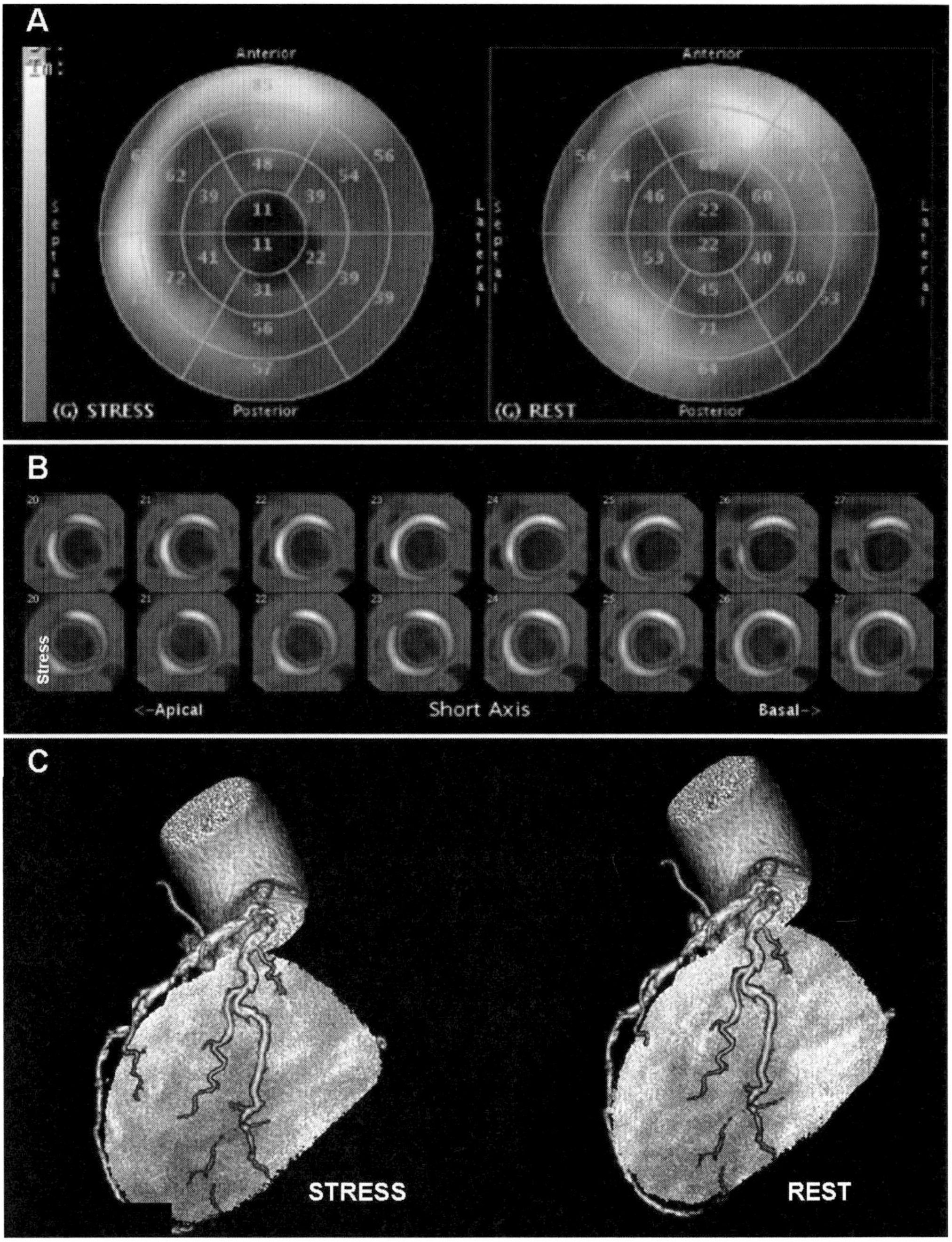

Figure 1. A and B: Assessment of myocardial viability: PET Perfusion images used in clinical routine showing a fixed perfusion defect apical i.e. scar and reversible perfusion defect in the neighboring areas (antero- and inferolateral) i.e. ischemia. C: Exemplary 3-dimensional PET-CT fusion images showing a reversible apical perfusion defect, i.e. ischemia. *Courtesy Prof. Ph. A. Kaufmann and Dr. M. Fiechter, Cardiac Imaging, University Hospital Zurich, Switzerland.*

In contrast the analysis also stressed the fact of a possible harm associated with revascularization if ischemia was not present. In patients with extensive scar (>10% total myocardium fixed) the role of ischemia was secondary to identify the optimal treatment strategy [38].

To assess myocardial viability SPECT, positron emission tomography (PET) and stress echocardiography are well established and known for their high sensitivity [36] (Figure 1). Various reports have suggested these methods as a reliable predictor for an improved left ventricular function following surgical revascularization [36]. The current evidence is mainly based on non-randomized, observational reports or meta-analyses. Only few prospective, randomized trials assessing the potential value of PET imaging are available [39, 40].

Rationale for OPCAB in Patients with Impaired Left Ventricular Function

Beside the organ protective qualities of hypothermia, CPB comes with an increased risk for major complications such as stroke [41] and renal failure [42] CPB and ischemic arrest is well established to have a damaging effect on the myocardium including an extended degree of myocardial injury [10,11] and inflammatory response [9]. In particular, the contact with the CPB circuit surface, the ischemia and reperfusion can cause the release of cytokines and inflammatory mediators [9] disturbing myocardial performance, particularly if the LV function is already severely impaired [12]. These deleterious effects particularly apply if the CPB run is prolonged [43].

Other factors known to contribute to myocardial damage after CPB are the direct damage to myocardial cells during manipulation and cannulation maneuvers as well as the impact of potassium, hypothermia, ischemia or transient fibrillation on cellular function and cell membranes [44]. In addition, it has also been demonstrated that on-pump surgery is associated with a more pronounced endothelial dysfunction and impairment of coronary artery vasodilatation [14].

Global ischemia and myocardial stunning in on-pump surgery lead to myocardial damage and ventricular dysfunction as compared to temporary regional ischemia induced during off-pump surgery [13]. More than a decade ago, Steed et al. have investigated the underlying mechanisms and studied subendocardial malperfusion during CPB45. In line with that, Akins and associates have also demonstrated off-pump surgery to better preserve normal septal motion, while on-pump CABG often results in paradoxical movement of the interventricular septum [46,47].

The use of intra-coronary shunts in off-pump surgery to maintain distal perfusion during the anastomosis may be beneficial in patients ILVF. Vassiliades et al. have elucidated the potential benefits and the efficacy of distal perfusion techniques during off-pump surgery. In a prospective design, patients were randomised to one of the following perfusion approaches including no coronary perfusion (NCP), passive coronary perfusion (PCP) or active coronary perfusion (ACP). The cardiac function was significantly better after ACP when compared to the PCP and NCP groups. Lower troponin levels in the perfusion groups (ACP and PCP) clearly indicated a better degree of myocardial preservation when compared to the NCP group [48]. Continuous ventilation of the lungs during off-pump surgery may also have a positive impact on cardiac performance.

Technical Aspects and Management of Patients with Ventricular Dysfunction

To perform OPCAB in patients with severe ventricular dysfunction a careful preoperative planning involving both the surgeons and anesthesiologists is mandatory. During the procedure, constant interaction between surgeon and anesthesiologist in order to improve cardiac positioning, exposure, and hemodynamics is necessary.

Anesthesiological Considerations

Judicious fluid administration is mandatory. Transesophageal echocardiography must be performed in all patients. In patients with decreased right ventricular function and/or pulmonary hypertension a Swan Ganz catheter can be inserted. Cardiac output is monitored continuously via a PiCCO™ catheter.

Preparation and Cardiac Exposure

The standard OPCAB procedure is carried out through a median sternotomy. Cardiac exposure should be obtained by pericardial stay sutures. The pericardium is opened in an inverted T fashion and if arterial T-grafts are planned the T-graft anastomosis is best performed at this point. Heparin is administered to obtain activated clotting time (ACT) in excess of 350 seconds and repeated if necessary. Next, epicardial atrial (in all) and ventricular (in some) temporary pace maker wires are placed. Cardiac positioning for LAD exposure is achieved with rolled up surgical swabs placed laterally to the heart if possible. Additional deep pericardial stitches are used to enhance exposure.

Preparation of Target Vessel, Shunt Insertion and Anastomosis

After stabilisation with a suction stabilization device (Figure 2), coronary arteriotomy is performed with a beaver blade. Thereafter, an intra-coronary shunt is inserted to maintain distal perfusion during anastomosis. If this is not feasible, vessel occlusion with a felt supported snare may be performed. Next, the anastmosis is performed with prolene 8/0 for all arterial anasotmosis and 7/0 or 8/0 prolene running suture when a venous graft is required, while a mister blower (with CO_2 and saline) is used to ensure that operative field is bloodlesss. If a proximal anastomosis is needed, a clamp-less 'no touch' technique, using clamp-less devices such as the Heartstring device (HEARTSTRING™ Proximal Seal System, Guidant, Indianapolis, USA) should be used [18]. The surgeon uses digital palpation to identify a healthy, non-calcified segment of aorta or epiaortic ultrasound [49]. An aortic-punch device is used to create a circular aortotomy. Thereafter, the hole is occluded with the finger before the coiled Heartstring device is inserted and opened to achieve a hemostatic seal against the aortic inner wall.

The anastomosis can then be carried out with a continuous 6-0 Prolene suture under clear vision without significant blood-loss while also using the blower mister. After completion of the anastomosis and before tightening of the suture the device is gently removed. Following that, coronary blood flow is measured and documented to confirm sufficient graft patency.

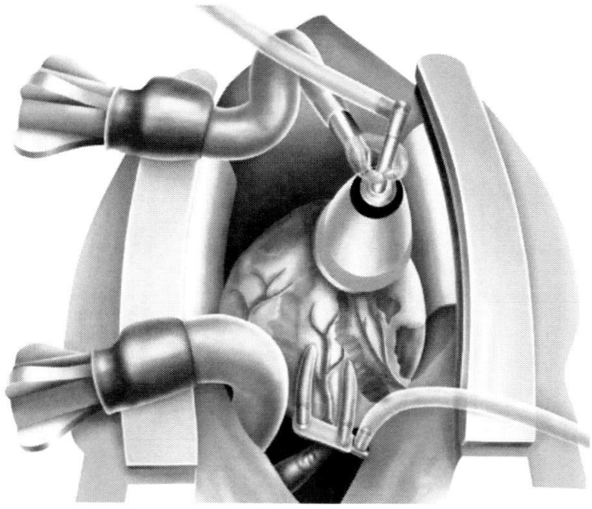

Figure 2. Apical suction device allows optimal cardiac exposure while avoiding repetitive re-positioning maneuvers which carry an increased risk for hemodynamic decompensation in patients with impaired left ventricular function.

Strategy for Revascularization

Surgical revascularization is started by LAD to LIMA grafting and followed by the right coronary system. And finally to better access the circumflex artery territory, the right pleural space can be widely opened to allow cardiac positioning into the right chest. In patients with LMD, the LAD and circumflex arteries are always grafted, regardless of the degree of stenosis. Other than that, all other vessels with significant stenoses (>70%) are identified on the preoperative angiogram and selected as targets for revascularization. Preoperative functional imaging should be used to guide the revascularisation strategy. In the setting of chronically occluded vessels, our strategy is to perform complete revascularisation whenever possible. For graft selection, LIMA is used in all patients when suitable. For patients under 70 years of age a total arterial revascularisation with bilateral IMA (skeletonized harvest) and radial artery is the preferred method.

Hemodynamic Management

Hemodynamic optimization is attempted by volume management, Trendelenburg positioning, atrial pacing and catecholamine administration. Volume overload should be avoided. Optimal hemodynamics can be maintained by using the Trendelenburg positioning which provides a sufficient venous return [34]. If catecholamine administration is necessary, it should be applied in an adjusted continuous fashion and not in the manner of bolus dosing. In addition, waiting approximately 2 to 3 minutes and intermittent removal of the stabilizer device often leads to normalization of the hemodynamic parameters allowing for completion of the anastomosis [50]. An intra-aortic balloon pump (IABP) can be inserted intra-operatively to achieve an increased coronary perfusion and afterload reduction. Standby cardiopulmonary bypass is mandatory in any case. If the patient remains unstable despite IABP support, initiation of cardiopulmonary bypass should be done in a semi-elective fashion before emergent conversion becomes necessary due to significant hemodynamic compromise. If conversion to CPB is necessary, most of the cases can then be continued in a beating heart fashion. On-pump beating heart surgery offers improved hemodynamic conditions while avoiding the myocardial ischemia associated with aortic cross-clamping and subsequent cardioplegic arrest [51,52].

Available Outcome Data and Current Status in Literature

For patients with ILVF, no randomized trials comparing on-pump CABG vs. OPCAB have been performed and among reports generally comparing high-risk patients [27, 53], only few, non-randomized reports for patients with ILVF are available [4,19,30,44,50,54-57] (Table 1).

In the largest series, Sharoni and colleagues analyzed 353 patients with an EF <35% who either underwent OPCAB (n=144) or on-pump (n=209) coronary surgery. There was no significant difference with regards to major postoperative complications or mortality; the authors concluded that OPCAB can be safely applied to patients with impaired left ventricular function. The authors observed an increase in the use of OPCAB over time, without any impact on morbidity or mortality [30].

Another study evaluating 478 patients with an ejection fraction ≤35% showed no detectable difference with regards to mortality and major adverse cardiac events including myocardial infarction, low cardiac output and stroke after propensity adjustment. Importantly, the authors demonstrated that patients undergoing off-pump surgery presented with a trend for less frequent occurrence of non-cardiac complications such as renal dysfunction, bleeding and respiratory failure.

In addition, the authors also addressed the important question if the OPCAB approach in patients with ILVF comes at price of less complete revascularization and were able to show that there was no significant difference between groups.

The authors concluded that OPCAB surgery may be safely applied to patients with severely decreased EF, may even benefit these patients with regards to non-cardiac complications and does not come at cost of less complete revascularization [19].

In general, the available studies demonstrate the principal feasibility and safety of OPCAB in patients with ILVF by providing a comparable overall mortality when compared to on-pump surgery.

Single reports are further indicative for a potential benefit with regards to overall morbidity and in particular the pulmonary outcomes. However, these retrospective studies displaying just trends and not hard facts may only be considered indicative. The real value of OPCAB in patients with ILVF can only be sufficiently explored by help of large, randomized prospective trials.

Table 1. Summary of available studies comparing OPCAB versus on-pump CABG in patients with impaired left ventricular function

Author	n	Type	Year	LVEF	Results	Conclusions and Comments
Sharoni [30]	353	r	2006	<35	1. The groups did not differ statistically in early (3% vs. 2%) or late mortality (8.3% vs. 7.7%) or major complications such as MI (0% vs. 1%) or stroke (1.4% vs. 1%). 2. OPCAB patients were more likely to undergo extubation earlier and had a lower tendency to develop new renal failure (p=ns).	1. OPCAB is feasible and potentially beneficial for patients with depressed LVEF.
Youn [57]	153	r, pm	2007	<35	1. Adjusted Mortality was comparable between groups (4% vs. 2%, p=ns). 2. The operation time, ventilation time, intensive care unit admission time and occurrence of respiratory failure were significantly lower after OPCAB. 3. The overall 6-year actuarial survival rates did not differ significantly (88.2% vs. 72.4%; p=ns) and there were no significant differences in 6-year rates of freedom from MACCE (p=ns).	1. OPCAB is safe in patients with decreased LVEF and offers superior outcomes with regards to respiratory failure. 2. At mid-term follow up both groups present with comparable outcomes.
Arom [50]	177	r	2000	<30	1. OPCAB and ONCABG were comparable with regards to mortality, stroke and major cardiac complications. 2. Blood loss and cardiac enzyme release was significantly lower among OPCAB patients. 3. The number of distal grafts was significantly lower after off-pump surgery.	1. OPCAB in patients with <30% LVEF and multivessel disease is feasible and may be beneficial with regards to blood loss and cardiac enzyme release. 2. OPCAB in patients with decreased LVEF may be at of less complete revascularization.

Table 1. (Continued)

Author	n	Type	Year	LVEF	Results	Conclusions and Comments
Attaran [44]	934	r, pm	2010	<30	1. Adjusted mortality and major postoperative complications were comparable between groups (p=ns), except MI (1.3% vs. 3.8%; p=0.04). 2. Unadjusted and adjusted mid-term and long-term survival rates were similar in both groups, while the re-intervention rate was found to be significantly higher after OPCAB (p<0.001). 3. After propensity matching, the mean number of distal grafts was comparable between groups.	1. There was no significant benefit for OPCAB with regards to in-hospital mortality, mid-term survival or long-term survival. 2. With sufficient myocardial protection in ONCABG and complete revascularization in OPCAB, comparable results can be achieved.
Emmert [19]	478	r, ps	2011	<35	1. There was no statistical difference (p=ns) between groups for mortality (2.3 vs. 4.1) and MACCE (13.7 vs. 17.6%) including myocardial-infarction (1.4 vs. 4.9%), low cardiac output (2.3 vs. 4.7%) and stroke (2.3 vs. 2.7%). 2. OPCAB patients presented with a trend to less frequent occurrence of a non-cardiac composite (12.1 vs. 22.1%; p=0.059) including renal dysfunction bleeding and respiratory failure. 3. Complete revascularization was achieved in similar levels for both groups (92.2 vs. 92.8%;p=ns)	1. OPCAB is feasible in patients with severely decreased LVEF and it may even benefit these patients in regard to non-cardiac complications 2. OPCAB does not come at cost of less complete revascularization.
Sternik [56]	117	r	1996	<35	1. Operative Mortality and major complications were comparable between groups. 2. One year and two year actuarial survival was better after off-pump surgery (91% vs. 79%; p= 0.03 and 86% and 65%; *p*=0.04).	1. OPCAB represents a valid alternative in patients with decreased LVEF and appears to improve the mid-term survival.

Author	n	Type	Year	LVEF	Results	Conclusions and Comments
Darwazah [54]	150	r	2006	<35	1. Mortality and major complications did not differ significantly between groups, whereas the overall morbidity was significantly higher in the ONCABG group (35.7% vs. 19.7%;p = 0.03). 2. Complete revascularization was significantly higher after ONCABG.	1. OPCAB in patients with decreased LVEF results in a comparable mortality, but lower overall morbidity. 2. OPCAB appeared to be at cost of less complete revascularization.
Maltais [55]	137	r, ps	2010	<35	1. Overall 30-day mortality was comparable between groups (1.5% EF >35% pts vs 2.9% in EF _35% pts; p=0.19). 2. Ten-year survival was lower in poor EF patients (44 % vs 762%), and remained significant even after adjusting for risk factors (p = 0.04). 3. Freedom from cardiac death for both groups was also significantly reduced in poor EF patients (p = 0.008), while freedom from the combined end point of cardiac or sudden death, myocardial infarction, repeat coronary revascularization, unstable angina, and cardiac failure was comparable in both groups (p = 0.5).	1. Off-pump coronary artery bypass surgery can be performed adequately and safely in patients with decreased LVEF. 2. However, overall and cardiac survival was decreased in this subset of patients with a comparable freedom from major cardiac adverse related events.

EF = ejection fraction; LVEF = left ventricular ejection fraction; MACCE = major adverse cardiac and cerebral events; MI = myocardial infarction; n = number; OPCAB = off-pump coronary artery bypass grafting; ONCABG = on-pump coronary artery bypass grafting; pm = propensity matched; ps = propensity score; r = retrospective.

CONCLUSIONS

In summary, OPCAB in patients with ILVF is feasible and can be safely performed yielding similar outcomes as achieved on the pump. The preoperative assessment of myocardial viability represents a key aspect in the process of decision-making for surgical revascularization and should be implemented into the clinical routine for these patients. Logistical key considerations of a successful OPCAB approach comprise of a careful patient selection and a sufficient preoperative planning.

A constant intra-operative interaction between the surgeon and the anesthesiologist in order to control and optimize the hemodynamic situation is required and stand-by cardio-pulmonary support is absolutely mandatory in case of cardiac decompensation. Although few, observational reports suggest a potential benefit of OPCAB in patients with ILVF with regards to improved morbidity, due to the small sample size and the retrospective design these data may only be considered as indicative. Large, randomized clinical trials are needed to assess if and to what extent OPCAB is beneficial for this subset of high risk patients.

REFERENCES

[1] Tarakji KG, Sabik JF, 3rd, Bhudia SK, Batizy LH, Blackstone EH. Temporal onset, risk factors, and outcomes associated with stroke after coronary artery bypass grafting. *JAMA* 305:381-90.

[2] Cooper EA, Edelman JJ, Wilson MK, Bannon PG, Vallely MP. Off-pump Coronary artery bypass grafting in elderly and high-risk patients - a review. *Heart Lung. Circ.* 2011;20:694-703.

[3] Eagle KA, Guyton RA, Davidoff R, et al. ACC/AHA 2004 guideline update for coronary artery bypass graft surgery: a report of the American College of Cardiology/American Heart Association Task Force on Practice Guidelines (Committee to Update the 1999 Guidelines for Coronary Artery Bypass Graft Surgery). *Circulation* 2004;110:e340-437.

[4] Task Force on Myocardial Revascularization of the European Society of Cardiology (ESC) and the European Association for Cardio-Thoracic Surgery (EACTS); European Association for Percutaneous Cardiovascular Interventions (EAPCI),Kolh P, Wijns W, Danchin N, et al. Guidelines on myocardial revascularization. *Eur. J. Cardiothorac Surg*. 2010;38 Suppl:S1-S52.

[5] Christakis GT, Weisel RD, Fremes SE, et al. Coronary artery bypass grafting in patients with poor ventricular function. Cardiovascular Surgeons of the University of Toronto. *J. Thorac. Cardiovasc. Surg*. 1992;103:1083-91.

[6] O'Connor GT, Plume SK, Olmstead EM, et al. Multivariate prediction of in-hospital mortality associated with coronary artery bypass graft surgery. Northern New England Cardiovascular Disease Study Group. *Circulation* 1992;85:2110-8.

[7] Nashef SA, Roques F, Michel P, Gauducheau E, Lemeshow S, Salamon R. European system for cardiac operative risk evaluation (EuroSCORE). *Eur. J. Cardiothorac. Surg.* 1999;16:9-13.

[8] Nesher N, Frolkis I, Vardi M, et al. Higher levels of serum cytokines and myocardial tissue markers during on-pump versus off-pump coronary artery bypass surgery. *J. Card. Surg.* 2006;21:395-402.
[9] Wan IY, Arifi AA, Wan S, et al. Beating heart revascularization with or without cardiopulmonary bypass: evaluation of inflammatory response in a prospective randomized study. *J. Thorac. Cardiovasc. Surg.* 2004;127:1624-31.
[10] Koh TW, Carr-White GS, DeSouza AC, et al. Intraoperative cardiac troponin T release and lactate metabolism during coronary artery surgery: comparison of beating heart with conventional coronary artery surgery with cardiopulmonary bypass. *Heart* 1999;81:495-500.
[11] Krejca M, Skiba J, Szmagala P, Gburek T, Bochenek A. Cardiac troponin T release during coronary surgery using intermittent cross-clamp with fibrillation, on-pump and off-pump beating heart. *Eur. J. Cardiothorac. Surg.* 1999;16:337-41.
[12] Stamou SC, Corso PJ. Coronary revascularization without cardiopulmonary bypass in high-risk patients: a route to the future. *Ann. Thorac. Surg.* 2001;71:1056-61.
[13] Calafiore AM, Di Mauro M, Contini M, et al. Myocardial revascularization with and without cardiopulmonary bypass in multivessel disease: impact of the strategy on early outcome. *Ann. Thorac. Surg.* 2001;72:456-62.
[14] Lockowandt U, Franco-Cereceda A. Off-pump coronary bypass surgery causes less immediate postoperative coronary endothelial dysfunction compared to on-pump coronary bypass surgery. *Eur. J. Cardiothorac. Surg.* 2001;20:1147-51.
[15] Mangano DT. Biventricular function after myocardial revascularization in humans: deterioration and recovery patterns during the first 24 hours. *Anesthesiology* 1985;62:571-7.
[16] Emmert MY, Salzberg SP, Seifert B, et al. Is off-pump superior to conventional coronary artery bypass grafting in diabetic patients with multivessel disease? *Eur. J. Cardiothorac. Surg.* 2011;40:233-9.
[17] Emmert MY, Salzberg SP, Seifert B, et al. Routine off-pump coronary artery bypass grafting is safe and feasible in high-risk patients with left main disease. *Ann. Thorac. Surg.* 2010;89:1125-30.
[18] Emmert MY, Seifert B, Wilhelm M, Grunenfelder J, Falk V, Salzberg SP. Aortic no-touch technique makes the difference in off-pump coronary artery bypass grafting. *J. Thorac. Cardiovasc. Surg.* 2011;142:1499-506.
[19] Emmert MY, Salzberg SP, Theusinger OM, Rodriguez H, Sundermann SH, Plass A, Starck CT, Seifert B, Baulig W, Hoerstrup SP, Jacobs S, Grunenfelder J, Falk V. Off-pump surgery for the poor ventricle? *Heart Vessels* 2011 May 17 [Epub ahead of print].
[20] Hueb W, Lopes NH, Pereira AC, et al. Five-year follow-up of a randomized comparison between off-pump and on-pump stable multivessel coronary artery bypass grafting. The MASS III Trial. *Circulation* 2010;122:S48-52.
[21] Moller CH, Perko MJ, Lund JT, et al. Three-year follow-up in a subset of high-risk patients randomly assigned to off-pump versus on-pump coronary artery bypass surgery: the Best Bypass Surgery trial. *Heart* 2011;97:907-13.
[22] Shroyer AL, Grover FL, Hattler B, et al. On-pump versus off-pump coronary-artery bypass surgery. *N. Engl. J. Med.* 2009;361:1827-37.

[23] Edelman JJ, Yan TD, Bannon PG, Wilson MK, Vallely MP. Coronary artery bypass grafting with and without manipulation of the ascending aorta--a meta-analysis. *Heart Lung. Circ.* 2011;20:318-24.
[24] Halbersma WB, Arrigoni SC, Mecozzi G, et al. Four-year outcome of OPCAB no-touch with total arterial Y-graft: making the best treatment a daily practice. *Ann. Thorac. Surg.* 2009;88:796-801.
[25] Patel NN, Angelini GD. Off-pump coronary artery bypass grafting: for the many or the few? *J. Thorac. Cardiovasc. Surg.* 2010;140:951-3.e1.
[26] Puskas JD, Kilgo PD, Lattouf OM, et al. Off-pump coronary bypass provides reduced mortality and morbidity and equivalent 10-year survival. *Ann. Thorac. Surg.* 2008;86:1139-46.
[27] Puskas JD, Thourani VH, Kilgo P, et al. Off-pump coronary artery bypass disproportionately benefits high-risk patients. *Ann. Thorac. Surg.* 2009;88:1142-7.
[28] Puskas JD, Williams WH, Duke PG, et al. Off-pump coronary artery bypass grafting provides complete revascularization with reduced myocardial injury, transfusion requirements, and length of stay: a prospective randomized comparison of two hundred unselected patients undergoing off-pump versus conventional coronary artery bypass grafting. *J. Thorac. Cardiovasc. Surg.* 2003;125:797-808.
[29] Sedrakyan A, Wu AW, Parashar A, Bass EB, Treasure T. Off-pump surgery is associated with reduced occurrence of stroke and other morbidity as compared with traditional coronary artery bypass grafting: a meta-analysis of systematically reviewed trials. *Stroke* 2006;37:2759-69.
[30] Sharoni E, Song HK, Peterson RJ, et al. Off pump coronary artery bypass surgery for significant left ventricular dysfunction: safety, feasibility, and trends in methodology over time--an early experience. *Heart* 2006;92:499-502.
[31] Mukherjee D, Rao C, Ibrahim M, et al. Meta-analysis of organ damage after conversion from off-pump coronary artery bypass procedures. *Ann. Thorac. Surg.* 2011;92:755-61.
[32] Mukherjee D, Ashrafian H, Kourliouros A, et al. Intra-operative conversion is a cause of masked mortality in off-pump coronary artery bypass: a meta-analysis. *Eur. J. Cardiothorac. Surg.* 2011 Jue 16. [Epub ahead of print]
[33] Mukherjee D, Ahmed K, Baig K, et al. Conversion and safety in off-pump coronary artery bypass: a system failure that needs re-emphasis. *Ann. Thorac. Surg.* 2011;91: 630-9.
[34] Keeling WB, Halkos ME, Puskas JD. Management of patients with a calcified aorta or low ejection fraction undergoing multivessel coronary revascularization. Semin. *Thorac. Cardiovasc. Surg.* 2010;22:250-2.
[35] Velazquez EJ, Lee KL, Deja MA, et al. Coronary-artery bypass surgery in patients with left ventricular dysfunction. *N. Engl. J. Med.* 2011;364:1607-16.
[36] Allman KC, Shaw LJ, Hachamovitch R, Udelson JE. Myocardial viability testing and impact of revascularization on prognosis in patients with coronary artery disease and left ventricular dysfunction: a meta-analysis. *J. Am. Coll Cardiol.* 2002;39:1151-8.
[37] Bonow RO, Maurer G, Lee KL, et al. Myocardial viability and survival in ischemic left ventricular dysfunction. *N. Engl. J. Med.* 2011;364:1617-25.
[38] Hachamovitch R, Rozanski A, Shaw LJ, et al. Impact of ischaemia and scar on the therapeutic benefit derived from myocardial revascularization vs. medical therapy

among patients undergoing stress-rest myocardial perfusion scintigraphy. *Eur. Heart J.* 2011;32:1012-24.

[39] Beanlands RS, Nichol G, Huszti E, et al. F-18-fluorodeoxyglucose positron emission tomography imaging-assisted management of patients with severe left ventricular dysfunction and suspected coronary disease: a randomized, controlled trial (PARR-2). *J. Am. Coll. Cardiol.* 2007;50:2002-12.

[40] Di Carli MF, Davidson M, Little R, et al. Value of metabolic imaging with positron emission tomography for evaluating prognosis in patients with coronary artery disease and left ventricular dysfunction. *Am. J. Cardiol.* 1994;73:527-33.

[41] Taylor KM. Central nervous system effects of cardiopulmonary bypass. *Ann. Thorac. Surg.* 1998;66:S20-4.

[42] Weerasinghe A, Athanasiou T, Al-Ruzzeh S, et al. Functional renal outcome in on-pump and off-pump coronary revascularization: a propensity-based analysis. *Ann. Thorac. Surg.* 2005;79:1577-83.

[43] Moshkovitz Y, Sternik L, Paz Y, et al. Primary coronary artery bypass grafting without cardiopulmonary bypass in impaired left ventricular function. *Ann. Thorac. Surg.* 1997;63:S44-7.

[44] Attaran S, Shaw M, Bond L, Pullan MD, Fabri BM. Does off-pump coronary artery revascularization improve the long-term survival in patients with ventricular dysfunction? *Interact. Cardiovasc. Thorac. Surg.* 2010;11:442-6.

[45] Steed DL, Follette DM, Foglia R, Maloney JV, Buckberg GD. Effects of pulsatile assistance and nonpulsatile flow on subendocardial perfusion during cardiopulmonary bypass. *Ann. Thorac. Surg.* 1978;26:133-41.

[46] Akins CW. Noncardioplegic myocardial preservation for coronary revascularization. *J. Thorac. Cardiovasc. Surg.* 1984;88:174-81.

[47] Akins CW, Boucher CA, Pohost GM. Preservation of interventricular septal function in patients having coronary artery bypass grafts without cardiopulmonary bypass. *Am. Heart. J.* 1984;107:304-9.

[48] Vassiliades TA, Jr., Nielsen JL, Lonquist JL. Coronary perfusion methods during off-pump coronary artery bypass: results of a randomized clinical trial. *Ann. Thorac. Surg.* 2002;74:S1383-9.

[49] Suvarna S, Smith A, Stygall J, et al. An intraoperative assessment of the ascending aorta: a comparison of digital palpation, transesophageal echocardiography, and epiaortic ultrasonography. *J. Cardiothorac. Vasc. Anesth.* 2007;21:805-9.

[50] Arom KV, Flavin TF, Emery RW, Kshettry VR, Petersen RJ, Janey PA. Is low ejection fraction safe for off-pump coronary bypass operation? *Ann. Thorac. Surg.* 2000;70:1021-5.

[51] Mizutani S, Matsuura A, Miyahara K, et al. On-pump beating-heart coronary artery bypass: a propensity matched analysis. *Ann. Thorac. Surg.* 2007;83:1368-73.

[52] Rastan AJ, Eckenstein JI, Hentschel B, et al. Emergency coronary artery bypass graft surgery for acute coronary syndrome: beating heart versus conventional cardioplegic cardiac arrest strategies. *Circulation* 2006;114:I477-85.

[53] Al-Ruzzeh S, Nakamura K, Athanasiou T, et al. Does off-pump coronary artery bypass (OPCAB) surgery improve the outcome in high-risk patients?: a comparative study of 1398 high-risk patients. *Eur. J. Cardiothorac. Surg.* 2003;23:50-5.

[54] Darwazah AK, Abu Sham'a RA, Hussein E, Hawari MH, Ismail H. Myocardial revascularization in patients with low ejection fraction < or =35%: effect of pump technique on early morbidity and mortality. *J. Card. Surg.* 2006;21:22-7.
[55] Maltais S, Ladouceur M, Cartier R. The influence of a low ejection fraction on long-term survival in systematic off-pump coronary artery bypass surgery. *Eur. J. Cardiothorac. Surg.* 2011;39:e122-7.
[56] Sternik L, Moshkovitz Y, Hod H, Mohr R. Comparison of myocardial revascularization without cardiopulmonary bypass to standard open heart technique in patients with left ventricular dysfunction. *Eur. J. Cardiothorac. Surg.* 1997;11:123-8.
[57] Youn YN, Chang BC, Hong YS, Kwak YL, Yoo KJ. Early and mid-term impacts of cardiopulmonary bypass on coronary artery bypass grafting in patients with poor left ventricular dysfunction: a propensity score analysis. *Circ. J.* 2007;71:1387-94.

In: Off-Pump Coronary Artery Bypass Grafting
Editors: S.G. Raja and M. Amrani
ISBN 978-1-62081-575-5

Chapter 27

Off-Pump Coronary Artery Bypass Grafting in Patients with ST-Segment Elevation Myocardial Infarction

Khalil Fattouch[1], Pietro Dioguardi[2], Francesco Guccione[2] and Giuseppe Bianco[1]

[1]Department of Cardiac Surgery
University of Palermo, Palermo, Italy
[2]GVM Care and Research
Department of Cardiac Surgery, Palermo, Italy

Abstract

Despite more than 30 years of experience with coronary artery bypass grafting (CABG), controversy still exists on the optimal timing of surgical revascularization after acute myocardial infarction (AMI). Systemic fibrinolytic treatment and primary percutaneous coronary intervention (PCI) are both effective and represent the first-choice treatment for acute ST-segment elevation myocardial infarction (STEMI), although several randomized studies have shown that primary PCI is superior to thrombolytic therapy achieving early reperfusion and reducing mortality. In the last 2 decades, CABG during AMI was performed only in patients with mechanical complications or refractory cardiogenic shock (high mortality and morbidity rates). Emergency CABG in patients with STEMI is still associated with high mortality and morbidity, and the early outcome is poor compared with the outcome in patients with stable angina. Furthermore, it may be advisable to delay surgery whenever possible. However, in patients with STEMI, early surgery (within the first hours) is indicated. Current indications for emergency CABG in patients with STEMI are limited to those presenting with evolving myocardial ischemia refractory to optimal medical therapy, presence of left main stenosis or 3-vessel disease, ongoing ischemia despite successful or failed PCI, complicated PCI, or cardiogenic shock accompanied by complex coronary anatomy.

Operative mortality for these patients using conventional OPCABG (On-pump coronary artery bypass grafting) is from 1.6% to 32% and strongly depends on the preoperative hemodynamic condition. The use of off-pump strategies for CABG is being still debated at present. Several retrospective studies have suggested the benefits of off-pump surgery in terms of in-hospital mortality and postoperative outcomes.

This chapter focuses on the impact of off-pump surgery in patients with STEMI who undergo urgent CABG.

Introduction

Acute myocardial infarction (AMI) is the clinical syndrome leading to sudden and prolonged occlusion of a coronary branch, which leads to the ischemic necrosis of myocardial cells. Despite enormous advances in the diagnosis and treatment, coronary artery diseases (CAD) still remain a major health problem in the Western world. Moreover, more than a million patients, only in the United States, are hospitalized with suspected AMI annually in coronary care units [1]. Over the years, progressive improvement in the treatment of patients with AMI has resulted in reduced mortality. It has evolved from "clinical observation" that characterized the first half of the 20th century, the "staged coronary unit" that began in the mid-70th and has played an important role in the study and treatment of arrhythmias through to the modern "era of reperfusion" introducing thrombolysis and later primary percutaneous transluminal coronary angioplasty (PTCA), stent implantation and coronary artery bypass grafting (CABG) [2].

Etiopathogenesis of Myocardial Ischemia

Almost all cases (>90%) of AMI are caused by atherosclerosis. Histological studies of the atherosclerotic plaques often reveal, as a triggering cause of the ischemic process, the sudden change in the morphology of the plaque, such as hemorrhage, erosion, ulceration, fissuring or rupture [2-5].

The platelets are in contact with subendothelial collagen, adhering to the vessel wall and releasing powerful aggregators such as thromboxane A_2, serotonin and platelet factors, which stimulate the vasospasm. At the same time released tissue thromboplastin, which activates the intrinsic pathway of coagulation, initiates clot formation. In most cases, within a few minutes, the thrombus occludes the lumen of the coronary vessel. The result of occlusion of arteries is the loss of blood supply to the myocardium downstream of the occlusion. The ischemic myocardium undergoes progressive changes in biochemical, functional and morphological properties, whose severity is related to the amount and duration of the flow interruption.

The main consequence of myocardial ischemia is anaerobic glycolysis, which produces an inadequate quantity of high-energy phosphates (creatine phosphate, adenosine triphosphate) and causes accumulation of potentially harmful catabolites such as lactic acid [6-7]. The function of the myocardium is affected immediately after (60 seconds) the acute event and causes a loss of contraction. The early changes are reversible and do not cause cell death in a short time. The irreversible ultrastructural changes of myocytes occurs after 20-40 minutes. This irreversible damage begins in the subendocardial region; if ischemia is more extensive cell necrosis spreads like a wave front to involve a larger thickness of the ischemic area [5-7].

The timing of the intervention to reverse ischemia therefore represents one of the factors favorable to the survival of patients. Within 6 hours, 70% of patients will develop a transmural AMI; this percentage reaches 100% after 24h. Therapeutic approach for this group of patients is early reperfusion so as to ensure limitation of the infarcted area; reduce the risk of ventricular dysfunction; and increase early and long- term survival.

SURGICAL MYOCARDIAL REVASCULARIZATION FOR AMI

The time between onset of symptoms and intervention is still the key of the treatment. The improvement of thrombolytic and PTCA therapies, and the reduction of mortality following AMI, has reduced the interest in CABG as a first choice for early reperfusion, relegating such a therapeutic approach only in well-defined conditions [8]. However, with the improvement of surgical techniques, anesthetic management and myocardial protection, the role for revascularization by CABG has evolved [9].

Until 30 years ago, CABG surgery in patients with a diagnosis of AMI was only indicated as a concomitant procedure while tackling acute mechanical complications of AMI. Mortality and morbidity in the short and long term for these patients were high, both for those who underwent surgery during the acute phase of the AMI as well as for those in whom surgery was delayed as a strategy to wait for evolution of the lesion.

In 1979 Steven Phillips et al. considered emergency CABG using saphenous vein bypass grafts as a possible technique of early reperfusion to effectively stop the progressive deterioration of the infarcted heart muscle. Authors found that patients operated within six hours after onset of symptoms have an increase in ejection fraction of 34%, a reduction in left ventricular end-diastolic pressure by 40% and a decrease volume of the infarcted area equal to 25% [10].

In the 1980's two different groups published retrospective studies: Spokane and Des Moines. They endorsed the possible use of CABG as early reperfusion therapy for AMI. The surgery was preferable to medical therapy, as associated with lower mortality in the short and long term.

De Wood et al. reported outcomes of 701 patients who underwent CABG surgery, within 24 hours after onset of symptoms of AMI, including 440 diagnosed with STEMI and 261 with a diagnosis of non ST-segment elevation myocardial infarction (NSTEMI). Authors found a hospital mortality of 5.2% for STEMI group and 3% for NSTEMI group.

The study also identified cardiogenic shock, critical preoperative state and left main stem disease as predictors of mortality [11]. Phillips et al. in 1986 published a retrospective study of 592 patients reperfused by CABG (261 patients) or PCI (331 patients), versus 146 treated medically.

The results obtained in terms of mortality were: 4.9% for patients undergoing reperfusion compared with 17% for patients treated with medical therapy alone.

Authors recommended the choice of thrombolysis and/or PTCA as the most appropriate method for early myocardial reperfusion for patients with single-vessel disease and CABG for patients with three vessels disease [12]. During the last 2 decade only few centers focused their research on preoperative stratification, predictors of outcomes and mortality, timing and management of surgery, in patients with AMI considered as candidates for CABG for early complete reperfusion.

Hochberg et al. performed a retrospective study of 174 patients. They reported a mortality rate for those operated within 1 week by 46% compared with 6% of those operated after 5 weeks. They showed that in the first group, 50% of patients who died were admitted in shock. Therefore they concluded that CABG was safe at any time provided that the ejection fraction (EF) was not less than 50% [13]. In 1986, Katz et al. performed another study on 145 patients identifying EF and cardiac shock as risk factors predictive of mortality. They concluded that waiting for surgery does not reduce the risk of ventricular dysfunction and mortality rate [14]. Kouchoukos et al. performed a prospective study of 240 patients operated within 30 days after onset of symptoms.

In this study EF and left main coronary artery disease were predictive of mortality. They further concluded that the timing and status of emergency CABG surgery were factors that increase the operative risk [15].

In 1989, Kennedy et al. published a retrospective study of 793 patients undergoing CABG within 30 days from diagnosis of AMI, compared with a group of patients undergoing elective CABG surgery. Authors found a mortality of 5.7% for the first group and 1.9% for the second, identifying EF, age and state of emergency as risk factors predictive of mortality [16]. Floten et al. analyzed 832 patients, with a diagnosis of AMI, focusing on the timing of surgery. They reported a mortality of 7.6% for surgery within 24hour from onset of symptoms and 4% for those between 1 and 7th days and concluded that delayed CABG does not provide benefit in the long-term survival and also exposes patients to increased risk of extension of AMI and mortality [17].

Between 1990 and 1993 Sintek et al. performed a prospective study of 530 patients, reporting a mortality of 4.4% for those undergoing surgery within 24hours, 2.1% for those operated on between the 3rd and 7th day and 1.4% for those operated between 1 and 4 week. They identified age, site and type of AMI as risk factors predictive of mortality.

They concluded that for patients with a diagnosis of AMI in non-emergency conditions, it is possible to perform CABG surgery at any time, without an increase in mortality [18]. Recently, Lee et al. published two retrospective studies of patients undergoing CABG, post-AMI. They reported a mortality rate of 11.8% for patients undergoing surgery within 6 hours after onset of symptoms, 9.5% for those operated between 6 and 24hours and 2.8% for patients who underwent surgery after 1 day. The authors concluded that CABG, performed with a diagnosis of AMI, is burdened by a high risk, with a higher mortality than the control group (treated with medical therapy).

These data confirmed that surgical intervention in patients diagnosed with AMI is legitimate. Lee et al. concluded that surgery can benefit, if delayed by at least 24 h, especially in the presence of an AMI [19]. All data from these studies confirm the effectiveness of CABG in patients diagnosed with AMI, compared to conservative treatment, especially as regards the long-term mortality.

Many authors think that CABG for patients with early diagnosis of AMI may be performed safely especially if the patient has a condition of hemodynamic stability.

OFF-PUMP CABG AS AN EARLY MYOCARDIAL REPERFUSION THERAPY

In the past two decade, the enthusiasm for emergency CABG in evolving AMI was dampened due to the advent of thrombolytic and PTCA therapies but the failure of these measures in several cases and the appearance of post-infarction angina revived the interest in CABG both with and without CPB in this cohort of patients. Recently, the use of off-pump beating heart surgery versus conventional on-pump surgery with cardioplegic cardiac arrest for myocardial revascularization is being intensively debated.

Theoretically, off-pump CABG seems to be an ideal procedure for patients with AMI because it preserves the coronary flow during surgery avoiding global myocardial ischemia characteristic of cardioplegic arrest period and post ischemia-reperfusion myocardial damage. Moreover, the superiority of off-pump technique versus conventional CABG in short-term cardiac outcome is well demonstrated by several randomized controlled studies [20-21]. However, it must be mentioned that most of these excluded emergency patients with AMI.

Currently, few reports are available on the postoperative outcomes of off-pump CABG in AMI patients. Mohr et al. [22] found in a group of 57 patients who underwent off-pump CABG within first week following AMI that CABG without cardiopulmonary bypass is a relatively low risk procedure. Locker et al. [23] in a series of 225 patients who underwent CABG within 7 days from onset of AMI showed that early mortality of patients operated within the first 48 hours with CPB was significantly higher compared to off-pump CABG (16.5% vs 4.3%, p=0.044) but the mortality rate in patients who underwent surgery after 48 hours became similar in both groups (5.8% vs 3.4%, p=0.44). They concluded that CPB can be used safely for most patients within the first week of AMI but for patients operated on within 48 hours from onset of symptom advocated avoiding CPB because it associated with high operative mortality.

In an another publication the same authors [24] found that emergency off-pump CABG for AMI results in lower mortality compared with conventional CABG (5% vs 24%); however, the long-term results of patients operated on without CPB were no better than the results of those operated with CPB, which might have been related to the incomplete revascularization or inferior patency rate of anastomoses performed on the beating heart. Rastan et al. [25] studied 638 consecutive patients with acute coronary syndrome who received emergency CABG (240 patients without CPB and 398 patients with CPB). These authors concluded that beating heart surgery was associated with improved in-hospital outcomes and comparable long term results for high-risk patients presenting with acute coronary syndrome with or without cardiogenic shock. Similarly, Sergeant et al.[26] found in 269 consecutive patients with AMI that CABG can be performed with acceptable early and long-term risk in selected patients with evolving myocardial infarction, whatever the hemodynamic state.

In our experience, overall in-hospital mortality rate was 4.7%. Five patients (7.7%) died in on-pump group and 1 patient (1.6%) died in off-pump group (p = 0.04).

We found that in-hospital mortality was significantly higher in on-pump versus off-pump group in patients with preoperative cardiogenic shock (27% vs 7.5%, p= 0.0018) and in those who underwent CABG within 6 hours from onset of AMI (23% vs 7.5%, p= 0.0026)[27].

Timing of Surgery

The optimal timing of operation after AMI remains controversial. Locker et al. [24] demonstrated that timing in itself is not a significant predictor of early mortality in off-pump CABG but it is a significant predictor in patients operated on with CPB.

Creswell et al.[28] reported that mortality rates of patients who underwent surgery within 6 hours after onset of AMI symptoms was 9.1%, 8.3% in those underwent surgery within 6 hours to 2 days, and 5.2% within 2 to 14 days after AMI. Lee et al.[19], in a multicenter analysis showed that hospital mortality decreased considerably with increasing time interval between CABG and AMI: 11.8%, 9.5% and 2.8% for less than 6 hours, 6 hours to 1 day, and longer, respectively. In a recent review Weis et al.[29] reported that patients undergoing CABG within 2 days of hospitalization for AMI experienced higher mortality rates than those undergoing CABG 3 or more days after AMI, independently of clinical condition and suggested that CABG may best be deferred for 3 or more days after admission for AMI in non-urgent cases.

In our experience, incidence of early mortality in all patients operated on within 6 hours from onset of AMI and 6 hours to 2 days was 15.5% (4/26pts) and 2% (2/101pts), respectively ($p<0.0001$).

In on-pump group incidence of early death in patients operated on within 6 hours and longer than 6 hours was 23% (3/13pts) and 3.8% (2/52 pts), respectively ($p=0.006$).

In off-pump group incidence of early death in patients operated on within 6 hours and longer than 6 hours was 7.5% (1/13 pts) and 0% (0/49 pts), respectively (p= ns) (27). Our results were in agreement with Locker et al.[24] and suggested that timing of surgery (< 6 hours) is a significant predictor of early death in on-pump group but not in patients who underwent surgery off-pump.

The poor outcomes in the cohort of patients undergoing CABG within few hours from onset of symptoms may depend on factors such as acute left ventricular dysfunction in the early evolving phase of AMI with hemodynamic instability, appearance of post reperfusion life-treating arrhythmias, presence of collaterals to ensure coronaries run-off after acute occlusion, fibrinolytic and glycoprotein inhibitor administration that can lead to severe postoperative bleeding specifically if patients undergo on-pump CABG.

Fortunately, most AMI patients are referred to the cardiac surgeons after the first 6 – 12 hours but for emergency patients operated on within 6 hours from onset of symptoms, we advocate avoiding CPB because it is associated with low incidence of in-hospital mortality and improved outcomes.

Impact of Preoperative Cardiogenic Shock

Impact of preoperative cardiogenic shock on early outcome in patients who undergo CABG after AMI is still controversial. Several authors [30-33] have shown that patients with AMI presenting in cardiogenic shock have poor outcome after CABG. On the other hand, Sergeant et al. [25] and Rastan et al. [26] reported that CABG can be performed with acceptable outcome in patients with evolving AMI, whatever the preoperative hemodynamic state. In our experience, incidence of early mortality for patients presenting with cardiogenic shock was 16.5% (4/24 pts) versus 1.9% (2/103 pts) for those without shock ($p<.0001$).

In on-pump group incidence of early death in patients presenting in shock and in patients without shock was 27% (3/11 pts) and 3.7% (2/54 pts), respectively (p=0.004). In off-pump group incidence of early death in patients presenting with preoperative shock and in patients without shock was 7.5% (1/13 pts) and 0% (0/49 pts), respectively (p= ns). Our data suggested that preoperative cardiogenic shock increase dramatically early mortality after CABG in patients with AMI specifically in those who underwent on-pump cardioplegic arrested heart CABG procedure [27].

Risk of Conversion and Postoperative Outcomes

In our experience, patients who underwent off-pump CABG needed less postoperative catecholamine drugs administration (p=0.02) and required shorter duration of inotropic support (p=0.001) than patients who had on-pump CABG.

Incidence of postoperative low cardiac output syndrome (p=0.001) and reoperation for bleeding (p=0.04) were significantly higher in on-pump group versus off-pump group. Moreover, patients in on-pump group had longer duration of mechanical ventilation support (p=0.006), intensive care unit (ICU) stay (p=0.01) and in-hospital stay (p=0.02) compared to patients in off-pump group [27, 34, 35].

Our data are in agreement with the work of Kerendi et al. [36] who reported that off-pump patients received fewer blood transfusions and had a significantly shorter postoperative ICU stay compared with on-pump patients.

In our experience, the significant improvement of myocardial contractility and reduction of postoperative serum cardiac troponin I (cTnI) release in the off-pump group compared to the on-pump group may indeed be attributed to avoidance of CPB, since complete and effective myocardial revascularization was performed in all patients in both groups (measured by intraoperative grafts flow) and all baseline characteristics of the two study groups were comparable with no statistically significant differences concerning preoperative extent of acute myocardial ischemia (measured by preoperative serum levels of cTnI and CK-MB), LVEF%, wall motion score index, and preoperative clinical presentation being present [27].

It is known that off-pump CABG is essentially associated with an acute conversion risk, which causes death and serious complications [37,38]. The conversion risks are difficult to quantify [39] and suggested predictors of conversion have included previous CABG, congestive heart failure, AMI, low ejection fraction and a surgeon with poor experience [37,40].

The reported conversion is from 0.4% to 2.8% [41,42]. In our study, one patient (1.6%) in off-pump group was converted to on-pump beating heart technique during revascularization of marginal ramus for severe systemic hypotension and CABG was completed on CPB with good result [27].

Graft Patency and Incidence of Cardiac-Related Events after Off-Pump CABG

Completeness of revascularization and long-term graft patency are important related to off-pump CABG. Some authors found an inferior graft patency rate and recurrent symptoms for patients who underwent off-pump CABG compared with the conventional technique. Several prospective randomized trials [21, 43, 44-46] comparing graft patency in on-pump versus off-pump surgery are available in the literature. A recent meta-analysis of those trials is reported by Takagi and colleagues who found a non-statistically significant benefit of conventional CABG over off-pump CABG for overall graft patency; a pooled analysis demonstrated a statistically significant increase in overall graft occlusion with off-pump CABG relative to on-pump [47]; a sub-analysis showed a significant increase in venous graft occlusion.

In our experience[34], we found that the overall grafts patency rate were 90.7% and 91% in on-pump versus off-pump groups, respectively. Furthermore, the patency rate was also similar between the two groups for arterials and saphenous vein grafts. In our series we did not observe any difference in terms of graft patency between off-pump and on-pump even of vein graft patency.

Our results are contrary to the conclusions of the two met-analyses that reported a reduction in postoperative patency of graft performed during off-pump CABG [47, 87]. Recently the ROOBY trial did not report any difference in terms of adverse events within 30 days between off-pump and on-pump CABG but at one year the composite outcome (reoperation, new mechanical support, cardiac arrest, stroke, and renal failure) was higher in the off-pump group and also the graft patency was inferior[49].

On the other hand, our data gives similar results compared with the results of trials published by Kobayashi and colleagues [50], Al-Ruzzeh and colleagues[44], and an updated trial published by Lingaas and colleagues [51] that showed same graft patency rates between off-pump and conventional CABG.

Recently, Kuss and colleagues published a systematic review and meta-analysis of propensity score analyses showing that off-pump surgery was superior to on-pump CABG in all of the assessed short-term outcomes [52]. Our early results for the present cohort of patients were in line with the collected evidence from the randomized trials included in this recent study. Finally our results were closer to Angelini's series that showed no differences between off-pump and on-pump CABG in terms of graft occlusion and similar long term health outcome [53].

Anesthetic Management and Surgical Technique

Monitoring

The patient is positioned on a water-heating mattress in the operating room. A 5-channel ECG is recorded. The combination of leads II/V4-V5 is continuously displayed and used for ST-segment trend analysis. Capillary pulse oximetry is recorded. After local skin infiltration, one peripheral line is inserted to secure intravenous access and arterial canulation of the radial artery is performed. A pulmonary artery catheter is inserted. After induction of general anesthesia the continuous cardiac output (CO) and mixed venous oximetry is monitored. Recorded variables include cardiac index (CI), mean arterial pressure (MAP), central venous pressure, mean pulmonary arterial pressure (mPAP), pulmonary capillary wedge pressure (PCWP), mixed venous oxygen saturation and heart rate. Hemodynamic data is obtained during conduits harvesting, after stabilizer tentacles positioning, and at 5 minutes-interval throughout the procedure. Central and peripheral temperatures are measured with nasal and rectal temperature probes. A urinary catheter is introduced to monitor urinary output.

Intraoperative transesophageal echocardiographic (TEE) control is performed in all patients to evaluate global and regional myocardial function. A 2-dimensional cardiac ultrasound from Hewlett Packard (Sonos 4500, Palo Alto, Calif) equipped with a transesophageal echocardiographic probe is used. Myocardial kinesia is evaluated in according to the guidelines of the American Society of Echocardiography.

Anesthesia

Standard anesthesia is induced with fentanyl (20–50 mg/kg), midazolam (0.1 mg/kg), and pancuronium bromide (0.1 mg/kg), and maintained with a continuous infusion of fentanyl (0.5–1 mg/kg/h) and propofol (50–200 mg/kg/h). Moderate dose of opioids is used to attenuate the operative stress response.

Surgical Management

Off-pump CABG is performed using a commercially available suction stabilizer (Octopus, Medtronic Inc, Minneapolis, Minnesota). To reach the anterior wall for left anterior descending or diagonal arteries grafting, the surgeon places 2 to 3 moistened gauze pads behind the left ventricle to elevate and to rotate the left ventricle into the midline. In some cases, this caused compression of the right heart, which is squeezed between the thick, bulky left ventricle and the right pericardium. These results in a drop in right ventricle output, which is reflected in a decrease of mPAP, MAP, and CO. Treatment consists of filling of the heart and Trendelenburg position. In some patients with AMI who undergo early off-pump CABG, the left ventricle function is very poor and acute filling may be dangerous. In this case, the right pericardium is opened to aid heart displacement into the right pleura. A vertical incision of the pericardium at the level of the right atrium to the inferior cava vein is also applied to avoid right atrial compression.

The most challenging site to graft on the beating heart and specifically in patients with acute ischemia is the posterior wall. In order to view this invisible area from sternotomy approach, the heart must be tilted out of the pericardial cradle. Slow manipulation of the heart is necessary to avoid ventricular arrhythmias and hemodynamic deterioration. Four Lima stitches are placed deeply in the pericardium from the left pulmonary veins to the diaphragm (in midline) to push up the heart avoiding complete heart verticalization that leads to hypotension. The same procedures for the anterior wall exposure must be performed in more pronounced way. A slow apical suction cardiac positioning device (Starfish, Medtronic Inc, Minneapolis, Minnesota) can be used for revascularization of the circumflex branch. During revascularization of the lateral/posterolateral wall TEE and SvO2 monitoring are necessary because the ECG ischemia monitoring is not of value since the amplitude is decreased by the loss of contact between the heart and pericardium. Compared with LAD and right coronary artery grafting, coronary circulation is only impaired in the circumflex territory as usually the other areas have already been bypassed. Normalization of MAP with judicious use of vasoconstrictors will restore residual myocardial blood flow, as well as flow through the grafts on the anterior and inferior wall, and the situation of acute low output syndrome will disappear. It is very important to avoid overshooting with inotropic drugs. This may compromise local cardiac wall stabilization, the accuracy of the anastomosis, and cardiac performance because of increase oxygen demand.

To allow a good surgical view of the right coronary artery and its distal branches, the operating table is placed in the head-down position. A slow right ventricle anterior wall suction, close to the acute margin of the heart, is applied to facilitate vessels exposure. The suction arms are placed around the target vessel and moved ventrally in order to elevate the target area 3 to 5 cm. This results in increase in the surgical view but it also caused some obstruction of the tricuspid orifice.

Transesophageal echocardiography as well as monitoring of right atrial pressure are helpful in identifying the limit of elevation in order to prevent tricuspid valve blockage or insufficiency. In this case, right pericardium may be opened to aid right heart displacement.

Intra-coronary shunts may be used for all anastomoses (Clearview, Medtronic Inc, Minneapolis, Minnesota). Temporary proximal occlusion of the target vessel is performed using 5-0 polypropylene sutures with Teflon pledgets. The first anastomosis is routinely performed between the left internal thoracic artery (LITA) and the LAD, but the right coronary or posterior descending artery (PDA) may be grafted first in patients with inferior AMI who undergo surgery within 12 hours from onset of symptoms. The second anastomosis is performed between the conduit and PDA and finally obtuse marginal artery is grafted.

Perioperative Hemodynamic Management

Grafting to the inferior and the posterolateral myocardium demands lifting of the heart partly out of the pericardium and out of the thoracic cavity. This maneuver compromises cardiac output and reduces mean arterial blood pressure. Hypotension upon dislocation of the heart is resolved by increasing preload by placing the patient in Trendelenburg position; however caution must be exercised in patients with severe acute left ventricular dysfunction due to AMI, because the acute rise in preload can lead to hemodynamic deterioration. The decrease of cardiac output and MAP are mostly caused by an outflow obstruction of the right ventricle. This is caused by a compression of the right atrium and ventricle by the displacement and torsion of the heart. This is projected in increase in central venous pressure, decrease or unchanged mPAP and decrease PCWP. This situation normally restores to acceptable hemodynamic levels without the use of vasoactive medication. Unfortunately, in patients with AMI often the hemodynamic condition deteriorates with decrease in mPAP and increase in PCWP necessitating vasoactive drug administration. Judicious use of alpha agonists may be necessary, despite the acute ischemic phase. Judgement must be made quite early on in such cases for conversion as emergency conversion may result in suboptimal outcome.

CONCLUSION

Off-pump CABG surgery appears to be the optimal treatment strategy for patients with STEMI whenever the preoperative conditions permit and CABG surgery is indicated. Although, CABG is still associated with high mortality and morbidity in patients who undergo surgery within the first 6 hours from onset of AMI symptoms and in those with cardiogenic shock, off pump surgery improves dramatically the results compared to on-pump revascularization. Maintaining native coronary blood flow during off-pump surgery avoids global myocardial ischemia, a hallmark of conventional CABG with cardioplegic arrest, and post CPB myocardial cell damage due to ischemia-reperfusion injury that can contribute to more postoperative left ventricular dysfunction and to poor postoperative outcome.

In our experience off-pump CABG has the same late mortality, major adverse cardiac related events, and grafts patency rate comparing to conventional CABG [34]. Furthermore, in our opinion urgent or emergent CABG for patients with STEMI can be done either way. Based on the evidence of our previous studies [27,34,35] showing reduced early mortality and morbidity rates for patients undergoing off-pump CABG and the current literature reporting a lower incidence of postoperative outcomes such as low cardiac output, bleeding and transfusion requirements we consider that off-pump CABG may have many advantages compared with on-pump surgery for this cohort of high-risk patients.

As an alternative to conventional CABG for patients with AMI, few centers have recently adopted on-pump beating-heart CABG. On-pump beating-heart CABG is an attractive technique that keeps heart beating with the aid of CPB but without aortic cross-clamping or cardioplegic arrest. Izumi and associates [54] demonstrated that on-pump beating-heart CABG reduces the mortality of patients with AMI and decreases the release of cTnI compared with conventional CABG.

Currently, in our opinion there are few absolute contraindications to off-pump surgery. The selection of patients should stem in large part from the operating surgeon's beating heart experience and comfort level.

Programs early in their off-pump experience should concentrate on patients with less demanding revascularization requirement. Optimal candidates for surgeons with limited experience typically include patients who are hemodynamically stable and require a limited number of bypasses located in easily accessible areas.

When surgeons start offering STEMI patients off-pump CABG, the patients' selection should include those with large target vessels free of diffuse calcified disease and hemodynamic stability despite ischemia and left ventricular dysfunction. With experience, higher risk patients with hemodynamic instability and technically more challenging procedures can be undertaken.

Difficult patients likely to benefit from off-pump surgery include those with severe left ventricular dysfunction, ischemic mitral insufficiency, or those grafted emergently after an acute myocardial infarction. Patients who are either severely hemodynamically or electrically unstable may not tolerate the manipulation required for off-pump bypass grafting, and therefore represent a population generally not considered candidates for off-pump CABG. However, this subset of patients may be safely operated performing pump-supported beating heart surgery.

REFERENCES

[1] Fang J, Alderman MH, Keenan NL, Ayala C. Acute myocardial infarction hospitalization in the United States, 1979 to 2005. *Am. J. Med.* 2010;123:259-66.

[2] Braunwald E (ed.). Heart Disease. WB Saunders Company, Philadelphia, 2003.

[3] The European Society of Cardiology/American College of Cardiology Committee. Myocardial infarction redefined. *Eur. Heart Journal* 2000; 21:1502-13.

[4] Boersma E, Mercado N, Poldermans D. Acute Myocardial infarction. *Lancet* 2003; 361: 847-58.
[5] Fuster V, Badimon L, Badimon JJ. The pathogenesis of coronary artery disease and the acute coronary syndromes. *N. Eng. J. Med.* 1992; 326:310-318.
[6] Rauch U, Osende J, Fuster V. Thrombus formation on atherosclerosis plaque. Ann *Intern. Med.* 2001;134:224-238.
[7] Ross R. Atherosclerosis an inflammatory disease. *N. Eng. J. Med.* 1999;340:115-126.
[8] Ryan TJ, Antman EM, Brooks NH, et al. 1999 update: ACC/AHA Guidelines for the Management of Patients with Acute Myocardial Infarction: Executive Summary and Recommendations: A report of the American College of Cardiology/American Heart Association Task Force on Practice Guidelines (Committee on Management of Acute Myocardial Infarction). *Circulation* 1999;100:1016-30.
[9] Lee DC, Ting W, Oz MC. Myocardial revascularization after acute myocardial infarction. In: Cohn LH, Edmunds LH Jr (eds.). *Cardiac Surgery in the Adult.* New York: McGraw-Hill, 2003:639-658.
[10] Phillips SJ, Kongtahworn C, Zeff RH, et al. Emergency coronary artery revascularization: a possible therapy for acute myocardial infarction. *Circulation* 1979;60: 241-6.
[11] Dewood MA, Spores J, Berg R, et al. Acute myocardial infarction: A decade experience with surgical reperfusion in 701 patients. *Circulation* 1983;68 (Suppl II):II8-16.
[12] Phillips SJ, Zeff RH, Skinner JR, Toon RS, Grignon A, Kongtahworn C. Reperfusion protocol and results in 738 patients with evolving myocardial infarction. *Ann. Thorac. Surg.* 1986; 41;119-125.
[13] Hochberg M, Parsonnet V, Gielchsinsky I. Timing of coronary revascularization after acute myocardial infarction. *J. Thorac. Cardiovasc. Surg.* 1984; 88:914-21.
[14] Katz NM, Kubanick TE, Ahmed SW, et al. Determinants of cardiac failure after coronary bypass surgery within 30 days of acute myocardial infarction. *Ann. Thorac. Surg.* 1986; 42; 658-63.
[15] Kouchoukos NT, Murphy S, Philpott P, et al. Coronary artery bypass graft surgery after acute myocardial infarction. *Circulation* 1988;79(suppl. I):I68-72.
[16] Kennedy JW, Ivery TD, Misbach G, et al. Coronary artery bypass after acute myocardial infarction. *Circulation* 1989;79;I73-78.
[17] Floten HS, Ahmad A, Swanson JS, et al. Long-term survival after post-infarction bypass operation: early versus late operation. *Ann. Thorac. Surg.* 1989;48: 752-62.
[18] Sintek CF, Pfeffer TA, Khonsari S. Surgical revascularization after acute myocardial infarction: does timing make a difference? *J. Thorac. Cardiovasc. Surg.* 1994;107:1317-21.
[19] Lee DC, Oz MC, Weinberg AD, Ting W, et al. Optimal timing of revascularization: transmural versus nontransmural acute myocardial infarction. *Ann. Thorac. Surg.* 2001;71:1198-1204.
[20] 20. Van Dijk D, Nierich AP, Jansen EW, et al. Early outcome after off-pump versus on-pump coronary bypass surgery: results from a randomised study. *Circulation* 2001;104:1761-6.
[21] Khan NE, De Souza A, Mister R, et al. A randomized comparison of off-pump and on-pump multivessel coronary – artery bypass surgery. *N. Engl. J. Med.* 2004; 350: 21-8.

[22] Mohr R, Moshkovitch Y, Shapira I, et al. Coronary artery bypass without cardiopulmonary bypass for patients with acute myocardial infarction. *J. Thorac. Cardiovasc. Surg.* 1999;118: 50-6.
[23] Locker C, Mohr R, Paz Y, et al. Myocardial revascularization for acute myocardial infarction: benefits and drawbacks of avoiding cardiopulmonary bypass. *Ann. Thorac. Surg.* 2003;76:771-7.
[24] Locker C, Shapira I, Paz Y, et al. Emergency myocardial revascularization for acute myocardial infarction: survival benefit of avoiding cardiopulmonary bypass. *Eur. J. Cardiothorac. Surg.* 2000;17:234-8.
[25] Rastan AJ, Eckenstein JI, Hentschel B, et al. Emergency coronary artery bypass graft surgery for acute coronary syndrome. Beating heart versus conventional cardioplegic cardiac arrest strategies. *Circulation* 2006:114 (Suppl I) I-477-485.
[26] Sergeant P, Blackstone E, Meyns B. Early and late outcome after CABG in patients with evolving myocardial infarction. *Eur. J. Cardiothorac. Surg.* 1997;11:848-856.
[27] Fattouch K, Guccione F, Dioguardi S,et al. Off-pump vs on-pump myocardial revascularization in patients with ST-segment elevation myocardial infarction: a randomized trial. *J. Thorac. Cardiovasc. Surg.* 2009;137:650-7.
[28] Creswell LL, Moulton MJ, Cox AL, Rosenbloom M. Revascularization after acute myocardial infarction. *Ann. Thorac. Surg.* 1995; 60: 19-26.
[29] Weis ES, Chang D, Joyce D, Nwakanma LU, Yuh DD. Optimal timing of coronary artery bypass after acute myocardial infarction. A review of California discharge data. *J. Thorac. Cardiovasc. Surg.* 2008;135:503-11.
[30] Kaul TK, Fields BL, Riggins SL, et al. Coronary artery bypass grafting within 30 days of an acute myocardial infarction. *Ann. Thorac. Cardiovascular Surg.* 2001;7:28-34.
[31] Yamagishi I, Sakurada T, Abe T. Emergency coronary artery bypass grafting after acute myocardial infarction. What influences early postoperative mortality? *Ann. Thorac. Cardiovasc. Surg.* 1998;4:28-33.
[32] Wasvary H, Shannon F, Basset J, O' Neill W. Timing of coronary bypass grafting after acute myocardial infarction. *Am. Surg.* 1997;63:710-5.
[33] Quigley RL, Milano CA, Smith LR, et al. Prognosis and management of anterolateral myocardial infarction in patients with left main disease and cardiogenic shock. The left main shock syndrome. Circulation 1993:88 (Suppl II) 65-70.
[34] Fattouch K, Runza G, Sampognaro R, et al. Graft patency and late outcomes for patients with ST-segment elevation who myocardial infarction underwent coronary surgery. Perfusion 2011;28:401-408.
[35] Fattouch K, Bianco G, Speziale G, et al. Benefits effects of C1 esterase inhibitor in ST-elevation myocardial infarction in patients who underwent surgical reperfusion: a randomized double-blind study. *Eur. J. Cardiothorac Surg.* 2007;32: 326-32.
[36] Kerendi F, Puskas JD, Craver J, et al. Emergency coronary artery bypass grafting can be performed safely without cardiopulmonary bypass in selected patients. *Ann. Thorac. Surg.* 2005;79:801-806.
[37] Edgerton JR, Dewey TM, Magee MJ, et al. Conversion in off-pump coronary artery bypass grafting: an analysis of predictors and outcomes. *Ann. Thorac. Surg.* 2003;76:1138-43.

[38] Légaré JF, Buth KJ, Hirsch GM. Conversion to on pump from OPCAB is associated with increased mortality: results from a randomised controlled trial. *Eur. J. Cardiothorac Surg*. 2005;27: 296-301.

[39] Reeves BC, Ascione R, Caputo M, Angelini GD. Morbidity and mortalità following acute conversion from off-pump to on-pump coronary surgery. *Eur. J. Cardiothorac Surg*. 2006; 29:941-7.

[40] Vassiliades TA Jr, Nielsen JL, Lonquist JL. Hemodynamic collapse during off-pump coronary artery bypass grafting. *Ann. Thorac. Surg*. 2002;73:1874-9.

[41] Hart JC, Spooner TH, Pym J, et al. A review 0f 1,582 consecutive octopus off-pump coronary bypass patients. *Ann. Thorac. Surg*. 2000;70:1017-20.

[42] Anyanwu AC, Al-Ruzzeh S, George SJ, et al. Conversion of Off-Pump coronary bypass without increased morbidity or change in practice. *Ann. Thorac. Surg*. 2002;73: 79-802.

[43] Puskas JD, Williams WH, Mahoney EM, et al. Off-pump vs conventional coronary artery bypass grafting: early and 1-year graft patency, cost, and quality of life outcomes: a randomized trial. *JAMA* 2004; 291:1841-1849.

[44] Al-Ruzzeh S, George S, Bustami M, et al. Effect of off-pump coronary artery bypass surgery on clinical, angiographic, neurocognitive, and quality of life outcomes: randomized controlled trial. *BMJ* 2006; 332:1365.

[45] Widimisky P, Straka Z, Stros P, et al. One year coronary graft patency: a randomized comparison between off-pump and on-pump surgery – angiographic result of the PRAGUE-4 trial. *Circulation* 2004;110:3418-23.

[46] Nathoe HM, van Dijk D, Jansen EW, et al; Octopus Study Group. A comparison of on-pump and off-pump coronary bypass surgery in low-risk patient. *N. Engl. J. Med.* 2003;348:394-402.

[47] Takagi H, Tanabashi T, Kawai N, Kato T, Umemoto T. Off-pump coronary artery bypass sacrifices graft patency: Meta-analysis of randomized trials. *J. Thorac. Cardiovasc. Surg*. 2007;133:e 2-3.

[48] Parolari A, Alamanni F, Polvani G, et al. Metanalysis of randomized trials comparing off-pump with on-pump coronary artery bypass graft patency. *Ann. Thorac. Surg*. 2005;80:2121-5.

[49] Shroyer AL, Grover FL, Hattler B, et al; Veterans Affairs Randomized On/Off Bypass (ROOBY) Study Group. On-pump versus off-pump coronary-artery bypass surgery. *N. Engl. J. Med.* 2009;361:1827-37.

[50] Kobayashi J, Tashiro T, Ochi M, et al; Japanese Off-pump Coronary Revascularization Investigation (JOCRI) Study Group. Early outcome of a randomized comparison of off-pump and on-pump multiple arterial coronary revascularization. *Circulation*. 2005;112(9 suppl): I 338-43.

[51] Lingaas PS, Hol PK, Lunblad R, et al. Clinical and radiological outcome of off-pump coronary surgery at 12 months follow-up: a prospective randomized trial. *Ann. Thorac. Surg*. 2006;81:2089-96.

[52] Kuss O, Salviati BV, Borgermann J. Off-pump versus on-pump coronary artery bypass grafting: A systematic review and meta-analysis of propensity score analyses. *J. Thorac. Cardiovasc. Surg*. 2010; 140: 829-35.

[53] Angelini GD, Culliford L, Smith DK, et al. Effects of on- and off-pump coronary artery surgery on graft patency, survival, and health-related quality of life: long-term follow up of 2 randomized trials. *J. Thorac. Cardiovasc. Surg.* 2009;137:295-303.

[54] Izumi Y, Magishi K, Ishikawa N, Kimura F. On-pump beating-heart coronary artery bypass grafting for acute myocardial infarction. *Ann. Thorac. Surg.* 2006;81:573-6.

INDEX

B

D

F

G

H

I

N

O

P

Q

R

S

T

U

V

W

Y